MASTERING THE BOARDS AND CLINICAL EXAMINATIONS IN INTERNAL MEDICINE IN GASTROENTEROLOGY

A. B. R. Thomson

www.giandhepatology.com

athoms47@uwo.ca

i

MASTERING THE BOARDS AND CLINICAL EXAMINATIONS IN INTERNAL MEDICINE IN GASTROENTEROLOGY

This book compliments

Mastering the Boards and Clinical Examinations in Internal Medicine in Hepatobiliary and Pancreatic Disease

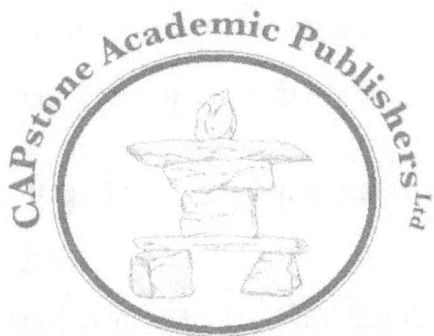

CAPstone (Canadian Academic Publishers Ltd) is a not-for-profit company dedicated to the use of the power of education for the betterment of all persons everywhere.

"For the Democratization of Knowledge"

 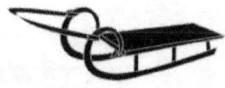

ARE YOU PREPARING FOR EXAMS IN GENERAL INTERNAL MEDICINE OR IN GASTROENTEROLOGY AND HEPATOLOGY?
See the full range of examination preparation and review publications from CAPstone on Amazon.com

For no cost viewing, please consult: www. giandhepatology.com

Gastroenterology and Hepatology

First Principles of Gastroenterology and Hepatology in Adults and Children – Volume I - Gastroenterology, 7th edition (ISBN: 978-1494345624)

First Principles of Gastroenterology and Hepatology in Adults and Children - Volume II - Hepatology and Paediatrics, 7th edition (ISBN: 978-1494345501)

GI Practice Review, 2nd edition (ISBN: 978-1475219951)
Endoscopy and Diagnostic Imaging Part I (ISBN: 978-1477400579)

Endoscopy and Diagnostic Imaging Part II (ISBN: 978-1477400654)

Scientific Basis for Clinical Practice in Gastroenterology and Hepatology (ISBN: 978-1475226645)

Guideline – Based Therapy in Gastroenterology and Hepatology

General Internal Medicine

Achieving Excellence in the OSCE. Part I. Cardiology to Nephrology (ISBN: 978-1475283037)

Achieving Excellence in the OSCE. Part II. Neurology to Rheumatology (ISBN: 978-1475276978)

Bits and Bytes for Rounds in Internal Medicine (ISBN: 978-1478295365)

Mastering the Boards and Clinical Examinations. Part I. Cardiology, Endocrinology, Gastroenterology, Hepatology and Nephrology (ISBN: 978-1461024842)

Mastering the Boards and Clinical Examinations. Part II. Neurology to Rheumatology (ISBN: 978-1478392736)

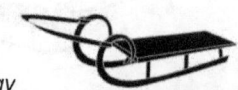

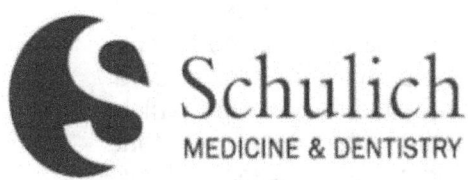 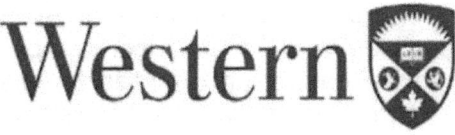

THE WESTERN WAY

DISCLAIMER

The primary purpose of this publication is education. The author, editor and publisher acknowledge that the development of new material opens to way for possible errors – what is correct today might not be the standard of care tomorrow. Readers are advised to ensure that the doses of drugs which they use are in compliance with their country's product information, and that the use of any therapeutic agent, be it a pharmaceutical or a technology, should be guided by local guidelines. There is often a wide diversity of professional opinion, and guidelines from one country are not always congruent with another.

The author, editor and publisher do not guarantee the safety, reliability, accuracy, completeness or usefulness of this material.

They disclaim any and all liability for damage and claims that may result from the use of information, publications, technologies, products, and for series provided in this publication.

We have made every attempt to trace the holders of copyright for material reproduced in this book. If by some oversight we have omitted a copyright holder, please contact us.

Thank you

A. B. R. Thomson

 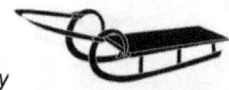

TABLE OF CONTENTS

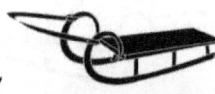

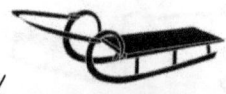

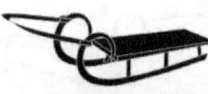

Mastering the Boards: Gastroenterology   A.B.R. Thomson

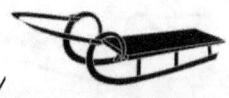

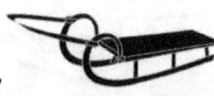

References: Please see Current and Classical Key References in Gastroenterology and Hepatology.

Available online at www.giandhepatology.com

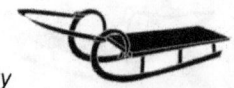

GI Practice Review and The CANMED Objectives

Medical Expert
The discussion of complex cases provides the participants with an opportunity to comment on additional focused history and physical examination. They would provide a complete and organized assessment. Participants are encouraged to identify key features, and they develop an approach to problem-solving.

The case discussions, as well as the discussion of cases around a diagnostic imaging, pathological or endoscopic base provides the means for the candidate to establish an appropriate management plan based on the best available evidence to clinical practice. Throughout, an attempt is made to develop strategies for diagnosis and development of clinical reasoning skills.

Communicator
The participants demonstrate their ability to communicate their knowledge, clinical findings, and management plan in a respectful, concise and interactive manner. When the participants play the role of examiners, they demonstrate their ability to listen actively and effectively, to ask questions in an open-ended manner, and to provide constructive, helpful feedback in a professional and non-intimidating manner.

Collaborator
The participants use the "you have a green consult card" technique of answering questions as fast as they are able, and then to interact with another health professional participant to move forward the discussion and problem solving. This helps the participants to build upon what they have already learned about the importance of collegial interaction.

Manager
The participants are provided with assignments in advance of the three day GI Practice Review. There is much work for them to complete before as well as afterwards, so they learn to manage their time effectively, and to complete the assigned tasks proficiently and on time. They learn to work in teams to achieve answers from small group participation, and then to share this with other small group participants through effective delegation of work. Some of the material they must access demands that they use information technology effectively to access information that will help to facilitate the delineation of adequately broad differential diagnoses, as well as rational and cost effective management plans.

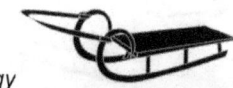

Health Advocate
In the answering of the questions and case discussions, the participants are required to consider the risks, benefits, and costs and impacts of investigations and therapeutic alliances upon the patient and their loved ones.

Scholar
By committing to the pre and post-study requirements, plus the intense three day active learning GI Practice Review with colleagues is a demonstration of commitment to personal education. Through the interactive nature of the discussions and the use of the "green consult card", they reinforce their previous learning of the importance of collaborating and helping one another to learn.

Professional
The participants are coached how to interact verbally in a professional setting, being straightforward, clear and helpful. They learn to be honest when they cannot answer questions, make a diagnosis, or advance a management plan. They learn how to deal with aggressive or demotivated colleagues, how to deal with knowledge deficits, how to speculate on a missing knowledge byte by using first principals and deductive reasoning. In a safe and supportive setting they learn to seek and accept advice, to acknowledge awareness of personal limitations, and to give and take 360^0 feedback.

Knowledge
The basic science aspects of gastroenterology are considered in adequate detail to understand the mechanisms of disease, and the basis of investigations and treatment. In this way, the participants respect the importance of an adequate foundation in basic sciences, the basics of the design of clinical research studies to provide an evidence-based approach, the relevance of their management plans being patient-focused, and the need to add "compassionate" to the Three C's of Medical Practice: competent, caring and compassionate.

"They may forget what you said, but they will never forget how you made them feel."

Carl W. Buechner, on teaching.

"With competence, care for the patient. With compassion, care about the person."

Alan B. R. Thomson, on Being a Physician.

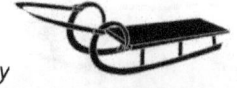

PROLOGUE

Like any good story, there is no real beginning or ending, just an in-between glimpse of the passing of time, a peek into a reality of people's minds, thoughts, feelings, and beliefs. The truth as I know it has a personal perspective which drifts into the soul of creation. When does life begin, when does an idea become conceived, when do we see love or touch reality? A caring, supportive, safe, and stimulating environment creates the holding blanket, waiting for the energy and passion of those who dream, invent, create – disrupt the accepted, challenge the conventional, ask the questions with forbidden answers. Be a child of the 60's. Just as each of us is a speck of dust in the greater humanity, the metamorphosis of the idea is but a single sparkle in the limitlessness of the Divine Intelligence. We are the ideas, and they are us. No one of us is truly the only parent of the idea, for in each of us is bestowed the intertwined circle of the external beginning and the end....

...during a visit to the Division of Gastroenterology at the University of Ottawa several years ago, the trainees remarked how useful it would be to have more than two hours of learning exchange, a highly interactive tutorial with concepts, problem solving, collegial discussion, the fun and joys of discovery and successes. Ms. Jane Upshall of BYK Canada (Atlanta, Nycomed), who had sponsored two of these visiting Professorships, encouraged the possibility of the development of a longer program. Her successor, Lynne Jamme-Vachon, supported the initial three day educational event for the trainees enrolled in the GI training program at the University of Ottawa. With her entrepreneurial foresight, wisdom, and enthusiasm, the idea began. Lynne's commitment to an event which benefited many of the future clinicians, who will care for ourselves and our loved ones, took hold. Then, thanks to the GI program directors in Ottawa and the University of Western Ontario, Nav Saloojee and Jamie Gregor, more trainees were exposed, future GI fellows talked with other trainees, and a grassroots initiative began. Had it not been for Nav and Jamie's willingness to take a risk on something new, had they not believed in me, then there would have been no further outreach. Thank you, Lynne, Nav, and Jamie. You were there at the beginning. I needed you.

By 2008, all but one GI program in the country gave their trainees time off work to participate in the three day event, GI Practice Review (GI-PR). The course is 90% unsponsored, and is gratis to the participants, (except for the cost of their enthusiastic participation!) I am happy to give back to the subspecialty that gave me so much for 33 years. I hope GI-PR is helpful to all trainees. I know that from these future leaders there will arise those who will continue to dedicate and donate their time, energy, and ability to the betterment of those who contribute to the continued improvement of our medical profession. The clinicians, the teachers, the researchers.

In the short span of eight years, more than 300 fellows, coming from all the 14 training programs in Canada, have participated in the small group

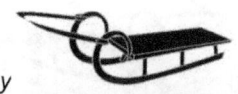

sessions in the GI practice review. I thank the training program directors who have supported GI-PR. Special appreciation as well to their many staff physicians who worked without their trainees for the three days of each program.

The idea for the electronic and hard copy summary of the "list of facts" came from the trainees who wished for an aide memoir. But the GI-PR is about more than lists and facts – it is about problem formulation, case discussions, review of endoscopy, histopathology, motility, diagnostic imaging. It is about having fun working together to learn. The subterfuge to gain interest in the basic sciences is the use of clinical scenarios to show the way to the importance of first principles. While the lists are here, the experience is in the performance.

The child will grow, the images will expand, the learning of all aspects of our craft will develop and flourish amongst persons of good will. Examinations will become second nature, as each clinical encounter, each person, each patient, becomes our test, the determination of clinical competence, of caring, of compassion. May these three C's become part of each of our life's narrative. And from this start comes Capstone Academic Publishing, an innovation for the highest quality and value in educational material, made available at cost, speaking in tongues, in the languages of many cultures, with the dialect of the True North strong and free, so that knowledge will be free at last.

Outstanding medical practice and true dedication to those from whom we receive both a privilege and pleasure of care, comes from much more than the GI-PR can give you, much more than Q & As, descriptions of diagnostic imaging or endoscopy stills or videos, histopathology or motility. True, we need all of these to jump over a very high bar. But to be a truly outstanding physician, you need to care for and care about people, and you must respect the dignity and rights of all others. You must strike a balance between love and justice, and you place your family and friends at the top of your wish-list of lifetime achievements.

For the skeptics who ask "What do you want from me?" I simply say "You are the future; I trust that in time you too will help young people to be the best they can be."

May good luck, good health, modesty, peace, and understanding be with you always. Through medicine, all persons of the world may come to share caring, respect, dignity, and justice.

Sincerely,

Alan Thomson

Emeritus Distinguished University Professor, U of A

Adjunct Professor, Western University, London, Canada

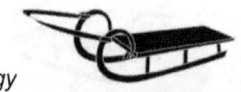

ACKNOWLEDGEMENTS

Patience and patients go hand in hand. So also does the interlocking of young and old, love and justice, equality and fairness. No author can have thoughts transformed into words, no teacher can make ideas become behavior and wisdom and art, without those special people who turn our minds to the practical – of getting the job done!

Thank you, Naiyana and Duen, for translating those scribbles (called my handwriting), into the still magical legibility of the electronic age. Sarah, thank you for your hard work and creativity.

My most sincere and heartfelt thanks go to the excellent persons at JP Consulting, and CapStone Academic Publishers. Jessica, you are brilliant, efficient, dedicated, and caring. Thank you most sincerely.

When Rebecca, Maxwell, Megan, Henry, Felix, Toby and Grady, ask about their Grandad, I will depend on James and Anne, Matthew and Allison, Jessica and Matt, and Benjamin to be understanding, generous, kind and forgiving. For what I was trying to say and to do was to make my professional life focused on the four C's and an "H"; competence, caring, compassion, and composure, as well as humour – and to make my very private personal life dedicated to family – to you all.

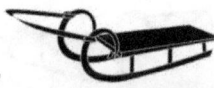

Mastering the Boards: Gastroenterology   A.B.R. Thomson

DEDICATION

Dedicated to Jeannette Rita Cécile Mineault

My life began when I met you:

Your wit, your charm, your laughter,

Your love for children, your caring, your common sense.

As always, all ways, thank you for saying I do.

– – – – – – – – – –

For the parents who gave us life.

For the children and grandchildren who give us hope.

For the teachers who gave us knowledge.

For the partners who give us confidence, encouragement and meaning.

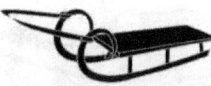

ESOPHAGUS

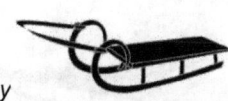

TABLE OF CONTENTS

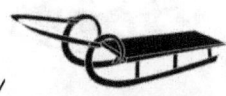

SWALLOWING

➢ Physiology

- Give the physiological mechanisms involved in swallowing.

- Mouth/tongue
  - The tongue, like the face and palate, has a bilateral upper motor neuron innervation in most people, so a unilateral upper motor neuron lesion often causes no deviation.
  - A clinically obvious upper motor neuron lesion of the twelfth nerve is usually bilateral and results in a small immobile tongue.
  - The combination of bilateral upper motor neuron lesions of the ninth, tenth and twelfth nerves is called pseudobulbar palsy.
  - A lower motor neuron lesion of the twelfth nerve causes fasciculation, wasting and weakness. If the lesion is bilateral, it causes dysarthria.
  - Movement disorders may affect the tongue.

  - Muscles of soft palate, tongue and pharynx shorten the lumen of the pharynx.

- Oropharynx
  - Complex coordinated transfer of bolus from mouth to upper esophagus
  - Affected by neurological disease affecting cranial nerves
  - Pharyngeal swallow
    - Coordination of patterned activation of motor neurons and muscles to transform the oropharynx from a respiratory pathway to an esophageal transfer pathway
    - From VFSA (video fluoroscopy swallowing assessment), there are several mechanical steps:
      - Nasopharynx-soft palate elevation and retraction
      - UES – opens
      - Larynx – closes
      - Tongue – becomes filled with food & fluid
    - Propulsion of bolus
      - Pharynx – constrictors clear the pharynx
      - UES pressure rises

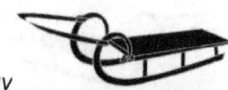

Mastering the Boards: Gastroenterology A.B.R. Thomson

- UES (upper esophageal sphincter)
  - Cricopharyngeus forms the 1 cm area of ↑pressure of the UES (upper esophageal sphincter)
  - UES pressure maintenance and coordination of relaxation of swallowing is achieved by vagal trunks from the nucleus ambiguous
  - ↑ UES pressure
    - Distention of esophagus
    - Stress
    - Inspiration swallowing

  - ↓ UES pressure
    - Belching (causes relaxation of UES and closure of the glottis)
    - Anesthesia
    - Sleep
  - GER (gastroesophageal reflex) – no effect on UES pressure

- Larynx
  - Inlet to the larynx closes

- Esophagus

Muscle	Site	Efferent Nerves (Motor)
o Striated	Proximal 5% Middle 35%	– Lower motor neurons cell bodies in nucleus ambiguous
		– Excitatory vagal innervations
		– Activation of motor units in a craniocaudal sequence through the release of Ach and stimulation of nicotinic cholinergic receptors on motor endplates of striated muscle cells
		– Peristalsis of striated muscle of esophagus is controlled by the medullary swallowing centre
o Smooth	Middle 35% Lower 60%	– Dorsal motor nucleus of the vagus
		– Excitatory ganglionic neurons predominate proximally, inhibitory ganglionic neurons dominate distally

4

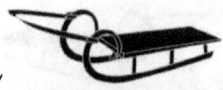

Muscle	Afferent (sensory)

- o High resolution esophageal pressure topography shows a transition zone between the skeletal and smooth muscle, characterized by

  - $\downarrow$ amplitude contractions

  - $\downarrow$ progression of peristalsis

  - $\uparrow$ likelihood of failed transmission

  – Superior laryngeal nerve, cell bodies in nodose ganglion

  – Recurrent laryngeal nerve, esophageal branches of vagus

- o ANS (autonomic nerve system)

  – Myenteric plexus between longitudinal and circular muscle layers

  – Meissner plexus between muscularis mucosa and circular muscle

- o **Peristalsis**

  – Primary (1°) wave – initiated by swallow 1° >2° wave pressure

  – Secondary (2°) wave – initiated by distention of esophagus (food, fluid, air; balloon)

  – A "milking" wave clears the esophagus from the top to the bottom

  – When the pressure of the 1°/ 2° peristaltic milking wave is low (<30 mmHg), the esophagus is less likely to be completely cleared

  – If there are two swallows made in rapid succession, in such a way that the first peristaltic wave is still in the esophagus, the inhibitory ganglionic neurons in the myenteric plexus rapidly cause hyperpolarization of the circular smooth muscle in the lower third of the esophagus

  – This hyperpolarization of the circular smooth muscle inhibits the peristaltic contraction of the first swallow (deglutitive inhibition)

  – There is no deglutitive inhibition in the longitudinal muscle layer

  – With contraction of the outer longitudinal and inner circular smooth muscle, the esophagus may shorten (about 1 inch, 2.5 cm)

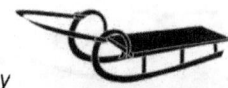

- There may be a central origin to deglutitive inhibition
- Thus, the esophageal clearance is less efficient with low pressure esophageal peristaltic waves, on with rapid swallowing causing deglutitive inhibition

- o Skeletal muscle
  - From the swallowing centre in the medulla, vagal efferent fibres are excited, and discharge in spike bursts during 1°/ 2° peristalsis
  - The Ach stimulates nicotinic cholinergic receptors on the motor end plates of the striated muscle cells
  - The medullary swallowing centre vagal efferent fibres discharge first the vagal fibres in the upper and then the middle of the esophagus
  - This sequential firing of skeletal muscle first in the proximal and then in the middle esophagus leads to peristalsis
  - These discharges leading to peristaltic muscle contraction are enhanced when the afferent sensory fibres are activated by the bolus passing along the esophagus
  - These vagal motor efferents are inhibited during the pharyngeal component of swallowing, or when the proximal esophagus is distended (deglutitive inhibition)

- o Smooth muscle
  - Vagus nerve also controls 1° peristalsis in lower esophagus (smooth muscle)
  - Stimulation of the vagal efferent (motor) may ↑ or ↓ the smooth muscle activity:
  - Control of peristalsis by smooth muscle – medullary swallowing centre
  - Stimulation by swallowing (vagus):
    - Longitudinal muscle
    - Depolarization with superimposed spike bursts
  - Circular muscle: hyperpolarization, then depolarization and spike bursts
    - Myenteric plexus – necessary for peristaltic propagation
  - Smooth muscle contraction caused by ganglionic cholinergic neurons in response to swallowing

6

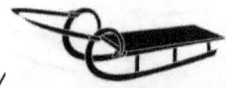

- This vagal nerve stimulation simultaneously reaches the ganglionic neurons in the middle and distal third of the esophagus
- There is a short (2 sec) latency in the proximal smooth muscle in terms of the time of the arrival of the nerve stimulation and muscle contraction
- There is a longer (5 to 7 sec latent period in the distal esophagus)
- This latent period may result "....from a neural gradient along the esophagus, where in excitatory ganglionic neurons dominate proximally and NO&VIP-releasing inhibitory ganglionic neurons dominate distally" (Feldman M., et al. Sleisenger and Fordtran's Gastrointestinal and Liver Disease. 9th Edition. Saunders/Elsevier, Philadelphia, 2010, page 682).

➢ **LES (lower esophageal sphincter)**
- The high pressure at the esophagogastric junction (EGJ) is caused by
  - LES (lower esophageal sphincter) pressure
    - 3-4 cm in length
    - Tonically contracted
  - Crural diaphragm
    - 2 cm length
    - ↑ in crural diaphragm contraction, with ↑ EGJ pressure
    - Inspiration (abolished by mechanical ventilation)
  - ↓ crural contraction, ↓ EGJ pressure
    - Distention of esophagus
    - Belching air, vomiting
  - Sling and clasp fibres of the middle layer of the musculature of the gastric cardia (including the angle of His)
- The high pressure in EGJ goes form 1-1.5 cm proximal and 2 cm distal to the SCJ (squamocolumnar junction)
- The LES is tonically contracted
- This myotonic LES tone"... varies directly with membrane potential and superimposed electrical spike activity that leads to an influx of Ca^{2+}." (Feldman M., et al. Sleisenger and Fordtran's Gastrointestinal and Liver Disease. 9th Edition. Saunders/Elsevier, Philadelphia, 2010, page 683).
- The spike activity with influences Ca^{2+} flux is itself regulated by K^+ - and Ca^{2+} - activated Cl^- channels
- Vagal (cholinergic input partially determines LES basal tone

7

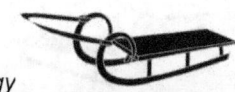

- o Adrenergic (sympathetic, acting through the myenteric neurons)
  - – Stellate and proximal thoracic ganglia – with
    - • splachnic nerve
    - • celiac ganglion
    - • α – adrenergic receptors on myenteric neurons (excitatory, as well as inhibitory)
- o Sympathetic (adrenergic, α – adrenergic receptors) activity
  - – ↑ excitatory neurons activity
  - – ↓ inhibitory neuron activity
  - – The net effect of α – adrenergic stimulation is
    - ↑ LES pressure
    - ↓ body muscle (relaxation)
- o Hormonal factors
- o Mechanical factors

- • Relaxation of LES

  - o An intramural process

  - o Mediated by post ganglionic nerves, ".... mediated by vagus"

  - o Caused by swallowing or distention of esophagus

  - o Post-ganglionic transmission is by way of nicotinic and muscarinic receptors

  - o Transmitters of post ganglionic neurons causing LES relaxation and ↓ LES pressure is mediated by NO (nitric oxide, produced from the amino acid L-arginine, by way of the enzyme NO synthase)

  - o Postganglionic deglutitive relaxation of the LES may also occur with other peptides such as VIP (prejunctional neurotransmitter acting on nerves containing NO synthase), as well as possibly PHI (peptide histidine isoleucine), CGRP (calcitonin gene-related peptide), galamin, and PACAP pituitary adenylate cyclase activation peptide)

- • Give myogenic factors which physiologically modulate LES pressure

  - o Membrane potential

  - o K^+ and Ca^{2+} - activated Cl^- channels

  - o Spike activity

  - o Ca^{2+} flux

  - o Pressure
    - – Gastric distention
    - – Intra-abdominal pressure (e.g., obesity, ascites)

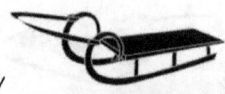

- Food
- Peptides
- Hormones
- Medications
- MMC (migrating motor complex (MMC phase III ↑ LES to 80 mmHg [NORM] resting LES pressure/ tone is 10 – 30 mmHg)
- Neurogenic factors
  - Vagal (cholinergic input partially determines LES basal tone
  - Adrenergic (sympathetic, acting through the myenteric neurons)

- Transient lower esophageal sphincter relaxation (tLESR) ED1340

- Give differences in the physiology of tLESR and swallow-associated declines in sLES pressure (sLESP).

	tLESR	sLESR
o Stimulus	o Distention of gastric cardia/fundus, even without swallowing or peristalsis	o Swallowing, or peristalsis
o Association with pharyngeal swallowing	No	Yes
o Associated with synchronized peristalsis	No	Yes
o Post-prandial	Yes	No
o Inhibition of crural diaphragm	Yes	No
o Contraction of distal esophageal longitudinal muscle	Yes	No
o Shortening of esophagus	Yes	No

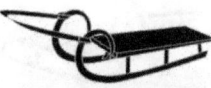

	tLESR	sLESR
o Afferent neural pathway	o Gastric afferents in the subdiaphragmatic vagus	o Pharyngeal and superior o Laryngeal nerves
o Central neural circuit	o Caudal dorsal motor nucleus	o Subnuclei of the medulla
o Efferent limb in the preganglionic vagal inhibitory pathway to LES	Yes	Yes

Abbreviation: tLESRs, Transient lower esophageal sphincter relaxations; sLESR, swallow-associated lower esophageal sphincter relaxations

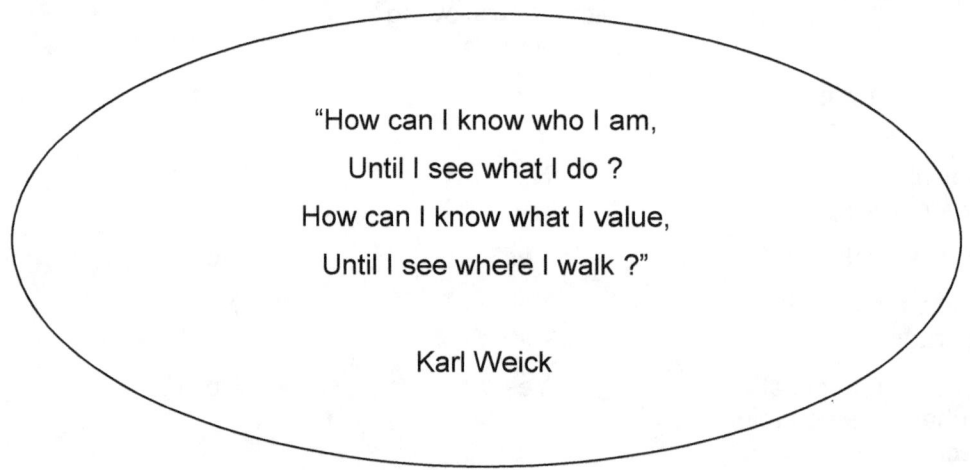

"How can I know who I am,
Until I see what I do ?
How can I know what I value,
Until I see where I walk ?"

Karl Weick

Dysphagia

- Clinical

- Give causes of oropharyngeal (transfer) dysphagia.

  - Peripheral and central nervous system (PNS and CNS)
  - Skeletal, muscular or neuromuscular
  - ENT
    - Xerostomia
    - Cancer, radiation to or surgery on cricopharynx or larynx
    - Tonsillar abscess
    - Foreign body

  - Esophagus
    - Intrinsic
      - Achalasia of UES
      - High esophageal rings, webs
      - Zenker diverticulum
    - Extrinsic
      - Thyromegaly
      - Spinal osteophytes
      - Senile Ankylosing hyperostosis
      - Rheumatoid cricoarytenoid arthritis
      - Cervical lymphadenopathy
      - Vascular abnormalities

  - Drugs
    - Anticholinergics
    - Antihistamines
    - Phenothiazine

Abbreviations: CNS, central nervous system; ENT, ear/nose/throat; PNS, peripheral nervous system; UES, upper esophageal sphincter

Adapted from: Cook IJ, and Shaker R. *2006 AGA Institute Postgraduate Course*: pg. 651.

11

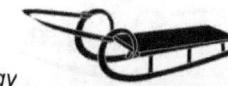

- Give symptoms of oropharyngeal dysphagia.

  - ENT
    - Difficulty in gathering or keeping bolus at the back of the tongue
    - Hoarse voice
    - Halitosis
    - Nasal regurgitation
    - Nasal speech and dysarthria
    - Swallow-related cough
    - Recurrent pneumonia
  - Esophagus
    - Food sticking in the throat (hesitation or inability to initiate swallowing; inability to propel food bolus caudad into pharynx)
    - Difficulty in swallowing solids
    - Frequent repetitive swallowing in attempts to clear the pharynx

- ➤ Investigations

- Give the "**Best test**" to evaluate
  - Oropharyngeal dysphagia
    - Videofluoroscopy, <u>not</u> ECD
  - The patient with symptoms of GERD
    - EGD + biopsy, <u>not</u> upper GI barium study
  - Any kind of esophageal or gastric symptoms in the patient over age 55.
    - EGD, EGD, EGD, even if a motility disorder is mentioned in the stem as a "red herring"
  - The patient < 55 years with no alarm symptoms has dyspepsia, and the MCQ asks you to choose between first doing a trial of PPIs, or to test and treat for H. pylori
    - The best test depends upon the pretest probability of the diagnosis. The symptoms of GERD are neither sensitive nor specific. If the MCQ stem suggest that the patient has a high pretest probability for an H. pylori infection (new Canadian from S. America or Middle East, or First Nation's person), then do T&T first. Otherwise, for persons with a low risk of H. pylori (prevalence in Canada overall is ~20%), then do EGD looking for esophagitis

12

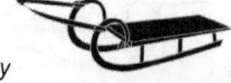

- ➢ Differential

- Because GERD (gastroesophageal reflux disease) is so common, and dysphagia occurs in some persons with GERD, it is useful to be mindful of the other causes besides GERD or cancer (squamous or adenomatous)
    - o Esophagitis
        - – Medications (pill esophagitis)
        - – Infections
            - ▪ CMV
            - ▪ HSV
            - ▪ candidiasis
        - – Eosinophilic esophagitis
    - o Dysmotility
        - – Achalasia (including Chagas disease from infection with T. cruzi)
        - – DES
        - – Hypertensive esophagus
        - – Scleroderma
        - – Post-polio syndrome
    - o Mechanical
        - – Cervical osteophytes
        - – Crircopharygeal bar
    - o MSK
        - – Dermatomyositis

Please see: Thomson ABR. Chapter 60. In: Therapeutic Choices. Grey J, Ed. 6th Edition, Canadian Pharmacists Association: Ottawa, ON, 2011, Table 2: Drugs used in GERD, page 810-812.

- ➢ Treatment
    - o Avoidance of social dining

- Give causes of dysphagia/odynophagia in patients with HIV/AIDS, which one related to their infection.
    - o Infections
        - – Candida albicans
        - – Cytomegalovirus (CMV)
        - – Herpes simplex (HSV)
        - – Histoplasma
        - – Mycobacterium avium complex (MAC)
        - – Cryptosporidium spp.
        - – PCP

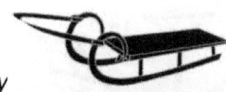

- o Neoplasm
  - – Kaposi sarcoma
  - – Lymphoma
  - – Squamous cell carcinoma
  - – Adenocarcinoma
- o Gastroesophageal reflux disease (increased frequency)
- o Pill-induced esophagitis
- o Idiopathic ulcerations

Abbreviations: CMV, cytomegalovirus; HSV, herpes simplex virus; MAC, myocobacterium avium complex

---

CLINICAL TIP

In the patient with dysphagia and a past history of polio, think about the possibility of the post-polio syndrome, even in the absence of bulbar symptoms/signs.

Dermatomyositis

Dermatomyositis involves the skeletal (striated) muscle of the upper third of the esophagus.

- Give clinical features of the patients with dysphagia which would raise the suspicion of dermatomyositis

  - o Eyes
    - – Red ring around eyes ("Helicotrope rash")

  - o Skin
    - – Red ring around neck ("shawl sign")
  - o MSK
    - – Gottron nodules knuckles

    - – Weakness of proximal muscle groups
  - o Laboratory
    - – ↑ ESR, ↑ CRP

14

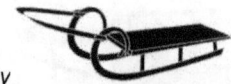

Systemic Sclerosis

➢ Clinical

• Give the conditions which develop in the GI tract in persons with systemic sclerosis.

- o Esophagus
  - – Severe esophagitis
  - – Strictures

- o Stomach
  - – Gastroparesis

- o Small bowel
  - – Mega-duodenum
  - – Chronic pseudo-obstruction
  - – SIBO (small intestinal bacterial overgrowth)
  - – Pneumatosis intestinalis

- o Colon
  - – Inertia (constipation)
  - – Wide-mouthed, R-sided diverticula

CLINICAL CASE

A 55 year old man develops solid food dysphagia. Careful physical examination shows pigmentation on the palms of his hands and soles of his feet.

• Give the anticipated findings on examination of his mouth, what is the likely cause of the dysphagia, and what is the management of this man's brothers and sisters?
  - o Hyperpigmentation of the palms and soles in a person with dysphagia suggests tylosis palmaris (aka H-E [Howel-Evans] syndrome).

  - o Oral leukoplakia is common.

  - o The condition is autosomal dominant, and 95% of patients develop esophageal squamous cell cancer by age 70.

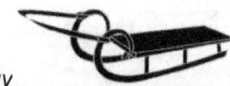

GASTROESOPHAGEAL REFLUX DISEASE (GERD)

➢ Clinical

- Give the "**Montreal definition**" of GERD and its constituent syndromes?

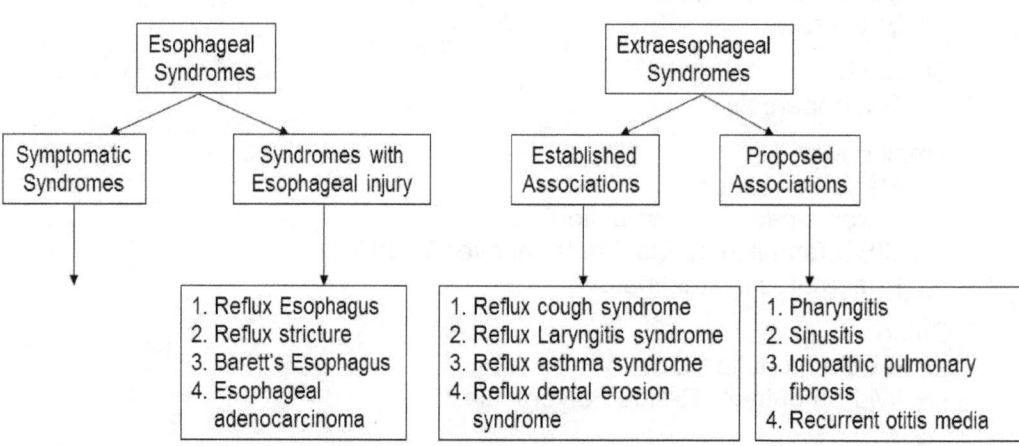

The overall Montreal definition of GERD and its constituent syndromes.

Abbreviation: GERD, gastroesophageal reflux disease

Printed with permission: Vakil N, et al. *Am J Gastroenterology* 2006;101(8):1900-1920.

- Give the **ENT/pulmonary (extraesophageal) symptoms** and ENT/ pulmonary signs of GERD.

Symptoms	Signs
o Pharynx, Sinuses – Throat clearing, throat mucus, globus, dysphagia, halitosis, acid regurgitation, waterbrash	- Sinusitis, Pharyngitis, Lingual Tonsillitis, Halitosis
o Larynx – Vocal fatigue, hoarseness (dysphonia)	- Posterior laryngitis, laryngeal carcinoma, vocal cord contact ulcers, granulomas, polyps, nodules, subglottic stenosis
o Ears – Ear pain	- Otitis media

16

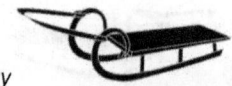

Symptoms	Signs
o Lungs – Interstitial pulmonary fibrosis (IPF), wheezing, asthma, chronic cough, aspiration	- Signs of pulmonary fibrosis - Wheezing
o Heart – NCCP, swallowing syncope	- Sinus arrhythmia
o Teeth – Tooth ache	- Dental carries
o Neck Pain – Muscle spasm	- Torticollis and muscle spasms

Abbreviations: ENT, ear nose throat; GERD, gastroesophageal reflux disease; IPF, interstitial pulmonary fibrosis

➤ Causes/associations

- Give the **non-dietary** causes/associations (not pathophysiology) of GERD.
  - o Hiatal hernia
  - o Scleroderma, Sjörgren syndrome
  - o Gastroparesis
  - o Zollinger-Ellison syndrome, G cell hyperplasia
  - o Pregnancy, ascites, obesity (increased BMI/ waist girth)
  - o Smoking, immobility, NG tube
  - o Medications (calcium channel blockers, theophylline, anticholinergics, nitrates, alpha adrenergic antagonists), Botox injections
  - o Vagotomy, gastrectomy, post dilation or myotomy for achalasia, bariatric surgery

Abbreviation: GERD, gastroesophageal reflux disease

➤ Pathophysiology

- Give a pathophysiology of GERD and GERD.
- Motility disorders
  - o Transient lower esophageal relaxations (TLESR)
  - o Lower esophageal sphincter
    - – Cholinergics (bethanecol)
    - – GABA receptor agonists [baclofen])
    - – Hiatus hernia
    - – Stomach (gastroparesis), obstructive sleep apnea
    - – Prokinetics

17

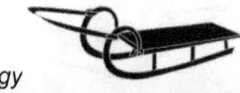

- o ↓ LES, ↑ LESR
- o Weak esophageal peristalsis
- o Scleroderma and CREST
- o Delayed gastric emptying

- Damaging factors
  - o Normal HCl secretion, but ↑ reflux of acid
    - − Alginate, antacids, H_2RAs, PPIs
  - o Increased gastric acid production
  - o Bile and pancreatic juice
    - − Sucralfate

- Resistance factors
  - o Reduced saliva, HCO_3^- and EGF production
    - − Chewing gum
  - o Diminished mucosal blood flow
  - o Growth factors (EGF)
  - o Protective mucus
  - o Normal epithelial mucosa and tight junctions
  - o Perception
    - − TCAs, SSRIs

Abbreviations: GERD, gastroesophageal reflux disease; H2RA, histamine 2 receptor antagonist; LES, lower esophageal sphincter; LESR, lower esophageal relaxations

Printed with permission: Murray JA. *Mayo Clinic Gastroenterology and Hepatology Board Review* 2008: pg. 3.

➢ Diagnosis
- Give the method to diagnose GERD.
  - o Compatible symptoms and signs
    - − Heartburn, dyspepsia, regurgitation
    - − "extraesophageal" conditions in ear, nose, throat, lungs
  - o Laboratory
    - − Iron deficiency ± anemia
    - − Absence of eosinophilia

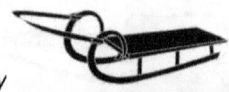

- o Diagnostic imaging
  - – Barium esophagogram
    - ▪ GER
    - ▪ Erosion/ulceration
    - ▪ Stricture
    - ▪ Hiatus hernia
    - ▪ Lower esophageal cancer
- o Endoscopy (white band)
  - – Who should have an EGD:
    - ▪ Depends upon which guideline is being followed
    - ▪ New symptoms age > 50 to 55 years
    - ▪ Alarm symptoms at any age
    - ▪ > 10 years of moderately severe symptoms occurring ≥ 3x per wk
    - ▪ Note: alarm symptoms have a very low PPV, but a NPV of ~98% for esophageal/gastric cancer
  - – Normal, or grades LA A to D esophagitis
  - – Complications
    - ▪ Stricture
    - ▪ Mass
    - ▪ Adenocarcinoma
  - – Exclude other causes for symptoms
    - ▪ Other causes of esophagitis, e.g., EoE (eosinophilic esophagitis) about 5% of persons with refractory GERD may have EoE
    - ▪ Peptic ulceration
    - ▪ Gastric ulceration
    - ▪ Gastritis outlet (e.g., H. pylori)
    - ▪ Gastric outlet obstruction
- o Physiological studies*
  - – Esophageal pH testing
  - – Esophageal manometry
    - ▪ 24 hr
    - ▪ 4 day BRAVO® study
  - – Esophageal pH and multichannel intraluminal impedence testing
  - – High resolution manometry

* under special circumstances

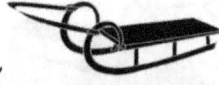

Mastering the Boards: Gastroenterology   A.B.R. Thomson

- Give the diagnostic tests for GERD.

❖ Tests to assess symptoms

   o Empirical trial of acid suppression

		Sensitivity %	Specificity %
- Heartburn and regurgitation	twice daily for 7 days	80	56
- Noncardiac chest pain	twice daily for 14 days	75	85

   o Intraesophageal pH monitoring with symptom association analysis

   o Bernstein test (acid infusion test to reproduce patient's typical symptoms)

   o Cortical sensing and motor control

   o Symptom-Association Indices

   o Request® questionnaire

❖ Tests to assess esophageal function

   o Esophageal manometry (normal or high resolution)

   o Esophageal impedance

   o VFSS

❖ Tests to assess reflux

   o Ambulatory intraesophageal pH monitoring

   o Ambulatory bilirubin monitoring (bile reflux)

   o Ambulatory esophageal impedance and pH monitoring

   o Barium esophagogram, video fluoroscopy swallowing study (VFSS)

   o Optical coherence manometry

   o Scintigraphy

   o Milk scan in infant

❖ Tests to assess esophageal damage

   o Endoscopy (optical white light EGD, capsule endoscopy [CE], EUS/FNA narrow band imaging [NBI] with zoom, chromoendoscopy)

   o Esophageal biopsy

   o Contrast radiography

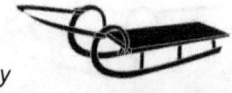

Abbreviations: CE, capsule endoscopy; EUS, endoscopic ultrasound; FNA, fine needle aspiration; GERD, gastroesophageal reflux disease; NBI, narrow band imaging; VFSS, videofluroscopy swallowing study

Adapted from: *Sleisenger & Fordtran's gastrointestinal and liver disease: Pathophysiology/Diagnosis/Management* 2016, pg. 744.; Printed with permission: Murray JA. *Mayo Clinic Gastroenterology and Hepatology Board Review*: pg. 11.; Thomson ABR. *Clinical Medicine Gastroenterology* 2008;1:pg. 11.; and Spechler SJ. *2008 ACG Annual Postgraduate Course book*: pg. 113.

- Give the uses of ambulatory 24 hr esophageal pH **impedence monitoring (EIM)**.
  - Acid reflux
    - Acid, non-acid, gas
  - Rumination
  - Bolus transit
  - Dysmotility (spasm)

Abbreviation: EIM, esophageal pH impedence monitoring

Adapted from: Murray JA. *Mayo Clinic Gastroenterology and Hepatology Board Review*: pg. 11.; and Printed with permission: Thomson ABR. *Clinical Medicine Gastroenterology* 2008;1:pg. 11.

- Give conditions that must be excluded before considering the diagnosis of GER-related cough.
  - No exposure to environmental irritants
  - Not a present smoker
  - Not on an ACE inhibitor
  - Normal or stable chest radiograph
  - No symptomatic asthma (i.e., cough not improved on therapy, or negative methacholine inhalation challenge test)
  - No upper airway cough syndrome due to rhinosinus diseases ruled out (i.e., cough not improved by first generation H_1-receptor antagonists and 'silent' sinusitis ruled out)
  - No non-asthmatic eosinophilic bronchitis (i.e., sputum studies negative or cough not improved by inhaled/systemic corticosteroids)

Abbreviations: ACE, angiotensin-converting enzyme; GER, gastroesophageal reflux

Printed with permission: Chandra KM and Harding SM. *Nat Clin Pract Gastroenterol Hepatol* November 2007;4(11): 606.

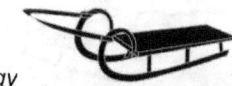

➢ Endoscopy

- Give diseases/ conditions associated with a higher risk for sedation-related complications in persons undergoing upper gastrointestinal endoscopy (EGD).

  o Morbid obesity

  o Short neck

  o Alcohol or substance abuse

  o Persons on high doses of psychotropic medications

  o COPD, asthma

  o Cervical neck lesions

  o Chronic liver/kidney/heart/lung disease

- Give clinical applications of high-resolution **narrow band imaging** (NBI), along the GI tract, from mouth to anus.

  o Oropharynx and hypopharynx
    - Detection of premalignant and early cancer in high-risk individuals

  o Esophagus
    - Detection of premalignant (Barrett esophagus) and early cancer in high-risk individuals
    - Detection of specialized intestinal metaplasia in patients with a short segment of columnar-lined esophagus
    - Detection of flat areas of high-grade intraepithelial neoplasia and early cancer in patients with Barrett esophagus under surveillance

  o Stomach
    - Detection of premalignant and early gastric cancer lesions
    - Delineation of the spread of premalignant and early gastric cancer lesions to facilitate endoscopic mucosal resection and endoscopic submucosal dissection

  o Duodenum
    - Detection of foci of adenocarcinoma in patients with ampullary adenomas
    - Diagnosis and classification of villous atrophy in celiac disease

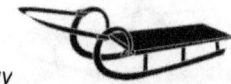

- o Colon
  - – Detection of flat and depressed lesions
  - – Differentiation of neoplastic and non-neoplastic colonic lesions
  - – Surveillance of patients with long-standing ulcerative colitis (UC) and hereditary non-polyposis colorectal cancer syndrome (Lynch syndrome)
  - – Screening colonoscopy

Abbreviations: NBI, narrow band imaging; UC, ulcerative colitis

Printed with permission: Larghi A., et al. *Gut* 2008;57:pg. 978.

- ➢ Histopathology
  - o Normal
  - o Reactive changes
  - o Erosion/ulceration
  - o Barrett epithelium (BE)
  - o Adenocarcinoma

- Give the **histological abnormalities** in GERD.
  - o Reactive epithelial changes
    - – Hyperplasia of the basal zone (3 layers or more)
    - – Elongation of papillae (>15% of total epithelial thickness)
    - – ↑ mitotic figures
    - – ↑ vascularization of the epithelium
    - – Loss of usual longitudinal orientation of the surface epithelium
    - – Balloon cells
  - o Erosions
    - – Epithelial loss
    - – Inflammatory infiltrates – lymphocytes, plasma cells, eosinophils, neutrophils
    - – Necrosis
  - o Barrett
    - – Intestinal metaplasia, dysplasia, adenocarcinoma
    - – Columnar cells
    - – Goblet cells (shown with combined hematoxyline and eosin-alcian blue PAS stains)
    - – Fibrosis, strictures
  - o Signs of eosinophilic esophagitis response to PPI

Abbreviation: GERD, gastroesophageal reflux disease

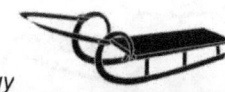

- Give the histological grading of GERD.

Grade	Inflammatory Infiltrates		Basal Cell Hyperplasia
	Definition	Cell Type	
0	0-6 cells/HPF	Lymphocytes, plasma cells	3 cell layers or less
0.5	Small areas >6 cells/HPF	Lymphocytes, plasma cells	3 cell layers or less
1	Slight focal infiltration	Lymphocytes, plasma cells	>3 cell layers, less than 1/3 epithelial thickness
2	Moderate diffuse infiltrate	Lymphocytes, plasma cells, eosinophils	>1/3 and <2/3 of epithelial thickness
3	Severe inflammation	Lymphocytes, plasma cells, eosinophils, neutrophils	>2/3 of epithelial thickness

Abbreviation: GERD, gastroesophageal reflux disease

Printed with permission: Vieth M. *Best Pract Res Clin Gastroenterol* 2008;22(4): pg. 629.

- Give the histological grading of GERD.

	Length of Papillae as % of Total Epithelial Thickness	Thickness of Basal Cell Layer as % of Total Epithelial Thickness
o Normal	<15%	1-2%
o Grade 1	15-33%	2-20%
o Grade 2	34-66%	21-50%
o Grade 3	>66%	>50%

Criticisms: Small number of patients; no interobserver variation; questionable control group

Abbreviation: GERD, gastroesophageal reflux disease

Printed with permission: Vieth M. *Best Pract Res Clin Gastroenterol* 2008;22(4): pg. 628.

24

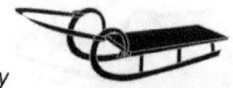

> Treatment

❖ Comorbidities
  o As in all medical conditions, psychological comorbidities need to be considered and managed where appropriate

❖ Lifestyle changes (LSC)
  o Evidence-based (EB)
    – Loss of excessive body weight
    – Elevation of head of bed (6 inches; or Styrofoam wedge under the mattess) for nocturnal or laryngeal
    – Diet
      ▪ Avoid reflux
        – Avoid reflux-inducing foods
        – Chocolate
        – Fatty foods
        – Peppermint
      ▪ Avoid symptom-aggravating foods (on an individual basis), e.g.,
        – Tomatoes
        – Citrus fruits
        – Colas
        – Red wine
        – Spices
      ▪ Avoid bedtime snacks/meals
      ▪ Avoid use of alcohol
    – Position
      ▪ Do not lie down for at least 2 hr after meals
    – Salvation
      ▪ Smoking – avoid tobacco products (↓ salvation)
      ▪ Chewing gum
      ▪ Oral lozenges

Abbreviations: BE, barrett epithelium; EB, evidence-based; EGD, esophagogastroduodenoscopy; GER, gastroesophageal reflex; GERD, gastroesophageal reflux disease; H2RA, H2 receptor antagonist; LESP, lower esophageal sphincter pressure; NAB, nocturnal acid breakthrough; Od, Rx given once a day; PPI, proton pump inhibitor; TG, therapeutic gain; TLESR, transient lower esophageal sphincter relaxation

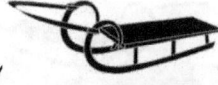

- Give lifestyle modifications for possible improvement of symptoms of gastroesophageal reflux (GER) and gastroesophageal reflux disease (GERD).
  - Weight loss if BMI is increased
  - Manage ascites
  - Smoking cessation
  - Elevate head of bed by 15 cm (6 inches)
  - Refrain from eating 2 hours before lying down (after meals and at bedtime)
  - Avoid a high-fat diet
  - Avoid foods that worsen GER symptoms (e.g., caffeine, carbonated beverages, chocolate, mint, citrus products, alcohol)
  - Avoid (if possible) medications that worsen GER symptoms e.g., (anticholinergics, benzodiazepines, beta-agonists, bisphosphonates, calcium-channel blockers, corticosteroids, estrogens, NSAIDs, opiates, progesterone, prostaglandins, theophylline)
  - Nasal CPAP if obstructive sleep apnea is present
  - Avoid exercise that may increase intra-abdominal pressure

Abbreviations: BMI, body mass index; CPAP, continuous positive airway pressure; GER, gastroesophageal reflux; GERD, gastroesophageal reflux disease

❖ Pharmaceutical measures

- Give classes of drugs used to treat GERD.
  - Sensation – TCA, SSRIs
  - ↑ saliva – chewing gum
  - ↑ LESP – cholinergic (bethanecol)
  - ↓ TLESP – (GABA receptor agonist [baclofen])
  - ↑ coating – alginate
  - ↓ acid – PPI, H_2RA, antacids, anti-cholinergics
  - ↑ gastric emptying – prokinetics (e.g., domperidone)
  - ↓ bile acids
    - Cholestyramine
    - Sucralfate

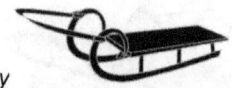

Mastering the Boards: Gastroenterology   A.B.R. Thomson

- ❖ Acute therapy
  - ○ Used in addition to tailor lifestyle changes
  - ○ ↓ **acid secretion** (to intragastric pH > 4 for ~ 14 hours)
    - – PPI > H2RA > antacids
      - ▪ TG 57% to 74% versus placebo for PPI, 10% to 24% for H2RA relief of heartburn and healing
      - ▪ Complete relief of heartburn, per week of Rx
    - – Start with standard dose of PPI, taken 30 min before the first meal of the day, for 8 weeks (11.5% healing per week, but LA grade C or D severe esophagitis may take longer to heal)
      - ▪ Lower response of symptom of regurgitation to PPI/H2RAs (0 to 35%)
        - – PPI   11.5%
        - – H2RA   6.4%
      - ▪ If symptom response to PPI is incomplete after 8 weeks of od therapy, increase to bid therapy, standard dose 30 min before breakfast and supper
      - ▪ The ↑ TG for doubling the dose of PPI is
        - – Symptom improvement 4%
        - – Healing 6%
      - ▪ In some persons, switching to another PPI may prove to be useful; the explanation for this phenomenon is not clear
  - ○ **Prokinetics** (↑ rate of gastric emptying / ↑ LES pressure)
    - – Use as adjunctive therapy of incomplete response to PPI bid for patients with possible delayed gastric emptying contributing to their poor therapeutic response
    - – There are concerns now of po domperidone causing ventricular arrhythmia and sudden cardiac death (SCD)
    - – Avoid in patients withHF or history of arrhythmias
    - – QTC (corrected QT) must be normal on ECG (no QT conduction defect through smooth muscle receptor) when using prokinetics
    - – Any drug potent enough to alter GI motility will affect the heart – same effects on smooth muscle
    - – Don't combine erythromycin and domperidone for gastroparesis (both CYP 3A4 inhibitors)
  - ○ ↓ TLESR
    - – Baclofen (gamma-aminobutyric acid agonist for the type B receptors) may be used in refractory GERD
    - – 10 mg bid, increasing slowly to 20 mg tid, or maximum benefit obtained without the development of CNS-related adverse effects

27

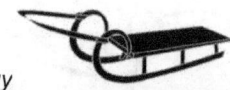

- o ↓ H. pylori
  - – Some algorithms for the management of uninvestigated dyspepsia support a therapeutic trial of empiric PPI therapy, or empiric anti-pylori therapy, or "test-and-treat" H. pylori infection.
  - – Without EGD plus biopsy, it is not possible to determine if the H.pylori-associated gastritis was
    - ▪ Increasing intragastric pH (hyposecretion as a result of pangastritis), or
    - ▪ Increasing intragastric pH (hypersecretion as a result of antral gastritis)

- ❖ Endoscopic therapy
  - o No longer widely practiced
  - o Radiofrequency energy delivery to the gastro-esophageal junction (the Stretta procedure) improves gastro-esophageal reflux disease (GERD) symptoms and quality of life.
  - o This was accompanied by a decrease in compliance of the gastro-esophageal junction.
  - o The decrease in compliance was not due to fibrosis, as it was reversible by smooth muscle relaxants.

Source: Arts J, et al. Am J Gastroenterol 2012; 107: 222-230.

- ❖ Maintenance therapy
  - o Rational: if a recurrence of symptoms occurs within 1 year, it will likely occur in < 3 months
  - o Continuous
    - – If recurrent typical symptoms in ' 3 months
    - – Use half the standard dose if od PPI was effective for acute Rx, and full single standard dose if bid PPI was necessary
  - o Repeat acute therapy
    - – If recurrent typical symptoms in 3 months
    - – This provides for a trial off medications, and to determine each person's individual natural history
  - o Intermittent
    - – Only for mild to moderate heartburn in the patient having had an EGD showing only mild or no esophagitis.

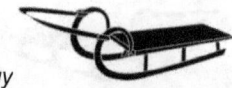

- Surgery
  - Surgery is an effective option for the management of GERD, but only in highly selected patients
  - The general standard of care is for the person with GERD who is being considered for a surgical procedure (e.g., fundoplication) to have at least esophageal manometry, and preferentially esophageal pH and multichannel intraluminal impedence testing.
- Pregnancy and lactation
  - PPIs and H_2RAs should only be used when life style changes fail do not confuse dyspepsia/heartburn with pregnancy-associated nausea
  - These drugs have category 'B' in the FDA classification, except for omeprazole, which is 'C'.

- Give the potential causes **of inadequate PPI response**.
  - Drugs
    - Not taking PPI for at least 4 wks
    - Non-adherence to PPI
    - PPI not given 30 minutes before breakfast (or first meal of the day if a shift worker)
    - Other medication (nitrites, calcium channel blocker, NSAIDs, ASA, tetracycline, bisphosphonates)
    - Rapid metabolism of PPI
    - Reduced bioavailabililty
  - Life style (dietary and non-dietary issues (please see above)
  - Large volume regurgitation and need for other drugs
    - Posture (bending, lack of head of bed elevation)
    - ↑ BMI/ascites/pregnancy
    - Previous myotomy, hemigastrectomy/ vagometry
  - Dysmotility
    - ↓ peristalsis
    - ↓ LESP, ↑ tLESR
    - Gastroparesis
    - DES
    - Achalasia
    - NCCP
    - Scleroderma
    - Myotomy
    - Vagotomy

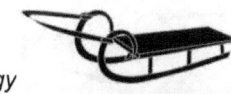

- o Other esophageal disease
  - – Non-acid GERD
  - – NERD
  - – NAB
  - – Functional esophagus
  - – Hypersensitive esophagus
  - – Pill esophagitis
  - – Esophageal cancer
  - – Eosinophilic esophagitis
  - – Infectious esophagitis (candida, HSV, CMV)
- o Non-esophageal conditions
  - – Stomach-- hypersecretory state, ,NAB gastroparesis
  - – Small intestine-- bile reflux
  - – Colon – GERD associated with IBS
  - – Skin disease with esophagitis (Epidermolysis dissecans, Mucocutaneous candidiasis)
  - – Other diagnoses (i.e., heart disease)

Abbreviations: CMV, cytomegalovirus; DES, diffuse esophageal spasm; GERD, gastroesophageal reflux disease; HSV, herpes simplex virus; IBS, irritable bowel syndrome; NAB, nocturnal acid breakthrough NCCP, non-cardiac chest pain; NERD, normal esophagus reflux disease; PPI, proton pump inhibitor

- Give indications for open or laparoscopic **surgical fundoplication** in the patient with GERD.
  - o GERD symptoms unsatisfactorily (partially) responding to PPI, (penalty for failure of PPI as an indication)
  - o Intolerance to PPIs
  - o Cost of PPIs
  - o Patient preference, desire for a "cure"
  - o Persistent large volume regurgitation
  - o Large symptomatic hiatus hernia
  - o Respiratory complications from recurrent aspiration
  - o Recurrent peptic strictures in a young person

Abbreviations: GERD, gastroesophageal reflux disease; PPI, proton pump inhibitor

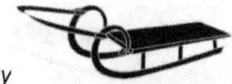

- Give the empiric medical trial for **GERD-related cough**.
  - ○ Twice daily PPIs 30-60 minutes before breakfast and dinner
  - ○ Consider adding a prokinetic agent initially if dysphagia is present or if cough does not improve with PPI
  - ○ Assess response to therapy within 1-3 months
  - ○ Lifestyle modifications (please see question 10, page 20)

Adapted from: Chandra KM and Harding SM. *Nat Clin Pract Gastroenterol Hepatol* 2007; 4(11): 606.

Peptic Strictures

- Give predictors of initial therapeutic failure of pneumatic dilation of benign esophageal strictures (i.e., repeated dilations required).
  - ○ Related to patient
    - – Age <40 years
    - – Male sex
    - – Dilated esophagus
  - ○ Related to procedure
    - – Inadequate dilation
      - ▪ Small size balloon (30 mm)
      - ▪ Lower esophageal sphincter pressure (LESP) >10 mm Hg post-treatment
    - – Poor esophageal emptying post-treatment

Adapted from: Boeckxstaens GEE. *Best Pract Res Clin Gastroenterol* 2007;21(4): 595.

- Give etiologies of benign, non-GERD related esophageal strictures.
  - ○ Congenital – Strictures, atresia
  - ○ Drugs and chemicals – Radiation, caustic, chemical, thermal, quinidine gluconate
  - ○ Webs, rings
  - ○ Sclerotherapy
  - ○ Acid and non-acid causes of esophagitis
  - ○ Surgery – Complicated reflux strictures (NG tube, ZE syndrome), ischemia, anastomotic (staples)
  - ○ Iatrogenic – EMR for BE, prolonged NG tube, therapy, PDT

Abbreviations: BE, Barrett epithelium; EMR, endoscopic mucosal resection; NG, nasogastric tube; PDT, photodynamic therapy; ZE, Zollinger-Ellison syndrome

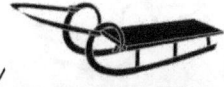

Non-Erosive Reflux Disease (NERD; aka Normal Esophagus Reflux Disease)

➤ Definition

o Persons with typical symptoms of gastroesophageal reflux disease (GERD) may have an endoscopically normal mucosa and be diagnosed as having nonerosive reflux disease (NERD).

➤ Classification

o This is sufficient for clinical practice, but in a research setting, NERD may be classified into three groups:

– Abnormal esophageal acid exposure (41% of NERD subjects)

– Hypersensitive esophagus (HE): normal esophageal acid exposure, positive symptom association with acid or non-acid reflux (32% of NERD patients)

– Functional heartburn (FH): normal esophageal acid exposure; negative symptom association with acid or non-acid reflux (27% of NERD patients).

o As defined by Rome III criteria, functional heartburn is defined as

– Burning retrosternal discomfort or pain; plus

– Absence of evidence of GERD as the cause of symptoms; plus

– Absence of histopathology-based esophageal motility disorders

– All 3 criteria fulfilled for the last 3 months prior to the diagnosis of functional heartburn

	Abnormal H+ Exposure	Symptom Association	PPI Respones	Normal EGD
o NERD	+	+	+	+
o HE	-	+	+	+
o FH	-	-	-	+

Abbreviations: FH, functional heartburn; HE, hypersensitive; NERD, non-erosive reflux disease

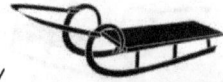

Refractory GERD

➢ Definition

- o GERD is said to be refractory if the patient's symptoms have not responded to their "satisfaction" after a 4 week course of PPI, taken once or twice a day.

- o The definition is based on subjective reporting of symptoms, and is not standardized in terms of which symptom(s), dose and duration of PPI use, naïve or pretreated patients, uninvestigated or investigated dyspepsia etc.

- o For example, the response rate of NERD (normal endoscopy reflux disease) to PPIs is only about 60% as that for erosive esophagitis.

- o Up to 58% of refractory GERD patients have "functional heartburn"

➢ Treatment

- Give the therapeutic option for refractory GERD, after confirming the diagnosis of GERD, and confirming that the patient is taking the PPI Rx 30 min before breakfast and dinner.

- o H2RA intermittently or on demand at bedtime

- o Antacids, barrier agents

- o Bile salt binders
  - – Sucralfate
  - – Cholestyramine

- o Prokinetics

- o Pain modulators (anti-depressants in low, non-mood-altering doses)
  - – SSRI (selective serotonin reuptake inhibitors)
  - – TCAs (tricyclic antidepressants)
  - – Trazodone

- o Baclofen

- o Acupuncture

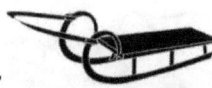

Nocturnal Acid Breakthrough (NAB)

➢ Definition

  o Intragastric pH<4 for >60 min during the night time

  o Exclude obstructive sleep apnea

➢ Demography

  o NAB may be more frequent in GERD plus BE

➢ Clinical

  o Poor correlation between NAB and nocturnal heartburn

➢ Treatment

  o In the occasional patient with nocturnal heartburn despite bid PPI may respond to the addition, as adjunctive therapy, of an H_2RA.

  o Because of high likelihood of the rapid development to an H2RA, if the patient continues to have symptoms at night despite PPI bid, H2RA may be helpful when given intermittently or on demand

---

Clinical Alert

When a patient is suspected as having NAB (nocturnal acid breakthrough), the PPI and the H_2RA must not be given concurrently, because this reduces the acid inhibitory effect of each.

Thoughtful reflections
"Discuss the ethical considerations relating to a nurse-based triage system for consultations from family physicians asking to see a gastroenterologist, using a protocol denying prompt access to persons with functional disorders or requesting a second opinion."

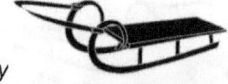

Rebound Acid Secretion

Persons treated with PPIs for > 6 months may be at risk of rebound of acid secretion, the development of recurrent acid-peptic symptoms when the PPIs are stopped, and a need for the dose of PPI to be slowly reduced (tapered) and not stopped suddenly.

- Give the likely physiological explanation for this rebound in acid secretion.
    - PPI → ↓ H+ → ↓ antral somatostatin → ↑ antral gastrin → ↑ parietal cell mass → ↑ H+ secretion when PPI stopped (until restoration of normal post-prandial pH-related feedback on gastric HCl secretion).

SO YOU WANT TO BE A GASTROENTEROLOGIST!

- Give mechanisms of action of gamma β receptor agonists (e.g.,baclofen) on the physiology of the esophagus and stomach which make this class of drugs potentially useful in persons with refractory GERD.
    - Gamma β receptor agonists have the following physiological effects
        - ↓ TLESR (~50%)
        - ↑ LESP (basal)
        - ↑ rate of gastric emptying
        - ↓ reflux episodes (~40%)

The H2RA (H2 receptor antagonists) are about 60% as effective as the PPIs in the reduction of gastric acid secretion, the amelioration of acid-related symptoms and the healing of acid-induced damage.
- Give the reasons why despite these data, histamine is considered to be the most dominant amongst the 3 other main stimuli of gastric acid secretion, acetylcholine and gastrin.
    - Histamine is released from the ECL (enterochromaffin-like) cells close to the parietal cells.
    - Histamine is released from the ECL cells in response to food in the stomach.
    - The release of histamine is magnified by gastrin, which also acts on the ECL cells.

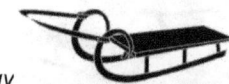

Acid-related Disorder Target Intragastric pHs

	pH (% pH ≥ n)	Duration of Treatment, wks
o DU*	3	4
o GERD	4	4-8
o H.pylori	5	1-2
o NVUGIB**	6	3 days

* the usual duration of treatment of DU is 4 weeks, and 8 weeks for gastric ulcer (GU), but the pH target (% pH ≥ n) is not known for GU.
** Initially IV PPI for 3 days, followed by oral for a period depending upon the etiology og the NVGIB

Abbreviations: DU, duodenal ulcer; GERD, gastroesophageal reflux disease; GU, gastric ulcer; NVUGIB, non-variceal upper GI bleed

xxxxxxxxxxxxxxxxxxxxxxxxxxxxxxxxxxxxxxxxxxxxxxxxxxx

SO YOU WANT TO BE A GASTROENTEROLOGIST!

- Give the influence of H. pylori infection on the PPI-associated risk of developing atrophic gastritis (gastric atrophy; atrophy of gastric glands) in the body of the stomach.

    o PPI user and annual incidence of atrophy of the mucosa of the gastric body

        – H. pylori
            ▪ Negative   0.7
            ▪ Positive   4.7
    Thus, practically (clinically speaking), the risk of gastric atrophy resulting from the long-term use of PPIs occurs mainly in persons who are H. pylori positive.

- Give the physiological explanation why some cardiac patients with congestive heart failure who are chronically taking PPIs require monitoring of their serum magnesium concentration.

    o PPIs lower the serum concentration management, as also do diuretics and digoxin, placing persons consuming these medications at risk of the adverse effects of hypomagnesemia.

xxxxxxxxxxxxxxxxxxxxxxxxxxxxxxxxxxxxxxxxxxxxxxxxxxx

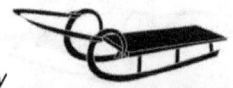

Proton Pump Inhibitors (PPI)

- ➢ Clinical

- • Give indications for the use of PPIs.

    - ○ Esophagus
        - – NERD
        - – GERD (symptoms and/or signs of damage from acid-related disorders), including BE
        - – Barrett epithelium (BE)
        - – Tracheopulmonary disorders associated with GERD
        - – Esophageal eosinophilia
        - – Motility disorders
            - ▪ Achalasia
            - ▪ Scleroderma
            - ▪ DES/hypertensive esophagus
        - – ↓ # of esophageal dilations needed to relieve dysphagia from benign (peptic) stricture
        - – Healing after EMR of BE
        - – Healing of post-banding or post-sclerotherapy ulcers
        - – Prevention of (reduction in damage) aspiration pneumonitis

    - ○ Stomach
        - – PUD (peptic ulcer disease, including GU [gastric ulcer] and DU [duodenal ulcer] and GU/DU caused by ASA/NSAIDs)
        - – H.pylori eradication
        - – Gastroparesis (with prokinetics)
        - – Hypersecretory states (e.g., ZES [Zollinger Ellison Syndrome])
        - – Nocturnal acid breakthrough
        - – Prevention of drug-induced damage to stomach
            - ▪ ASA
            - ▪ NSAIDs
            - ▪ COXIBs
        - – Upper GI bleeding
        - – Prevention of stress ulceration
        - – ↓ drainage gastric GI fistula

    - ○ Small bowel
        - – Short bowel syndrome (↓ small bowel output)
        - – Duodenal Crohn disease

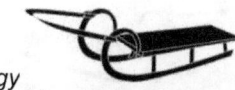

- o Pancreas
  - – Pancreatic insufficiency
    - ▪ Non-coated pancreatic replacement treatment
    - ▪ Pain control

- ➢ Metabolim
  - o The proton pump is comprised by the H^+ - K^+ - ATPase in the canalicular membrane at the apical surface of the parietal cell.
  - o The H^+ - K^+ - ATPase is a member of the P2 family of ion motive transport enzymes.
  - o The secretory canaliculus is an acidic space in a slightly invaginated area of the apical membrane of the parietal cell.
  - o The absorbed PPIs accumulate in this acidic space in the secretory canaliculus.
  - o The PPIs are weakly protonatable pyridines, with values of pKa ~4, depending on the individual PPI.
  - o The higher the value of the pKa, the faster the PPI undergoes an acid-catalyzed conversion to the active agent, a thiophilic sulfonamide.
  - o The thiophilic sulfonamide forms a non-reversible disulfide bond with cysteine 813 in the activated H^+ - K^+ - ATPase in the canaliculus and apical membrane of the parietal cell.
  - o Cysteine 813 is in the catalytic alpha-subunit of the H^+ - K^+ - ATPase.
  - o While all PPIs bind to cysteine 813, some PPIs may bind to additional cysteine molecules (e.g., pantoprazole also binds to cysteine 822).
  - o The resulting non-competitive inhibition in the final common pathway of the parietal secretion of HCl lasts until new pumps and produced in new parietal cells.
  - o This explains why the biological and pharmacodynamics T½ (~ 60 min).
  - o There are differences between PPIS in terms of their pKa, rate of absorption and metabolism, including differences in PK (pharmacokinetics) and PD (pharmacodynamics) properties.

Caucasian race	CYP2C19 gene	Polymorphisms	Duration of ↓ H^+
5%	Inactivating mutation	Slow (↓ rate)	Long
~65%	Wild type gene	Rapid (↑ rate)	Short

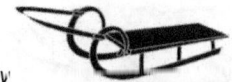

- Give the regimens for "hepatic dosing' or "renal dosing" of PPIs in persons with cirrhosis or renal insufficiency, and in persons on certain HIV protease inhibitors.
  - PPIs do not require either hepatic nor renal dosing
  - PPIs reduce the absorption of some HIV protease inhibitors

✕✕

SO YOU WANT TO BE A GASTROENTEROLOGIST!

- In the context of PPIs, give the advantages and disadvantages of polymorphisms for a mutation in CYP2C19.

	Clinical Advantage	
	H.pylori Eradication	GERD
Homozygous CYP2C19 mutation (slow metabolizers)	100%	85%
Heterozygotes	60%	68%
Homozygous, wild type (rapid metabolizers)	29%	96% (overall) 16% (severe)

  - CYP2C19 mutation and saturation
    - Adverse interactions with
      - Warfarin
      - Diazepam
      - Theophylline
      - Clopidogrel
      - Phenytoin

- Give the explanation why the PPI rabeprazole has many fewer adverse effects than omeprazole, and why pantoprazole has even lower risks.

  - Omeprazole is metabolized by CYP2C19, and depending upon whether the patient is a deficient or saturated phenotype, the PPI may interfere with the metabolism of many drugs.

  - Rabeprazole has affinity for CYP2C19 plus CYP3A4, so the risk of adverse effects from drug interactions is less.

  - Pantoprazole is rapidly sulfated after CYP2C19 methylation, so it does not induce CYP3A4 or CYP1A.

✕✕

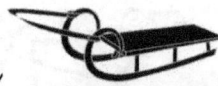

SO YOU WANT TO BE A GASTROENTEROLOGIST!

The acid inhibitory effect of a single dose of PPI is less than the inhibitory effect which occurs after multiple dosing.

- Give the explanation for this **steady-state phenomenon**.

  - When food enters the stomach, not all the parietal cells become active.

  - PPIs only bind to the cysteine 813 of H^+ - K^+ - ATPase when the H^+ - K^+ - ATPase is active.

  - Over several days, more and more parietal cells will have been stimulated, resulting in more and more proton pump being activated and subsequently inhibited by the PPI.

  - In the same manner as the effect of the progressively increased recruitment of H^+ - K^+ - ATPase and its inhibition by PPIs, the acid inhibitory effect of the PPIs may last 1 to 2 days after the PPI has been stopped.

Adverse Effects of PPIs

- Give long-term adverse effects of PPI therapy.

<u>Risk Possible/Magnitude Consequence</u>

❖ Associated with hypergastrinemia

  - Hypergastrinemia-induced carcinoid tumours
    – Not demonstrated in humans

  - Accelerated progression of atrophic gastritis/gastric cancer with concomitant *H. pylori* gastritis
    – No documentation of an increase in atrophic gastritis and no basis to recommend testing or treatment for *H Pylori* before long-term PP use

  - Formation of gastric fundic gland polyps
    – Odds ratio of 2.2 for developing Fundic gland polyps within 1-5 years, negligible, if any, risk of dysplasia

  - Acid rebound (hypochlorhydria)

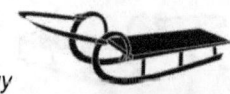

<u>Risk Possible/Magnitude consequence</u>

❖ Malabsorption

    o Vitamin B12 malabsorption
        – Nested case-control study of UK patients older than 50 years; adjusted odds ration of 1.44 (95% confidence interval, 1.30-1.59) of hip fracture with PPI use longer than 1 year

    o Calcium malabsorption
        – While there is an ↑ relative risk of metabolic bone disease in persons who used PPI > 2 years, the absolute ↑ risk was small
        – Absolute risk of hip fractures per 1000 person-years

PPI Non-Users	Regular PPI Users
1.51	2.02

	OR
– Fractures	
▪ Hip*	1.30
▪ Spine	1.56
▪ All sites	1.16

* Hazard ratio was higher in current and former smokers, 1.51

    o Iron malabsorption
        – Poor response to oral iron supplement absorption in 2 iron-deficient individuals improved after cessation of omeprazole; no clear clinical relevance

❖ Infection

    o ↑ risk of enteric infections in persons on PPI, including C.difficile, Campylobacter, Salmonella, and Travellers' Diarrhea

    o ↑ risk of development of SBP (spontaneous bacterial peritonitis) in patient with ascites

    o ↑ risk of C difficile colitis
        – PPI use is independent risk of C difficile diarrhea in antibiotic users, odds ratio of 2.1 (95% confidence interval, 1.2-3.5)
        – Associated with the use if PPIs occurs even in persons who have not previously taken antibiotics
        – Use of PPIs (or odds ratio)

	OR
– C.difficile infection	
▪ Incident	1.7
▪ Recurrent	2.5

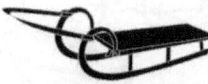

Risk Possible/Magnitude Consequence

- o ↑ risk of community-acquired or nosocomial pneumonia (presumably aspiration)
  - – Nested case-control analysis, adjusted odds ratio for pneumonia with PPI use of 1.73 (95% confidence interval, 1.33-2.25)

OR

	OR
– CAP/HCAP	1.27

- ❖ Cancer
  - – Data on PPI use and increased gastric *N*-nitrosamine remain uncertain and the risk of cancer is speculative
  - – Based on 345 accidental exposures compared with 787 controls, no observed increased teratogenicity

- ❖ Safety in pregnancy
  - – FDA category B
- ❖ Other GI conditions
  - – Collagenous colitis (lansoprazole)
  - – Pancreatitis

- ❖ No GI conditions
  - – CNS   ▪ Dementia
  - – CVS   ▪ Cardiovascular risk
  - – Kidney   ▪ Interstitial nephritis
  - – Anaphylaxis

- ❖ Drug-drug interactions; PPIs metabolized by cytochrome P450 and may induce or inhibit drug metabolism (phenytoin, warfarin, Plavix®) [clopidogre]

  - o Clinically significant PPI drug-drug interactions are rare (<1/million prescriptions); clinical significance of some PPIs reducing effectiveness of Plavix is uncertain
  - o Possible increased risk of gastric cancer theoretical consideration: Gastric colonization with bacteria that convert nitrates to carcinogenic *N*-nitroso compounds that then reflux

Abbreviations: CAP, community acquired pneumonia; HCAP, healthcare associated pneumonia

Printed with permission: AGA Technical Review. *Gastroenterology* 2008;135: pg. 1392-1413.

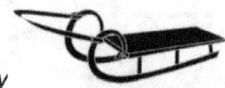

- Give the **FDA category** for the safety of drugs used to treat GERD in pregnancy and recommendations for breastfeeding.

Drugs	FDA Category	Recommendations for Breastfeeding
o *Antacids*		
– Aluminum-, calcium or magnesium-containing antacids	None	– Most are safe for use during pregnancy and for aspiration prophylaxis during labour because of minimal absorption – Avoid long-term, high-dose therapy in pregnancy
– Magnesium trisilicates	None	– **Not** safe for use in pregnancy, as causes fluid overload and metabolic alkalosis
– Sodium bicarbonates	None	– No teratogenecity in animals. – Generally regarded as acceptable for human use because of minimal absorption
o *Mucosal protectant*		
– Sucralfate	B	– A prospective, controlled study suggests acceptable for use in humans
o *Histamine2-receptor antagonist (H2RA)*		
– Cimetidine	B	– Same as above
– Ranitidine	B	– Ranitidine is the only H2RA whose efficacy during pregnancy has been established
– Famotidine	B	– Same as cimetidine, but paucity of safety data in humans
– Nizatidine	B	– Not recommended during pregnancy. In animals, spontaneous abortion, congenital malformations, low birth weight and fewer live births have been reported. Little data in humans.

Drugs	FDA Category	Recommendations for Breastfeeding
o *Proton-pump inhibitors*		
– Omeprazole	C	
– Lansoprazole	B	– For all PPIs, no teratogenicity or harm, but only limited human pregnancy data
– Rabeprazole	B	
– Pantoprazole	B	
– Esomeprazole	B	
o *Promotility agents*		
– Cisapride	C	– Embryotoxic and fetotoxic in animals. Prospective controlled study in human suggest acceptable in pregnancy, but was removed because of cardiac arrhythmias
o Metoclopramide	B	– No teratogenic effects in animals or humans reported – Embryotoxic and fetotoxic in animals. Case reports in human suggest similar concerns. Possible cardiac damage.

Printed with permission: Ali RAR, and Egan LJ. *Best Pract Res Clin Gastroenterol* 2007;21(5): 799-803.

"Praise improves work ethic and motivation.

When were you last given this kind of praise on your annual assessments?"

"Praise may be more effective than rewards."

(Bribes, money)

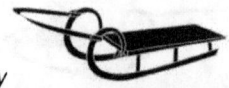

BARRETT ESOPHAGUS (BE)

➤ Definition

    o BE is defined as intestinal metaplasia of the distal esophagus, in which normal squamous epithelium is replaced by columnar epithelium.

➤ Demography

    o Barrett persons with a high pre-test probability of Barrett epithelium include middle-aged Caucasian males, or a person with a long (>5 year) history of moderate/severe heartburn occurring more than 3 times per week).

    o Compared to the risk in the general population, the relative risk of adenocarcinoma among patients with BE was 11.3 (95% CI, 8.8-14.4), with an annual risk of esophageal adenocarcinoma of 0.12% (95% CI, 0.09-0.15).

    o This risk is much lower than the previously reported figure of 0.5%.

    o Detection of low-grade dysplasia on the index endoscopy was associated with an incidence rate of ~$500/10^5$ person-years.

    o The incidence rate among patients without dysplasia was $100/10^5$ person-years.

    o The progression of BE to ECa is 0.09% per person year, (not 0.5%).

    o SSIM (subsquamous intestinal metaplasia) can be detected in some patients with BE following long-term treatment with PPIs, and either before or after endoscopically ablation therapy.

    o SSIM may exist in the absence of endoscopically visible columnar epithelium characteristic of BE, or may coexist with endoscopically visible BE.

    o SSIM possesses unique biological properties compared with surface epithelium.

    o Distinct biological properties from BE and normal squamous epithelium:
        – Reduced rates of crypt proliferation
        – No aneuploidy following PDT
        – ↑ KI-67, COX-2, BCL-2 (than squamous epithelium)

Source: Nvid-Jenson et al. NEJM 2011; 365: 1375-1383 and Wani S, et al. Gastroenterol 2011; 141: 1179-1186.

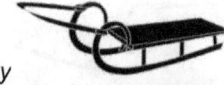

➤ Genetics

- Give molecular tests which may suggest the presence of dysplasia in BE.
  - DNA aneuploidy
  - Ki67 (proliferation) – increased expression on immunohistochemistry
  - Oncogenes – cyclin D1, TGFα, EGFR, Rus, B-catenin
  - Tumour suppressors genes
  - Anti-apoptosis genes
  - Anti-senescence markers – telomerase

Printed with permission: Flejou JF. *Best Pract Res Clin Gastroenterol* 2008; 22(4): pg. 680.

Useful background: Differences in the genetics of Familial Barrett esophagus (BE), hereditary diffuse gastric cancer (HDGC) and Tylosis Palmaris

Genetics	Familial Barrett Esophagus	Hereditary Diffuse Gastric Cancer	Tylosis Palmaris
○ Pattern of inheritance	Proposed autosomal dominant with incomplete penetrance	Autosomal dominant	Autosomal dominant
○ Chromosome	Unknown	Chromosome 16q22	Chromosome 17q25
○ Genetic basis	Linkage analyses ongoing	Mutations in E-cadherin/CDH1 gene	Downregulation of cytoglobin gene
○ Cancer risk	Up to 31% risk of adeno-carcinoma	70% of lifetime risk of diffuse gastric cancer	40-95% lifetime risk of squamous esophageal cancer
○ Clinical strategies	Consider family history in assessment of GERD	Genetic testing for CDH1 -Endoscopic surveillance -Prophylactic gastrectomy	Endoscopic surveillance

Abbreviations: BE, Barrett esophagus; GERD, gastroesophageal reflux disease; HDGC, hereditary diffuse gastric cancer

Printed with permission: Robertson E and Jankowski J. *Am J Gastroenterol* 2008;103: 445.

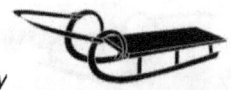

- ➤ Clinical

  - o The presence of alarm symptoms/signs such as vomiting, anemia/bleeding, dysphasia or weight loss have a relatively low sensitivity and specificity to identify the persons with a high probability of having dysplasia or cancer, and therefore requiring an EGD in the management of their symptoms.

  - o About two-thirds of persons with alarm symptoms/signs have a normal EGD, and less than 10% of dyspeptic persons with alarm symptoms will have a neoplasia (Zoggari et al., AJG 2010; 105; 105; 565-71).

Subtypes of Barrett epithelium

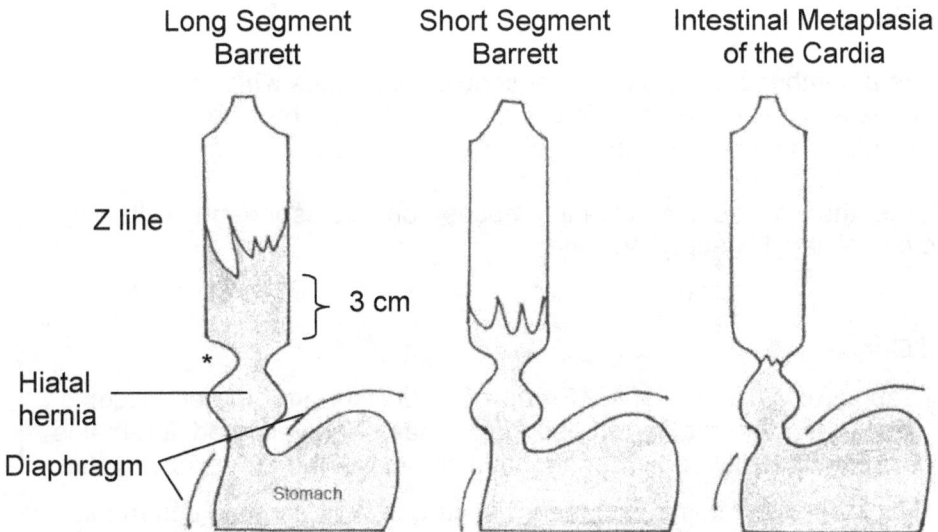

  - o Patients with long segment or short segment Barrett esophagus have salmon-coloured mucosa extending up into the tubular esophagus.

  - o Biopsy shows intestinal metaplasia with goblet cells

  - o If intestinal metaplasia with goblet cells is found at a normally located zig zag line (Z line), the patients has intestinal metaplasia of the cardia, which confers a lower cancer risk.

*End of tubular esophagus and beginning of stomach.

Abbreviation: SSIM, subsquamous intestinal metaplasia

Source: Yachimski P, et al. Clin Gastroenterol Hepatol 2012; 10: 220-224.

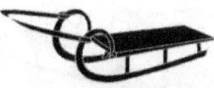

➢ Endoscopy
  ○ High frequency miniprobes
    – Provide better visualization and resolution of the mucosa than does EUS and therefore to T-staging in BE, but gives poorer visualization of deeper areas, and thus less reliable N-staging.
    – The deeper depth of the HGD/EC, the greater the likelihood of metastasis to lymph nodes.

  ○ EUS
    – Has greater value for identifying lymph node involvement (metastasis) (N (nodal)-staging)
    – NPV (negative predictive value) > 95%

Clinical Pearl

There are a number of expensive endoscopic techniques which may increase the accuracy of diagnosis of Barrett epithelium by highlighting sites of higher likelihood for obtaining "positive histopathological diagnosis.

Don't forget the simplest trick clearing mucus from the esophagus with water flushes containing 1% acetylcysteine.

Clinical Gems

  ○ Sapphire: While use of the Praque C & M criteria for the endoscopic grading system for Barrett esophagus has been validated, it remains to be confidently confirmed that this has more than descriptive value.

  ○ Nonetheless, if this is a standard of care in your practice community, "go with the flow".

  ○ Emerald: Most BE neoplasia is at the 12 to 6 o'clock in the endoscopic view with the patient in the left lateral position, so take a good second look in this area.

  ○ Even with the new high-frequency mini-probes, the accuracy of endoscopic ultrasound (EUS) in distinguishing T1sm (submucosal disease) is only 75-85%.

  ○ Low pressure spray cryoablation using liquid nitrogen gives premise for modular and non-nodular HGD and early esophageal cancer (Johnston MH, et al. *Gastrointest Endosc* 2005: 62: 842-8).

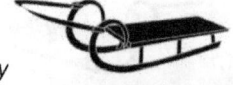

- Give recommendations for endoscopic surveillance of persons with Barrett esophagus (BE).
    - Patient
        - Middle-aged (> 50 yr)
        - Caucasian
        - Male
        - ↑ BMI
        - Smoker
    - GERD symptoms
        - > 3x per wk
        - > 5 / > 10 yr
        - Severe

American College of Gastroenterology recommendations for surveillance by esophageal gastroduodenoscopy (EGD)

Dysplasia	Documentation	Follow-Up EGD
o None (metaplasia)	– 2 EGDs with biopsy (4 quadrant, q 2 cm, separate jars) – Confirm by two expert pathologists	3 - 5 years
o LGD	– Repeat EGD with biopsy, when erosive esophagitis healed, confirm by two expert pathologists – Confirm with #3 EGD plus biopsies to exclude HGD/esophageal cancer	q 1 year until no dysplasia
o HGD – Focal (<5 crypts)	– Repeat EGD with biopsy to rule out cancer/document HGD, expert pathologist confirmation	
o HGD – Multifocal (>5 crypts)	– Consider endoscopic therapy ▪ Radiofrequency ablation, (RFA) ▪ PDT, cryosurgery, EMR, esophagectomy in surgical candidate	q 3 months and q 1 cm, 4 quadrant

* Recent dilation has focused on considering treatment at these stages

Abbreviations: BE, Barrett epithelium; EGD, esophageal gastroduodenoscopy; EMR, endoscopic mucosal resection; EUS, endoscopic ultrasound; GERD, gastroesophageal reflux disease; HGD, high grade dysplasia; LGD, low grade dysplasia; PDT, photodynamic therapy

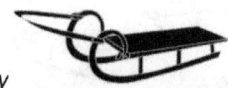

➤ Histopathology

• Give the **Seattle protocol** which is recommended for taking esophageal mucosal biopsies for Barrett esophagus (BE).

  ○ Visible abnormalities – Multiple biopsies to be targeted to this area

  ○ All other areas – Four-quadrant biopsies from the top of the gastric folds, proximally for every 1 cm to the squamocolumnar junction (the upper most part of the BE)

Note:
- Taking esophageal mucosal biopsies at 2 cm rather that at 1 cm intervals will miss half of the neoplasias.
- Targeted biopsies will yield ~80% of BE lesions.

T-N-M staging of high grade dysplasia and esophageal cancer

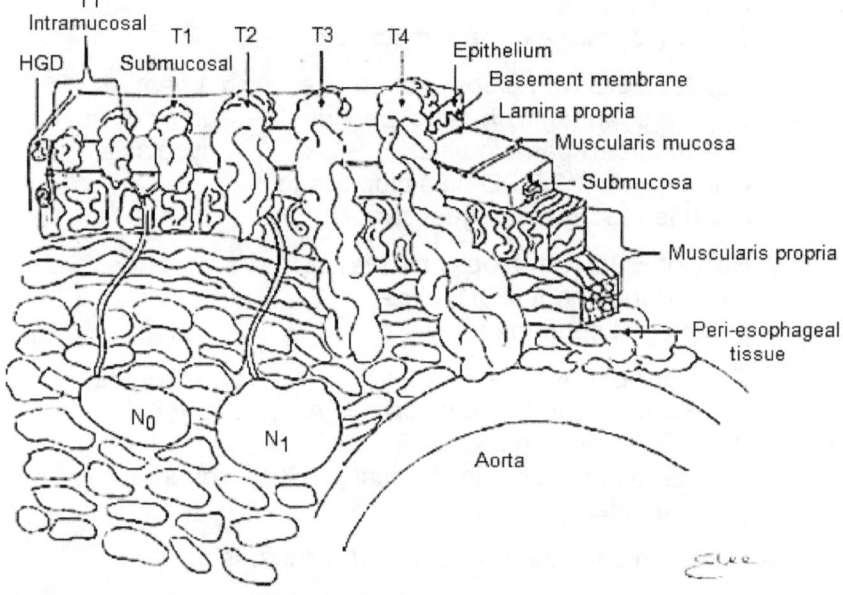

Abbeviation: HDG, high grade dysolasia
Adapted from: Mayo GI, Figure 7, page 31.

Useful background: The terminology of early neoplastic lesions in BE, using Riddell's and Vienna classification, and clinical consequences.

Category	Terminology
1	Negative for dysplasia
2	Indefinite for dysplasia
3	Low grade dysplasia
4	4.1 High grade dysplasia; 4.2 Non-invasive carcinoma (carcinoma in situ) ; 4.3 Suspicion of invasive carcinoma
5	Invasive neoplasia; intramucosal carcinoma; Submucosal carcinoma or beyond

Abbreviation : BE, Barrett esophagus

Adapted from: Flejou JF. *Best Pract Res Clin Gastroenterol* 2008; 22(4): 679.

SO YOU WANT TO BE A GASTROENTEROLOGIST!

- Give the explanation for the possible difficulty in distinguishing histopathologically between M3 and SM1 BE tumours.

  - M3 invades into but not through the muscularis mucosa (MM)

  - In BE, there may be both a superficial and a deep layer of the MM!

  - Infiltration through the superficial MM layer is M1, and only infection through the deeper SM layer represents invasion of the SM, and is therefore SM1.

  - The 5 year survival rate for EMR alone, or EMR plus PDT for early stage esophageal cancer is 97%, and minimally invasive endoscopic therapies may be comparable to esophagectomy for early stage esophageal cancer (ASGE Technology Committee. *Gastrointest Endosc* 2008: 11-18.; Das A, et al. *Am J Gastroenterol* 2008:1340-5).

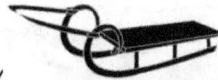

Staging

Using the T-N-M Classification system, mucosal (M) and submucosal (SM) tumours may be differentiated further:

	Subclassification		Tumour
(T1a)	M	1	Limited to epithelium
		2	Invades the LP (lamina propria)
		3	Invades into but not through MM (muscularis mucosa)
(T1b)	SM	1	Penetration into up to 1/3 of SM (< 500 microns)
		2	2/3
		3	3/3

Shown in brackets is AJCC stage definition.

It is recommended that mucosal (M1 and M2, and possibly M3) tumours be treated by one form of EMR, and that he submucosal (SM1, SM2, and SM3) tumours be treated by esophagectomy.

➢ Treatment

• Give endoscopic therapies for Barrett esophagus (BE) with high grade dysplasia (HGD) or early mucosal cancer (EMC).
   o Submucosal lifting, followed by endoscopic resection-cap technique (radical ER)
   o "suck-band-and ligate" (snare)
   o MBM (multiband mucosectomy Endoscopic mucosal resection (EMR)
   o Endoscopic submucosal resection (ESR)
   o Radiofrequency ablation (RFA)
   o Nd: YAG laser
   o Argon plasma coagulation (APC)
   o Photodynamic therapy (PDT) with porfimer or 5-aminolevulinic acid (5-ALA)
   o Cryotherapy
   o Esophagectomy in surgical candidate

Note: Consider using standard dose PPI bid for 3 to 6 weeks after ER to allow for regrowth of squamous epithelium.

Abbreviations: 5-ALA, 5-aminolevulinic acid; APC, argon plasma coagulation; BE, Barrett esophagus; EMC, early mucosal cancer; HGD, high grade dysplasia.

Printed with permission: Curvers WL, Kiesslich R, Bergman JJ. *Best Prac Res Clin Gastroenterol* 2008; 22(4):687-720.

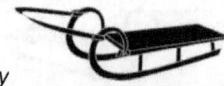

Endoscopic Mucosal Resection (EMR)

- Give the management of antiplatelets and anticoagulant drug before and after EMR.

  - General – Avoid aspirin and all nonsteroidal anti-inflammatory medications for the next 2 weeks

    – Advise patients to monitor for symptoms of overt gastrointestinal bleeding, consider prophylactic deployment of hemostatic clips to secure hemostasis, although this is unproven.

  - Warfarin – Stop Warfarin 5 days before the EMR

    – An INR level less than 1.5 is used as an arbitrary cut off value to proceed with EMR

    – Resume Warfarin 24 hours after the procedure with the usual daily dose

    – Check INR levels 1 week later to ensure adequate anticoagulation

    – In patients deemed to be at high risk of thrombosis, Warfarin cessation is bridged with low molecular weight heparin

  - Clopidogrel – Discontinue Clopidogrel 7 days before endoscopy in patients with high risk cardiac conditions

    – Cessation of Clopidogrel is performed after discussion with the cardiologist

    – This may entail deferring the EMR, where feasible, until a suitable time period after the insertion of coronary stents

Abbreviation: INR, international normalized ratio

Printed with permission: Namasivayam et al. Clin Gastro Hep 2010;8:743-754.

- Give the risk of serious complications of EMR for BE, when performed by experienced endoscopists.

  - Bleeding – 0% to 46%

  - Perforation – 1% to 5%

  - Strictures – 2% to 88%

  - Depending on C & M criteria (e.g., if BE > 50% of circumference of esophagus, or for stricture is 4;2) and possibly also on the use of tobacco products

53

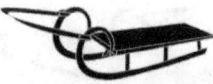

o Treat any esophageal ulceration

o The multiband mucosectomy devise may be superior to the injection/CAP EMR (endoscopic mucosal resection) method for high grade dysplasia in Barrett epithelium, in terms of procedure time and cost (Pouw RE, et al. *Gastrointest Endosc* 2008; 67:AB75).

o Radiofrequency ablation (RF) with the Hab ablation system give a >90% cure rate for low and high grade dysplasia (LGD, HGD), in flat, non-nodular BE tissue (Waye JD, et al. Gastrointest Endosc. 2010;71(3):551-6).

o The morbidity of esophagectomy includes strictures (20-40%), leaks (3-39%), left recurrent laryngeal nerve paralysis (3-16%), gastroparesis, regurgitation of gastric contents, and mortality of 2-10%.

o Photodynamic therapy (PDT) with porfimer-Na, when exposed to non-thermal red laser light, yields singlet oxygen which results in ischemic necrosis in metaplastic and dysplastic BE.

o The complications of PDT include stricture in 40% (8% severe), chest pain, mediastinitis, pleural effusion, chest pain and vomiting.

Abbreviations: EMR, endoscopic mucosal resection; EUS, endoscopic ultrasound; HGD, high grade dysplasia; LGD, low grade dysplasia; PDT, photodynamic therapy; RF, radiofrequency ablation

➢ Success of ER (esophageal resection) for BE

| | Complete Eradication | |
Timing	Neoplasia	Metaplasia
Initial	98%	85%
Follow-up (19 to 49 months)	95%	81%

o Recommended surveillance
  – First year after ER q 3 month
  – Subsequently q 1 year

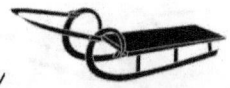

- Give the factors which influence the rate of remission after endoscopic resection for HGD or EC, as well as those factors which influence the rate of recurrence (or development of metachronous malignancies).

❖ Higher rate of remission (59% to 99%)

- o Macroscopic characteristics   Type
  - Protruded   I
  - Flat, elevated   IIa
  - Flat   IIb
  - Flat, depressed   IIc
  - Success: I > IIa > IIb > IIc

- o Size
  - < 20 mm

- o Differentiation
  - Well to moderate differentiation > poor differentiated (univariate, but not multivariate analyses)

❖ High rate of recurrence (7% to 30% within 5 years)

- o Lesion   – Macroscopic features
  - ↑ diameter of lesion
  - ↑ length of BE
  - – Microscopic
    - Residual dysplasia
    - Multifocal neoplasia

- o Treatment   – Piecemeal resection
  - – Monotherapy (ER without adjunctive ablative therapy)
    - PDT (photodynamic therapy)
    - APC (argon plasma coagulation)
    - RFA (radiofrequency ablation)
  - – > 10 month to achieve remission

"The decisions of our present are the architects of our present."

Dan Brown

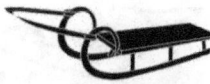

ESOPHAGEAL MOTILITY DISORDERS (EMD)

- ➢ Definition
  - ○ A patient is said to have an esophageal motility disorder if their findings on motility study are two standard deviations beyond normal.

- ➢ Classification
  - ○ Esophageal motility disorders may be primary or secondary to (associated with) another disease process.

- • Give a simple classification of esophageal motility disorders (EMD).

Primary EMD	Secondary EMD	Manometric Variants
○ Achalasia (three subtypes)	– Pseudoachalasia	▪ Hypertensive peristalsis
○ Diffuse esophageal spasm	– Chaga disease	▪ Hypertensive LES
○ Nutcracker	– Scleroderma esophagus	▪ Ineffective esophageal motility
○ Absent peristalsis	– Parkinson disease	
○ Gastroesophageal reflux disease (GERD)	– Infiltrative disorders	

- • Give the classification esophageal motor abnormalities based upon conventional manometry.

Upper Esophageal Sphincter (UES)	Esophageal Body (EB)	Lower Esophageal Sphincter (LES)
↑ Contraction	↑ Contraction	↑ Pressure
○ Zenker diverticulum	– Nutcracker esophagus	▪ Isolated hypertensive LES
	– Achalasia (compartmentalized pressurization)	▪ Achalasia

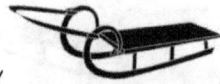

Mastering the Boards: Gastroenterology

A.B.R. Thomson

Upper Esophageal Sphincter (UES)	Esophageal Body (EB)	Lower Esophageal Sphincter (LES)
<u>↓ Contraction</u> ○ MCTD (e.g., scleroderma) ○ Oculopharyngeal dystrophy	<u>↓ Contraction</u> – Ineffective esophageal motility (IEM) – Aperistalsis (e.g., scleroderma)	<u>↓ Pressure</u> ▪ Hypotensive LES ▪ GERD (↑ tLESR) ▪ Scleroderma
<u>↓ Co-ordination</u> ○ Achalasia (complicated) ○ Parkinson disease ○ Cricopharyngeal bar ○ Belch dysfunction	<u>↓ Co-ordination</u> – Diffuse esophageal spasm (DES) – Achalasia (absent or simultaneous contractions)	<u>↓ Co-ordination</u> ▪ (relaxation*) ▪ Achalasia, type I ▪ Atypical LES relaxation (pseudo-achalasia) ▪ Post-fundoplication gas-bloat syndrome contraction, or impaired retrograde inhibition

* relaxation, or inadequate swallow-induced inhibition

Abbreviations: EB, esophageal body; IEM, ineffective esophageal motility; LES, lower esophageal sphincter; MCTD, mixed connective tissue disease; UES, upper esophageal sphincter

- Give the advantages of high resolution esophageal manometry (HREM), and high resolution esophageal pressure topography (HREPT).
    - High quality, uniform format
    - Greater reproducibility
    - Viewing simultaneous contractions of the entire esophagus
    - Standardized objective metrics
    - Topographic patterns easily learned and recognized
    - Allows for subclassification of achalasia, and of DES.

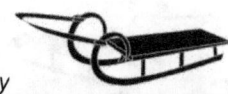

Mastering the Boards: Gastroenterology   A.B.R. Thomson

- **Give classification of** esophageal motor abnormalities based on high-resolution manometry.
  - Normal
    - Normal EGJ pressure (10-35 mm Hg) and relaxation (see below)
    - Peristaltic velocity <8 cm/s in >90% of swallows
    - ↑ intra-bolus pressure at <8 cm/s to <30 mm Hg in > 90% of swallows
    - Normal velocity, <8 cm/s in > 90% of swallows; normal peristaltic amplitude; (≥7 peristaltic contractions with an intact wave progression [amplitude >30 mmHg])
    - Mean distal contractile index (DCI) <5000 mm Hg·s·cm**
  - Peristaltic dysfunction
    - Mild
      - 3-6 swallows with failed peristalsis or
      - >2 cm defect in the 30 mm Hg
      - Isobaric contour of the distal esophageal peristalsis (15 mm Hg in proximal-mid esophagus)
    - Severe
      - 7 swallows with either failed peristalsis or
      - >2 cm defect in the 30 mm Hg isobaric contour of distal esophageal peristalsis (15 mm Hg in proximal-mid esophagus)
    - Aperistalsis
      - Contractile pressure <30 mm Hg throughout mid-distal esophagus in all swallows (*Scleroderma* pattern: aperistalsis with LES pressure <10 mm Hg)
      - Absent or simultaneous contractions (<30 mmHg)
  - Hypertensive dysfunction
    - Peristaltic velocity <8 cm/s in >80% of swallows
    - Mean distal contractile index (DCI) >5000 mm Hg·s·cm**
      - *Hypertensive peristalsis*: mean DCI >5000-8000 mm Hg·s·cm
      - *Segmental hypertensive peristalsis*: hypertensive contraction restricted to mid- or distal esophagus
      - LOS after-contraction: mean DCI 5000-8000 mm Hg·s·cm

- ❖ Spastic esophageal motility disorders
  - Nutcracker esophagus
    - Nutcracker esophagus may be a hypercholinergic condition which leads to a loss of the normal synchrony between the inner circular and other longitudinal smooth muscle layers of the esophagus.
    - Average peristaltic amplitude >180 mmHg over pressure sensors 3 and 8 cm above LES
    - Modest ↑ amplitude → better transit (less dysphagia) plus NCCP

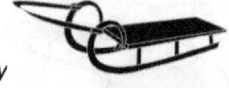

- ≥ 20% simultaneous contractions with an amplitude of > 30 mm Hg
- 1/3 of DES patients also have ↑ LES pressure a ↓ LES relaxation
- This latter subgroup of DES may actually have achalasia (on HREPT, distal latency plus DES may be spastic achalasia).
- Barium sallow in DES
  - May be normal, or show corkscrew esophagus
  - Low sensitivity and specificity
- The average amplitude in the distal 10 cm of esophagus from ≥ 10 5 mL liquid swallows, ≥ 220 mm Hg
- HREPT defines 2 subgroups of nutcracker esophagus, based on the DCI
- DCI (distal contractile integral) is an integration of the amplitude, duration and length duration of a contraction.
- DCI is expressed as mm Hg.s.cm
- Values of DCI on HREPT
  - Normal ≤ 5000 mm Hg.s.cm
  - Nutcracker 5000 to 8000 mm.Hg.s.cm
  - Spastic nutcracker 8000 mm.Hg.s.cm
- May be associated with ↑ LESP pressure and ↓ LES relaxation.
- The manometric diagnosis of a motility disorder may change if it is performed at a time the patient is having symptoms.
- Hypertensive LES (lower esophageal sphincter)
  - Resting LES > 45 mm Hg
  - ~ 50% have ↓ LES (> 35 mm Hg on HREPT) relaxation and ↑ amplitude distal esophageal contraction amplitude, as high as ≥ 220 mm Hg.
- The relationship between a manometric event and the patient's symptoms may be poor, and association indices have been developed to establish the probability of a cause and effect relationship between a motility event, e.g., gastroesophageal reflux or DES, and patient symptoms, e.g., heartburn or NCCP (non-cardiac chest pain).

- o Esophageal spasm (rapidly propagated contractile wavefront)
  - Peristaltic velocity >8cm/s in ≥20% of swallows ± raised DCI
    - *Diffuse esophageal spasm:* rapid contractile wavefront throughout the distal esophagus
    - *Segmental esophageal spasm:* rapid contractile wavefront limited to mid or distal esophageal segment

59

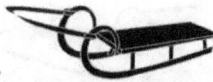

- o Rapid elevation of intra-bolus pressure (increased resistance to flow due to functional or structural obstruction in the esophagus or at the esophago-gastric junction [e.g., stricture, post-fundoplication, eosinophilic esophagitis, poorly coordinated contractions])
  - – Rapid elevation of intra-bolus pressure to >15 mm Hg in >8 cm/s in ≥20% of swallows
    - ▪ Mild: Intra-esophageal bolus pressure (15 to 30 mm Hg) with ≥80% preserved peristalsis
    - ▪ *Severe*: Intra-esophageal bolus pressure (>30 mm Hg) with ≥20% failed peristalsis
    - ▪ The nutcracker esophagus and a hypertensive LES may be seen in persons with GERD
- o Hypertensive peristalsis ("nutcracker esophagus") is defined by high-amplitude peristaltic contractions, and can be associated with dysphagia and/or chest pain.
- o Nutcracker esophagus is a relatively common heterogeneous condition encountered in normal controls, dysphagic patients, and patients with reflux disease.
- o Esophageal hypercontractility is defined in esophageal pressure topography (EPT) by the occurrence of propagated swallow-induced contractions with distal contractile integral (DCI) > 8,000 mm Hg-s-cm (a magnitude never encountered in control subjects).
- o Hypercontractility, ("Jackhammer Esophagus") is associated with multi-peaked contractions, is rare, and is usually associated with dysphagia.
- o Subsets of patients with "Jackhammer Esophagus" had this as an apparent primary abnormality of hypercontractility or in association with EGJ outflow obstruction or reflux disease.
- o DES (diffuse [or distal] esophageal spasm)
  - – In DES (distal or diffuse esophageal spasm), there is an uncertain relationship between symptoms and the DES motility changes
  - – Contractile velocity >8 cm/s mmHg over pressure sensors 3 and 8 cm above LES in ≥2 swallows

Abbreviations: DES, distal or diffuse esophageal spasm; DSRS, distal splenorenal shunt; EHT, endoscopic hemostatic therapy; LES, lower esophageal sphincter; MCTD, mixed connective tissue diseases; MII, multichannel intraluminal impedence; TIPS, transjugular intrahepatic postoperative shunt; tLESR, transient lower esophageal sphincter relaxation

Adapted from: Pandolfino et al. *AJP* 2008;103: pp 28.; and Printed with permission: Sifrim D and Fornari F. *Best Pract Res Clin Gastroenterol* 2007;21(4): pg. 575-576.

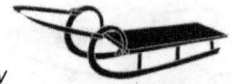

Achalasia

➢ Definition

   o Primary achalasia is associated with loss of ganglion cells in the myenteric plexus of the esophagus.

   o Complete absence of peristalsis (One peristaltic contraction rules out achalasia)

   o In order to make the diagnosis of achalasia, there must be standard manometric or HREPT evidence of
      – Loss of relaxation ± opening of LES (lower esophageal sphincter), plus
      – Loss of peristalsis in distal esophagus (GBA)
      – There may also be ↑LES pressure (not required for diagnosis)

   o Impaired deglutative EGJ relaxation and/or opening

   o ↑ intra-esophageal bolus pressure due to resistance to flow at EGJ
      – *Classic:* aperistalsis with no identifiable contractile activity
      – *Vigorous:* with persistent contractile activity (spasm) or gross elevation of intra-esophageal bolus pressure, with or without esophageal shortening
      – *Variant:* with preserved peristalsis in the distal esophagus in ≥20% swallows

Abbreviations: DCI, distal contractile index; EGJ, esophagogastric junction; LES, lower esophageal sphincter

Printed with permission: Fox MR, and Bredenoord AJ. *GUT* 2008;57: pg. 419.

➢ Types

● Distal segment, impaired EGJ relaxation

   o Classic achalasia (Type I)

   o Achalasia with esophageal compression (Type II)

   o ≥ 20% test swallows with esophageal compression (Type III)

Abbreviation: EGJ, esophagogastric junction

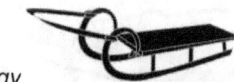

- Give subtypes of achalasia made by high-resolution manometry (HRM), and compare the treatment responses with each type.

	Type I (Classic)	Type II (Compression)	Type III (Chicago)
o Peristalsis			
– Absent peristalsis	+		
– Compartmentalized pressurization		+	
– Spastic contraction			+
o Response to treatment			
– Heller myotomy	67	100%	0
– Pneumatic dilation	38	73%	9
– Botulinim toxin	0	86%	22
o Subsequent interventions			
– Number of interventions	1.6 $\pm$ 1.5 1.2 $\pm$ 0.4	2.4 + 1.0	1.8 $\pm$ 0.7
– Successful last intervention	56% 96%	29%	71%

Printed with permission: Pandolfino et al. *Gastroenterology* 2008;135: pg. 1526-33.

➤ Causes

- Give causes of secondary achalasia (**pseudoachalasia**).
  - o Infection/Infiltration
    - – Sarcoidosis
    - – Sjogren syndrome
    - – Amyloidosis
    - – Fabry disease
    - – Chagas disease (Trypanosoma cruzi)
  - o Cancer
    - – GI
      - ▪ Squamous cell carcinoma of the esophagus
      - ▪ Adenocarcinoma of the esophagus
      - ▪ Hepatocellular carcinoma
      - ▪ Pancreatic adenocarcinoma
    - – Non-GI (Paraneoplastic syndrome)
      - ▪ Lung carcinoma (non-small cell)
      - ▪ Metastatic prostate carcinoma

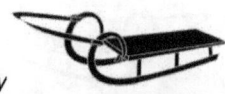

- Metastatic renal cell carcinoma
- Breast adenocarcinoma
- Leiomyoma
- Lymphoma
- Reticulum cell sarcoma
- Lymphangioma
- Mesothelioma

- Motility abnormalities
  - Achalasia with associated Hirchsprung disease
  - Familial achalasia
  - Fundoplication
  - Hereditary hollow visceral myopathy
  - Parkinson disease

- Surgical
  - Post-fundoplication
  - Post-vagotomy

- Miscellaneous
  - Allgrove syndrome (AAA syndrome) – (Alacidygia, Addisons disease, Achalasia)
  - Hereditary cerebellar ataxia (HCA)
  - Autoimmune polyglandular syndrome type II
  - MEN IIb (Sipple Syndrome)

Adapted from: *Sleisenger & Fordtran's gastrointestinal and liver disease: Pathophysiology/Diagnosis/Management* 2016, 10th edition, page 721.

SO YOU WANT TO BE A GASTROENTEROLOGIST!

Achalasia is rare, and an even rarer condition is achalasia secondary to a tumour (e.g., small cell lung cancer).

- Give the molecular basis for the paraneoplastic syndrome which may case secondary achalasia, gastroparesis, small intestinal pseudo-obstruction, or colonic intertia.

  - An epitope on the cancer forms an antibody (anti-Hu) which attaches to the myenteric plexus of different portions of the GI tract, resulting in dysmotility.

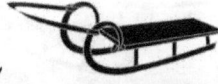

- High-resolution manometry (HRM) allows for better definition of esophageal motility disorders, including achalasia.
- Using HRM achalasia has been classified into three subtypes: type I (classic achalasia), type II (esophageal compression), and type III (spastic achalasia).
- Response to achalasia treatment appears to vary by subtypes.
- There is some variability in distinguishing between type I and type II achalasia.
- Thus, clarification of the criteria for type I and type II achalasia might improve the reliability of the classification.

Source: Hernandez et al. Am J Gastroenterol 2012; 107:

- ➤ Diagnostic imaging
  - Esophageal dilatation
  - Poor esophageal emptying
  - Bird-beak deformity of EGJ
  - Absent gastric air bubble

- ➤ Treatment
  - Smooth muscle relaxation (relaxants taken 15 to 30 min before meals)
    - Nitrates
    - Calcium channel blockers
      - Nifedipine
    - Botulinum toxin injection into the area of LES
      - Inhibits the acetylcholine-releasing excitatory neurons innervating the smooth muscle of the LES (lower esophageal sphincter), which thereby lowers the LES pressure.
  - Smooth muscle damage
    - Esophageal dilation
      - Bougie
      - Forceful balloon dilation (tears some of the smooth muscle fibres)
      - Success rates

Months	%
6	74%
12	~75%
24	86%
≥ 36	58%

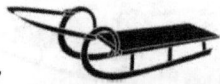

A.B.R. Thomson

- Post-procedure
  - Perforation 2 to 4%
  - Heartburn 45%
  - Repeated dilations if dilation approaches fail (there may be risk of complications from subsequent surgical myotomy)
  - Especially if patient < 40 years
  - 25% to 50% within 5 years

- Surgical myotomy (Heller myotomy, thoracic, or abdominal approach)
  - Success rate higher (70% to 90%), and recurrence rate lower at 10 years, 70% to 85%; 20-30 years, 65% to 75% lower than forceful pneumatic dilation
  - Short-term complications
    - Esophageal perforation ~5%
    - Mortality $< 1/10^3$
  - Long-term complications include
    - GER (gastroesophageal reflux) (heartburn, strictures, BE and adenocarcinoma of esophagus)
    - With fundoplication, risk of GER falls from 32% to 9%
- The 5 year likelihood of being asymptomatic after laparoscopic myotomy for achalasia is 87%.
- Laparoscopic myotomy

- Give the influence (approximate %) of endoscopic procedures performed for achalasia (pneumatic dilation or injection of botulinum toxic) which fail and are followed by surgical myotomy, as compared with surgical myotomy not proceed by endoscopic treatment.

Adverse Outcomes	Surgical Myotomy Alone	Surgical Myotomy Proceeded by Endoscopic Therapy
Complications		
– Intraoperative	4%	10%
– Post-operative	5%	10%
Persistent or recurrent symptoms	10%	20%

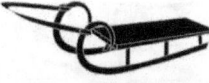

- Give the pre-operative factors which are associated with a higher risk of failure from laparoscopic myotomy.

  o LES pressure > 30 mm Hg (high)

  o Dilated S (sigmoid) shape esophagus

  o Chest pain

  o Endoscopy (POEM, peroral endoscopic myotomy [a form of NOTES: natural orifice transluminal endoscopic surgery])

    – Peroral endoscopic myotomy (POEM) has been demonstrated to be a highly effective treatment resulting in a more than 90% clinical success rate, improved Eckhard symptom score, as well as improved manometry outcomes.

Source: von Rentein D, et al. Am J Gastroenterol 2012; 107: 411-417.

- Compare the primary treatments for idiopathic achalasia under the headings: response (early, late) morbidity (minor, major).

- Pharmacological

Comparative Feature	Smooth Muscle Relaxants	Botulinum Toxin Injection
o Response		
– Early (<1 yr)	- 50%-70%	▪ 90% at 1 mo
– Late (>1-5 yr)	- <50%	▪ 60% at 1 yr
o Morbidity	- Headache, hypotension (30%)	▪ Rash ▪ Transient chest pain (20%)
o Advantage	- Rapidly initiated, well accepted	▪ Low morbidity ▪ Modest response durability ▪ Well accepted
o Disadvantage	- Inconvenient side effects - Tachyphylaxis - Poor effect on esophageal emptying	▪ Repeat injection often required within 1 yr ▪ fibroinflammatory reaction at LES

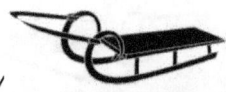

- Endoscopic/surgical

		Pneumatic Dilation	Open Myotomy	Laparoscopic/ Myotomy
o	Response			
	– Early (< 1 yr)	– 60%-90%	– >90%	– >90%
	– Later (> 1-5 yr)	– 60%	– 75% (at 20 yrs)	– 85%
o	Morbidity	– Rare – Techinique-related – 3%-5% perforation	– <10% at 1 yr – Symptomatic reflux (<10 % at 1 yr) – Dysphagia (10%) Mortality (<2%)	– Symptomatic reflux (10%) – NR
o	Advantage	– Good response durability	– Best response rate and durability	– Avoids thoracotomy, result is likely equivalent to openmyotomy technique
o	Disadvantage	– See Morbidity	– Thoracotomy required – Severe reflux may develop	– Long-term outcome unknown, small conversion to open procedure

Abbreviations: LES, lower esophageal sphincter; NR, not reported

Adapted from: Clouse RE, and Diamant NE. *Sleisenger & Fordtran's gastrointestinal and liver disease: Pathophysiology/Diagnosis/Management* 2006:pg. 879.

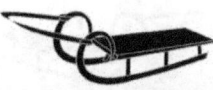

Diffuse Esophageal Spasm, Nutcracker Esophagus, and Hypertensive LES

➢ Treatment of DES, nutcracker esophagus and hypertensive LES

- o Generally small and less than ideal studies
- o Calcium channel blocker
  - – Diltiazem 60 mg to 90 mg po qid
- o Anti-depressive
  - – Trazodone 100 mg to 150 mg/day
  - – Imipramine 50 mg/day at bedtime
- o Anticholinergic
  - – Bethanechol
- o Anti-phosphodiesterase
  - – Sildenafil (50 mg prn); tadalafil; vardenafil
- o Nitrates
  - – Isosorbide 10 mg
- o Peppermint oil
- o Botulinum toxin endoscopic injection
  - – 20 units/mL injection at the Z-line 5 circumferential injections
  - – Inhibits the acetylcholine-releasing excitatory neurons innervating the smooth muscle of the LES, which thereby lowers the LES pressure.
- o Warm/hot water
- o Pneumatic dilation management of any associated psychological symptoms
- o Surgical myotomy

Source: Roman S, et al. Am J Gastroenterol 2012; 107: 27-45.

Zenker Diverticulum (ZD)

➢ Definition

- o A protrusion of the mucosa of the upper esophagus through Killian triangle (oblique muscle of the inferior pharyngeal constrictor muscle and the cricopharyngeal sphincter), producing a false diverticulum with its neck proximal to the cricopharyngeal muscle.

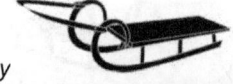

- ➢ Pathophysiology
  - ○ Motor abnormalities of upper esophagus
    - – ↑ degeneration of muscle fibres in upper esophagus
    - – ↑ replacement of degenerated muscle with fibrous and adipose tissue
    - – ↓ opening of UES (upper esophageal sphincter)
    - – ↑ intrabolus pressure upon swallowing
    - – ↑ hiatus hernia (possibly from ↑ GER)
    - – ↑ GER (gastroesophageal reflux > 50%,
      - ▪ BE [Barrett epithelium] in ~20%)
      - ▪ ↑ risk of squamous cell carcinoma in the diverticulum

---

Clinical Alert

While videofluoroscopy may be a good test to detect a small ZD, video capsule endoscopy is not!

Why? Because the device may become trapped in the pseudodiverticulum.

- ➢ Diagnostic imaging
  - ○ Cricopharyngeal bar
    - – A prominent cricopharyngeal bar from hypertrophy the cricopharyngeal muscle may occur in patients with Zenker diverticulum, and contribute to the symptoms of the diverticulum.
    - – However, a crycopharyngeal muscle may appear to be prominent on an upper GI barium swallow performed in persons with a variety of neuromuscular disorders.
      - ▪ CVA (stroke)
      - ▪ MS (multiple sclerosis)
      - ▪ ALS (amptrophic lateral sclerosis)
      - ▪ MG (myasthenia gravis)
      - ▪ Myopathies
- ➢ Treatment
  - ○ Endoscopic (flexible) or surgical (internal) myotomy of crycopharyngeal muscle (sphincterotomy), plus diverticulopexy
  - ○ ESED (endoscopic stapler esophagodiverticulostomy)
  - ○ One-or-two-step excision of ZD
  - ○ External sphincterotomy

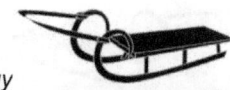

Scleroderma Esophagus

- Give the effects of scleroderma (systemic sclerosis [SSc] on the GI tract.
  - Mouth xerostomia
    - Facial exercises (small mouth)
    - Artificial hygiene
  - Esophagus
    - SSc associated loss of LES and 1% peristalsis leads to ↑ risk of symptoms and esophagitis, including severe (LA C-D) disease
    - Treat the GERD as per usual (non-SSc), remembering the higher risk of:
      - Need for higher dose PPI
      - NAB (nocturnal acid breakthrough)
      - Strictures
      - ENT complications, especially aspiration
      - Pill-associated esophagitis
  - Stomach
    - Delayed gastric emptying (may worsen GERD) bleeding from telangiectasia
  - Small intestine
    - SIBO (small intestinal bacterial overgrowth)
      - Slow small intestinal transit in SSc from ↓ MMCs (migrating motor complexes) leads to SIBO
      - Antibiotic therapy (7 to 10 days); intermittent, episodic, continuous, or rotational
        - Tetracycline 250 mg po qid
        - Trimethoprim 200 mg po bid
        - Amoxicillin-clavulanate po tid
        - Metronidazole 250 mg to 500 mg tid to qid
    - Dysmotility, pseudo-obstruction, nutritional risk
      - Octreotide
      - TPN (total parenteral nutrition)
      - HPN (home parenteral nutrition)
      - PEE/PEJ (percutaneous endoscopically-placed gastrostomy or jejunostomy feeding tube)
  - Colon
    - Constipation
    - Fecal incontinence
    - Wide-mouthed colonic diverticula
  - Liver
    - PBC (primary biliary cirrhosis)

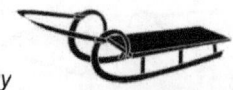

ESOPHAGEAL EOSINOPHILIA (EE) **AND EOSINOPHILIC ESOPHAGITIS** (EOE)

➢ Demographics

- o Eosinophilic esophagitis (EoE) is more common among males and Caucasians.

- o Caucasians are
  - Older at diagnosis with eosinophilic esophagitis (EoE) than African Americans
  - Less likely to present with failure-to-thrive
  - More likely to have esophageal rings

- o Males were more likely to be diagnosed in childhood and more frequently report dysphagia or food impaction.

➢ Clinical

• Give the typical presentation of eosinophilic esophagitis.

- o Young adult

- o Male to female ration of 3:1

- o Intermittent dysphagia, sometimes severe; food impaction

- o Failed treatment with proton pump inhibitor (PPI) therapy for presumed GERD – Note: PPI-sensitive EoE is now recognized as a subtype

- o Chest pain with odynophagia

- o Peripheral eosinophilia is common

- o Atopic diseases

Printed with permission: Attwood SEA, and Lamb CA. *Best Pract Res Clin Gastroenterol* 2008;22(4): 641.

• Give complications of eosinophilic esophagitis.

- o Dysphagia

- o Food impaction

- o Sloughing of mucosa (mucosal eosinophils)

- o Stricture

- o Mucosal tear

- o Perforation
  - EGD (esophagogastroduodenoscopy)
  - Spontaneous (Boerhaave syndrome) (transmural inflammation)

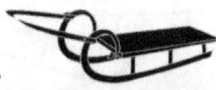

> Causes/associations

- Give causes/associations of eosinophilic gastrointestinal diseases (EGIDs).
  - Idiopathic
    - Eosinophilic syndromes
  - Infection
    - Fungal, parasitic and non-parasitic
  - Inflammation
    - GSE
    - IBD
    - MC
    - GERD
  - Neoplasia
    - Hodgkin lymphoma
    - Esophageal
    - Leiomyomatosis
  - Immune
    - Autoimmune
    - GVH disease
    - Connective tissue disease (e.g., scleroderma)
    - Hypersensitivity
    - Allergy (e.g., foods)
    - Allergic vasculitis
    - Post-transplant
  - Iatrogenic
    - Drugs (e.g., gold, azathioprine)

Abbreviations: EGID, eosinophilic gastrointestinal diseases; GERD, gastroesophageal reflux disease; GSE, gluten-sensitive enteropathy; GVH, graft-versus-host disease; IBD, inflammatory bowel disease; MC, microscopic colitis

Adapted from: Mueller S. *Best Pract Res Clin Gastroenterol* 2008;22(3): pg. 427.; and Atkins D, et al. *Nat Rev Gastroentol Hepatol* 2009;6(5): 267-278.

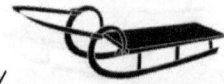

- ➢ Diagnosis

- • Give the diagnostic work-up for eosinophilic gastrointestinal diseases (EGIDs)

  - o Without associated eosinophilia
    - - Infection evaluation (stool, intestinal aspirates, and blood analyses)
    - - Total and allergen-specific IgE (immunoassays and skin tests)
    - - Differential blood cell count
    - - Microscopic evaluation of biopsy samples from the affected and non-affected gastrointestinal parts (histological and immunohistological analysis) T-cells , mast cells
    - - Granule protein and cytokine measurements (immunoassays using blood, feces, or urine)
    - - Immunophenotyping of blood cells (surface marker staining and subsequent flow cytometric analysis)

  - o With associated hypereosinophila
    - - In addition to the above, determine causes of EGID and peripheral eosinophilia
    - - Immunophenotyping of blood cells (in particular T cells and eosinophils)
    - - Bone marrow analysis (cellularity, dysplastic eosinophils, spindle-shaped mast cells, cytogenetic abnormalities, etc.)
    - - Measurements of vitamin B12, tryptase, IL-5, and TARC in blood
    - - Genetic analysis for the presence of a FIPILI-PDGFRA gene fusion
    - - Eosinophil granule protein measurements

Abbreviation: EGID, eosinophilic gastrointestinal diseases

Printed with permission: Conus S, and Simon HU. *Best Pract Res Clin Gastroenterol* 2008;22(3): pg. 443.

- ➢ Diiferential

- • Give the differentiated diagnosis of the causes of food impaction.
  - o Schatzki ring
  - o Peptic strictures
  - o EOE (eosinophilic esophagitis)

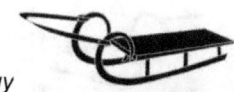

- ➢ Endoscopy
- • Give changes on EGD in the patient with eosinophilic esophagitis (EoE).
  - o Corrugation (multiple rings; feline esophagus; trachealization)
  - o Longitudinal furrows
  - o Mucosa featureless, fragile (crepe paper)
  - o White surface vesicles (eosinophilic microabscesses)
  - o Proximal or mid-esophageal stenosis/stricture (single, or multiple)
  - o Small calibre esophagus
  - o Food impaction
  - o EGD may be normal

Abbreviations: EoE, eosinophilic esophagitis; EGD, esophagogastroduodenoscopy

- ➢ Histopathology
  - o Esophageal mucosal biopsies
    - – From lower and mid esophagus
  - o Basal cell hyperplasia is more common in EoE than in GERD
  - o Eosinophils ↑ closer to surface of esophagus in EoE than in GERD
  - o Eosinophilic microabscesses, ≥ 4 eosinophils in aggregation
  - o Eosinophilic esophagitis, ≥ 15 eosinophils in 2 HPFs (high power fields)

- ➢ Treatment
- • Give the comparison the advantage and disadvantages of current medical and nutritional treatment strategies for eosinophilic esophagitis.

Treatment	Advantages	Disadvantages
o Viscous budesonide (<10 y, 1 mg daily; >10 y, 2 mg daily)	– Easier to swallow – Theoretically can reach more distal areas of esophagus – Shown to reduce symptoms and normalize esophageal mucosa	▪ Cumbersome to mix ▪ Theoretical risk of candidal esophagitis ▪ Long term efficacy unknown
o Prednisone* (1-2 mg/kg/day: maximum 60 mg)	– Rapid relief of symptoms	▪ Significant systemic side effects ▪ Prompt recurrence when discontinued

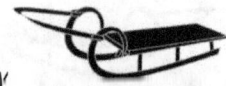

Treatment	Advantages	Disadvantages
o Swallowed fluticasone (children, 440-880 µg/day; adolescents/adults, 880-1769 µg/day)	– Minimal systemic steroid absorption – Shown to relieve symptoms – Normalizes esophageal mucosa	▪ Risk of candidal esophagitis ▪ Small amount systemically absorbed ▪ Long term efficacy unknown, but prompt recurrence when discontinued ▪ Difficult for small children and developmentally delayed patients to swallow ▪ Not for maintenance
o Elemental diet	– 92%-98% effective – Resolution of symptoms in 7-10 days – Histologic remission within 4-5 weeks	▪ Poor palatability ▪ Usually requires nasogastric or gastrostomy tube ▪ Very expensive ▪ Socially isolating
o Montelukast (20-40 mg daily) (leukotriene D4 receptor inhibitor)	– Symptomatic relief has been shown at high doses (100mg) – No significant adverse effects	▪ Not recommended because of lack of reduction of eosinophilic infiltration in the esophageal mucosa ▪ Inadequate studies

o Elimination diet
- Evidence for benefit in adults, similar to benefit in children
- Use skin prick testing to diagnose Type 1 IgE-mediated sensitivity, and skin patch testing for Type IV Th-2 delayed hypersensitivity reactions
- Most common food allergies are dairy, eggs, wheat, soy, peanuts, fish/shellfish

---

CLINICAL CHALLENGE

We all recognized that recurrent vomiting may cause a tear of the mucosa of the lower esophagus, with bleeding, and called a Mallory Weiss tear.

- Give the clinical features which suggest that the Mallory Weiss tear is complicated by Boerhaave syndrome.

  o Boerhaave syndrome is a tear of the esophagus which goes through the wall (transmural), and may be associated with
    - Subcutaneous crepitus
    - Mediastinal air
    - Typically, left-sided effusion

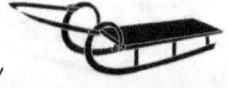

A.B.R. Thomson

Strictures in EoE

- A benign appearing stricture is seen. You suspect esophageal eosinophilia (EE). Give the steps in management.
  - Confirm EE by biopsy of lower and mid esophagus, >15 eosinophils
  - If positive for EE, treat for 4 weeks with PPI
  - If symptoms/endoscopic signs persist despite 4 wk of PPI, consider diagnosis to be eosinophilic esophagitis (EoE)
  - Do not do initial empiric dilation of stricture until EoE disproven, or proven by biopsy and treated
  - Dilate gently and progressively only after treatment of EoE
  - Use generous sedation
  - If perforation occurs, try to avoid surgery, since wall does not hold sutures well; may need to do Esophagectomy
  - Dietary elimination in children

Abbreviation: EoE, eosinophilic esophagitis

> "To be gentle, tolerant, wise and reasonable
> requires a goodly portion of toughness."
>
> Peter Ustinov

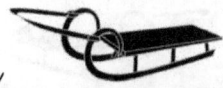

INFECTIOUS ESOPHAGITIS

➢ Causes/associations

MCQ Trick

- o Infectious esophagitis often causes odynophagia when an immune-suppressed patient has odynophagia.

- o If the stem of MCQ states that the examination of the mouth is normal → think candidiasis, CMV or HSV infection in the esophagus, even though there are no signs of infection in the mouth.

- Give causes of infectious esophagitis, and for each give the recommended antimicrobial therapy.

❖ Fungal
- o Candida Albicans
- o Aspergillosis
- o Blastomycosis   — Fluconazole or itraconazole
- o Cryptococcosis
- o Histoplasmosis

❖ Viral
- o CMV
  - – Pathology
    - ▪ Vasculitis, thrombosis of arterioles and
    - ▪ Intranuclear inclusion bodies ("owl's eyes" appearance)
  - – Endoscopy
    - ▪ A few long, deep, serbiginous, discreep, clean-based ulcers
  - – Treatment
    - ▪ Ganciclovir
    - ▪ Foscarnet
    - ▪ IV ganciclovir foscarnet

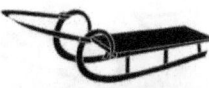

- o HSV (usually HSV type-1)
  - – Associations
    - ▪ Immunosuppression (may occur in immunocompetent persons)
    - ▪ Transplantation setting
    - ▪ During acute rejection
  - – Source of infection
    - ▪ Oropharyngeal HSV, directly to esophagus
    - ▪ Reactivation, indirect spread of HSV along vagus to esophagus
  - – HSV esophagitis may occur together with CMV

➢ Endoscopy
  - o Multiple, small, round ulcers with raised borders and central exudate ("volcano-like")
  - o "ground class nuclei"
  - o Multinucleated giant cells
  - o Eosinophilic "Cowdry bodies"

➢ Treatment
  - o Oral acyclovir or famciclovir

Candidiasis

➢ Risk factors

- • Give risk factors for the development of candidiasis.
  - o Drugs
    - – Corticosteroids
    - – Antibiotics, broad spectrum
    - – Chemotherapy
    - – Immunosuppressives
  - o Catheters
    - – TPN
    - – Hemodialysis
  - o Hospitalizations
  - o Pancreatitis
  - o Malignancy
  - o Transplantation
  - o Recent surgery
  - o AKI (acute kidney injury)
  - o Neutropenia
  - o HIV-infection, CD4 < 100 cells/µL

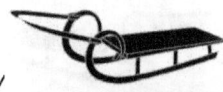

- Clinical: microabscesses in virtually any organ but especially
  - Eye   – White exudates
  - Skin   – Painless papules/pustules on red base
  - MSK   – Bone
                         – Joints
  - GI   – Peritoneum
  - GU   – UTI

➢ Diagnosis
  - Culture
    - Blood "gold standard"
    - Negative blood culture does not exclude systemic candidiasis
    - Positive culture from any normally sterile area
    - "Candidiasis species that is obtained from a blood culture should never be considered a contaminant but instead should initiate investigation for a course" (MKSAP 16, Infectious disease 2012, page 39).
  - Tissue from skin lesion, or any involved organ

Note: Since candida pneumonia is very rare, sputum culture is usually not done

➢ Treatment
  - Non-immunocompromised
    - Spontaneous remission is usual before 2 weeks;
    - Acyclovir 200 mg po 5x/day, or 400 mg pot id for 7 to 14 days for faster symptom relief
  - Non-neutropenic
    - Fluconazole
      - First choice for C. parapsilosis
      - If no/poor response, switch to
    - Echinocandin
      - Caspofungin
      - Anidulafungin
      - Micafungin
      - If echinocandin used first for empiric therapy and response is poor, may switch to Fluconazole if patient is stable
      - First choice empiric therapy for Candida glabrata
    - If echinocandin fails when used for C. glabrata, perform susceptibility testing before using
      - Fluconazole, or step-down
      - Voriconazole

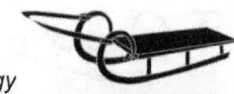

- Treat for 2 weeks after
    - Loss of symptoms
    - Clearance of fungemia
- Remove possibly causative catheters, central lines
- Neutropenic
    - Echinocandin, or
    - Voriconazole, or
    - Amphotericin B, echinocandin, or
    - Voriconazole
- Immunocompromised
    - HIV-seropositive
        - HAART therapy
            - Restoration of CD4 counts > 100 cells/μL helps to ↓ risk of recurrent disease
            - Recurrent disease, moderate-to-severe infection, or CD4 < 100 cells/μL (at risk for esophageal candidiasis)
                - Fluconazole po 200 mg loading dose, followed by 100 mg to 200 mg a day for 7 to 14 days.
    - Symptom relief: viscous xylocaine/lidocaine, gargle/swallow ~ 300 mg/dose, ≤ 8x/day
    - For severe disease (odynophagia, dysphagia, or unable to swallow):
        - Acyclovir 5 mg/kg IV q 8 h for 7 to 14 days
        - Acyclovir-resistant (cross-resistance of valacyclovir and famcyclovir to mutations of thymidine kinase or DNA polymerase): use foscarnet
- Asymptomatic cystitis
    - Treat with fluconazole, if patient
        - Neutropenic
        - Having urologic surgery
- Focal infections
    - Meningitis
    - Endophthalmitis
    - Do not use echinocandins
- Systemic/Invasion Candidiasis
    - Candidemia
    - Disseminate candidiasis
    - Focal organ involvement
    - Hepatosplenic (chronic disseminated)

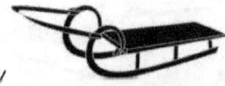

- ❖ Oropharyngeal candidiasis
  - ○ Local
    - – Nystatin swish and swallow 400,000 to 600,000 units qid for 7 to 14 days only for mild disease; clotrimazole or fluconazole higher relapse rate
    - – Cotrimazole: one 10 mg trouche dissolved slowly 5 times a day may be first-time Rx when risk factors (e.g., steroids, chemotherapy) continue ↓ no/poor response
  - ○ Systemic
    - – Fluconazole
      - ▪ 200 mg loading dose, followed by 100 mg to 200 mg a day for 7 to 14 days
      - ▪ Prophylaxis: 100 mg po od
  - ○ Risk factors for oropharyngeal candidiasis
    - – CD4 < 200 cells/µL
    - – Prior colonization or infection with C. albicans

Clinical Gems and Pearls

- ○ The presence of oropharyngeal candidiasis ↑ risk of esophageal infection, but Candida esophagitis may occur in the absence of oropharyngeal disease.

- ○ An immunosuppressant patient who develops odynophagia/dysphagia, with or without oropharyngeal candidiasis, may be treated empirically with fluconazole.

- ○ If a 3 day course of fluconazole does not relieve the esophageal symptoms, perform EGD to determine
  - – Other causes of esophagitis
    - ▪ Pill esophagitis
    - ▪ HSV
    - ▪ GERD
  - – Fluconazole-resistant strains

- ○ When esophageal candidiasis is associated with HIV-seropositivity with CD4 < 100 cells/µL don't forget to mention HAART therapy to restore CD4 levels to reduce the risk of recurrent disease.

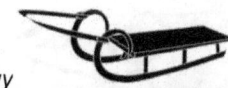

- o First infection, mild infection or CD4 > 100 cells /μL
  - – Oral nystatin or clotrimazole trouches
  - – Fluconazole po 200 mg
  - – 97% favourable response loading dose, followed by 100 mg to 200 mg a day

- ➤ Adverse drug effects
  - o Azoles
    - – Hepatotoxic
    - – Teratogenic in pregnancy
    - – All equally effective
    - – Multiple drug interactions (CYP450)
    - – ↑ risk of drug resistance
  - o Fluconazole
    - – Secondary prophylaxis, 100 mg to 200 mg per week, for
      - ▪ Risk of cryptococcosis
      - ▪ No immune reconstitution on HAART Rx – frequent/severe candidiasis
    - – Same dose as for oropharyngeal candidiasis, but treatment duration 7 to 14 days
    - – May be given IV
  - o Itraconazole oral solution
    - – 10 mg/mL, 200 mg daily for 7 to 14 days
    - – Nausea in > 10%
  - o Posaconazole
    - – 200 mg bid
    - – Transient visual disturbance in 23%
  - o Echinocandins are given IV for esophageal candidiasis refractory to azoles
    - – Caspofungin   50 mg IV per day for 7 to 21 days
    - – Micafungin   100 mg to 150 mg IV per day
    - – Anidulafunfin   100 mg IV per day
  - o Amphotericin B
    - – Indications
    - – Treatment of candidiasis during pregnancy (azoles –teratogenic)
    - – Resistance to azoles or echinocandins
  - o Dosage
    - – 0.3 to 0.7 mg/kg per day

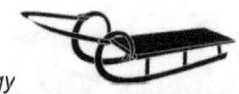

ESOPHAGEAL OBSTRUCTION

- Give the use of a plain film in the patient with suspected foreign body in the esophagus.
    - 47% false negative
    - If it's positive, of course it helps

- Give when it is recommended to do an EGD within 2 hours after the ingestion of a foreign body.
    - Sharps
    - Disc batteries
    - Unable to swallow salivary secretions
    - > 6 cm long and 2.5 cm wide
    - Leaving food bolus → risk of pressure necrosis
    - Treatment in addition to EGD removal: "urban myths" (no proof of efficacy)
        - Glucagon no better than placebo
        - Papain not effective, and may cause perforation
        - Coca-cola

Source: Sperry SLW, et al. Am J Gastroenterol 2012; 107: 215-221.

xxxxxxxxxxxxxxxxxxxxxxxxxxxxxxxxxxxxxxxxxxxxxxxxxxx

SO YOU WANT TO BE A GASTROENTEROLOGIST!

- In the context of the adult patient with regurgitation and dysphagia, define **dysphagia lusoria**, give its anatomy, the diagnostic imaging changes seen on barium swallow, and describe the cardiovascular sign observed at the time of endoscopy.

> Definition
    ○ Dysphagia lusoria (DL) is the term given for symptoms arising from vascular compression of the esophagus by an aberrant right subclavian artery

> Anatomy
    ○ In DL, the aberrant "right" subclavian artery (ARSA) arises from the left side of the aortic arch, distal to the left subclavian artery and the left common carotid artery

    ○ The ARSA courses from the aortic arch upwards and to the right, either behind (80%) or in front of the esophagus (20%)

> Barium swallow
    ○ Diagonal indentation of esophagus is seen from the lower left to upper right of esophagus, at the level of the T3/T4 vertebrae

> CVS sign
    ○ At EGD, compression by the endoscope on the ARSA causes the right radial pulse to weaken or disappear.

83

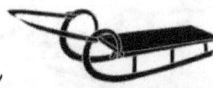

Foreign Body

On a very bizarre night on call, you are called by the Emergency physician with 4 different foreign bodies found by x-ray to be in 4 adult patients' stomachs. The patients are all adults who are asymptomatic. Which of these objects will you come in and retrieve? (Write YES for those you would come in for, and NO for those you wouldn't)

a) A quarter (25 cent piece) – *no*

b) A toothpick – *yes*

c) The plastic cap of a pen (2.0 cm long by 4 mm wide) – *no*

d) A razor blade – *yes [General rule of thumb: long objects (>5cm), wide objects (>3cm), or particularly sharp objects should be retrieved.]*

Rumination Syndrome

o Rumination syndrome is characterized by the "effortless, often repetitive regurgitation of recently ingested food into the mouth".

o The regurgitated material can be chewed and swallowed again or is spat out.

o Retrograde flow of gastric contents into the esophagus is due to contracting the abdominal muscles and subsequent increase in intragastric pressure.

Esophageal Rings and Webs

• Give features distinguishing type A (**Schatzki ring**) from type B esophageal ring.

	Type A	Type B
o Endoscopy		
– Encircle the lumen	– Yes	– Yes
– Esophageal vestibule	– Proximal	– Distal
– Thickness	– Thick, ~ 5 mm	– Thin ~ 2 mm
– Aperture	– < 13 mm	– ≥ 13 mm
– Presence of hiatus hernia	– Occasional	– Always
– Location	– Upper end, LES	– Lower end, LES*
o Histopathology		
– Composition	– Muscular	– Mucosa and submucosal
– Mucosal covering	– Squamous, upper & lower	– Squamous – upper – Columnar – lower
– Frequency	– Rare	– 4%
o Symptoms	– No	– Yes

Abbreviation: LES, lower esophageal sphincter

*junction of the vestibule of the esophagus, and the gastric cardia

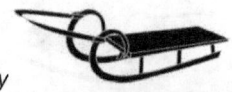

SO YOU WANT TO BE A GASTROENTEROLOGIST!

It is recognized that some patients with a Schatzki ring have symptomatic gastroesophageal reflex disease (GERD), almost all have a hiatus hernia, but only a proportion have erosive esophagitis.

- Give the explanation for this observation.

    o The ring in the lower esophagus prevents acid exposure to the more proximal portions of the esophagus, reducing the risk of mucosal damage.

- Give the role of PPI therapy in the patient with a Schatzki ring.

    o PPIs reduce the need for repeat esophageal dilation by 40% over 35 months.

- Give the anatomical difference between an esophageal ring (ER) and an esophageal web (EW).

	ER	EW
o Location	– Cervical esophagus	▪ Esophageal vestibule
o Encircle the lumen	– Yes, including posterior wall	▪ No (anterior wall of esophagus, extending to lateral but not to posterior wall)
o Symptomatic	– 95%	▪ May be asymptomatic
o ↑ risk of cancer	– Yes, adenocarcinoma	▪ Yes, squamous cell carcinoma

- In the setting of the patient with the sensation of a lump in their throat (globus), define **heterotropic gastric mucosa** (HGM) (inlet patch), and reasons for biopsy.

    o HGM is a small, clearly defined patch of salmon-pink mucosa seen taking a mucosal just below the upper esophageal sphincter

    o It is comprised of gastric fundic or antral-type mucosa

    o When the HGM is lined by chief or parietal cells, it may be infected by H. pylori, may ulcerate, may cause a web or stricture, or be complicated by adenocarcinoma

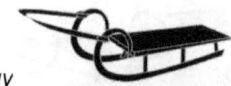

Mastering the Boards: Gastroenterology   A.B.R. Thomson

ESOPHAGEAL TUMOURS

- Give the **Vienna Classification** of esophageal neoplasia based on the internationally accepted histopathologic evaluation of endoscopic mucosal biopsies.

Category		Histopathology
1	–	No dysplasia
2	–	Indefinite for dysplasia
3	–	Low-grade dysplasia/adenoma (aka high-grade intraepithelial neoplasia)
4	–	High-grade dysplasia/adenoma (aka high-grade intraepithelial neoplasia, non-invasive carcinoma, non-invasive epithelial neoplasia suspicious for invasive carcinoma)
5	–	Invasive epithelial neoplasia Intramucosal carcinoma (5.1) Submucosal carcinoma (5.2)

Note: there is high inter-observer variability (as reflected by low kappa [k] statistic) distinguishing category 4 from 5.1, and 5.1 from 5.2

```
                k                    k
              0.42                 0.71
4 |-----------------------------5.1-----------------------------| 5.2
```

- Give the differential diagnosis of benign and malignant esophageal epithelial and non-epithelial tumours.

<u>Epithelial Tumours</u>

- o Malignant
  - Squamous cell
  - Adenocarcinoma of the esophagus and esophagogastric junctrion
  - Verrucuos carcinoma
  - Carcinosarcoma
  - Small cell carcinoma
  - Malignant melanoma

- o Benign
  - Squamous papilloma (2%)
  - Adenoma (1%)
  - Inflammatory fibroid polyp (20%)

<u>Nonepithelial Tumours</u>

- o Malignant
  - Lymphoma
  - Sarcoma
  - Gastrointestinal stromal tumour
  - Metastatic carcinoma

- o Benign
  - Leiomyoma (50%)
  - Granular cell tumour
  - Fibrovascular tumour* (3%)
  - Hemangioma (2%)
  - Hamartoma
  - Lipoma (2%)
  - Cyst (10%)
  - Neurofibroma (1%)

*also known as fibrovascular polyp, myxoma, angiofibroma, fibrolipoma, pedunculated lipoma, fibroepithelial polyp.

Adapted from: *Sleisenger & Fordtran's gastrointestinal and liver disease:* 2016, 10th edition, pg. 787-788.

86

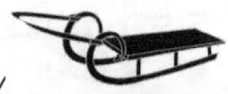

Mastering the Boards: Gastroenterology   A.B.R. Thomson

- ➢ Daignostic imaging
- • Give causes of multiple filling defects in the esophagus seen on barium swallow.
  - o Foreign body
    - – Effervescent granules
  - o Infection
    - – Candidiasis
  - o Tumour
    - – Squamous cell cancer
    - – Candidiasis
    - – Papillomatosis
  - o Blood vessels
    - – Varices

- ➢ Endoscopy
- • Give endoscopic imaging modalities for detecting/staging esophageal neoplasia.
  - o High resolution/high-definition/magnification endoscopy – White light high resolution endoscopy (HRHDME)
  - o Chromendoscopy (CE) (combined with HRHDME) – Lugal's sphincter, toludine blue, methylene blue, indigo carmine, acetic acid, crystal violet
  - o Narrow band imaging (NBI)
  - o FICE (Fuijnon intelligent chromendoscopy; computed interval chromendoscopy)
  - o Point spectroscopy – Fluorescence, elastic scattering, RAMAN, multimedial
  - o Autofluorescence imaging (LIFE, light -induced fluorescence endoscopy [FE]), drug-induced FE, video autofluorescence imaging)
  - o Optical coherence tomography (OCT; micro CT)
  - o Confocal endomicroscopy
  - o EUS

  Abbreviations: CE, chromendoscopy; CIC, computed interval chromendoscopy; EUS, endoscopic ultrasound; FE, fluorescence endoscopy; FICE, Fuijnon intelligent chromendoscopy; HRHDME, white light high resolution endoscopy; LIFE, light -induced fluorescence endoscopy; OCT, optical coherence tomography

  Printed with permission: Curvers WL, Kiesslich R, Bergman JJ. *Best Prac Res Clin Gastroenterol* 2008; 22(4):687-720.

87

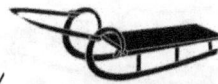

Endoscopic Ultrasound (EUS)

➢ Advantages
- o Endosonography allows distinction between intramural and extramural lesions by examination to a depth of ~20 mm (gut wall is about 4 mm thick).
- o Allows localization of intramural lesion to a specific layer of intestinal wall.
- o Provides the means to obtain tissue for pathological examination by way of FNA (fine needle aspiration) or trucut biopsy for cytological examination.
- o Miniprobes may be passed through the working channel of a standard EGD, and provide more detail, but only for flat lesions or lesions < 1 cm.
- o Describe the EUS image
  - − Size
  - − Vascularity
  - − Echogenicity
    - ▪ Hyperechoic
      - − Bright
      - − Intensity of similar to or greater than that layers
        - ▪ 1 mucosa (superficial)
        - ▪ 3 submucosa
        - ▪ 5 serosa
    - ▪ Hypoechoic
      - − Dark
      - − Intensity similar to or lower than that of layers
        - ▪ 2 LP (lamina propria)
        - ▪ 4 M (muscularis propria)
    - ▪ Anechoic
      - − Black, no internal echo
      - − Intensity of water
      - − Acoustic enhancement (a brighter echo behind a black fluid filled cyst, vessel or gallbladder

    - ▪ Light, hyperechoic

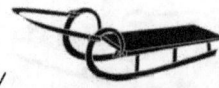

➢ Pathology

• Give the histological counterpast of the 5 layers of the wall of the GI tract seen on EUS (endoscopic ultrasound).

	Histology	Colour	EUS Layer
o Epithelial layer			
– Superficial	Mucosa	W white (hyperechoic)	1
– Deep	M. mucosa	B black (hypoechoic)	2
	Submucosal	W white	3
	M. propria	B black	4
	Serosa	W white	5

1	2	3	4	5
Mucosa	MM	Submucosa	MP	Serosa

▪ Dark, hypoechoic

Abbreviation: MM, muscularis mucosa; MP, muscularis propria

    – Overall accuracy of layer and location of tumour ~80%

    o Localization of tumour by EUS may suggest its diagnostic pathology, e.g.,
        – (white) hyperechoic (1,3,5)
           ▪ Usually a
               – Lipoma (especially when in Layer 3)
               – Duplication cysts in layer 3

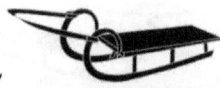

- – (dark) hypoechoic (2,4)
  - ▪ Usually a
    - – GIST (especially in 4)
    - – Leiomyoma (especially in layer 4)
    - – Cyst, filled with mucin, debris
    - – Carcinoids (usually layer 2)
    - – Aberrant pancreas
    - – Pancreatic pseudocysts
- – Note: Esophageal varices (EV) are seen in layers 2 and 4.
- – Anechoic
  - ▪ Black
  - ▪ Often associated with acoustic enhancement
  - ▪ Misclassifications in ~50% of hyoechoic tumour

- • Give the EUS layers and the tumours which are most common in each layer.

EUS layer	Tumour
1	o Lipoma
2	o GIST
	o ECL (granular cell)
3	o Lipoma
	o ECL (granular cell)
	o Duplication cyst
	o Esophageal varices
4	o GIST (gastrointestinal stromal tumours)
	o Leiomyoma
	o Glomus
	o Schwannoma

Lipoma	1, 3
GIST	2, 4
EV	2, 4

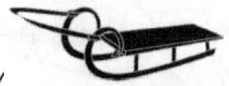

- Give ways to increase the depth of an EGD biopsy (e.g., for a submucosal lesion).

  - EGD   - tunnel biopsy (take a second biopsy from an initial biopsy site)
  - EMR   - unroof the mucosa, biopsy submucosal tissue
  - EUS   - FNA, or trucut biopsy
  - Overall accuracy for determining malignant GIST
    - EUS   78%
    - EUS + FNA   91%
    - EUS + FNA + KL-67   ~100%
  - ESD   - endoscopic submucosal dissection, including use of IT (insulated tip) knife for en bloc dissection

- Heterogeneous appearance of lesion on EUS

  - Especially when large and in esophagus – likely
    - Leiomyosarcoma
    - Lieomyoblastoma
  - May be due to associated
    - Liquefaction necrosis
    - Hyaline degeneration
    - Connective tissue
    - Cystic generation

- EUS features

- Suggestive of malignant tumour

  - Irregular Extraluminal margins
  - Cystic space (heterogeneous)
  - Associated large lymph nodes

# of above EUS findings (suggestive of malignancy)	Sensitivity	Specificity	PPV
1	91%	88%	93%
2	-	-	100%

Abbreviation: PPV, positive predictive value

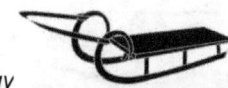

- o Benign tumour
  - – Regular margins
  - – Homogeneous
  - – Size ≤ 3 cm
  - – If all 3 above signs present , ~99% likelihood the GIST is benign
  - – Note: GISTs > 1 cm have the potential to be malignant, so even if A > 1 cm GIST looks benign on EUS, perform annual EUS surveillance for change in size, or development of malignant EUS features

➤ Esophageal varices on EUS

  - o Anechoic

  - o Layers 2 and 3

  - o Distinguish from esophageal duplication cyst, using Doppler colour ultrasound

---

SO YOU WANT TO BE AN EUS Expert!

On EUS of the esophagus, a **duplication cyst** (DC) is anechoic, homogeneous, has regular margins, and is usually seen in EUS layer 3.

- Give the name of a much more common anechoic lesion than DC seen on EUS of the esophagus, and name the diagnostic imaging test which helps to distinguish between these two lesions.
  - o Esophageal varices are also anechoic and are seen in layers 2 and 3 on EUS
  - o Dopper colour ultrasound will show flow in varices, but not in a duplication cyst.

- Give the clinical circumstance when EUS may be falsely negative for demonstrating esophageal varices (EV).
  - o Small EV may be compressed and made obscure by the EUS endoscope, or by the balloon of the transducer.

Duplication cysts (DC) are usually in the submucosal (EUS layer 3), and are anechoic, homogeneous and have regular margins.

- Give the complications of a DC which may make it difficult on EUS or on CT scan to distinguish a duplication cyst from a solid malignancy.
  - o A DC is, as the name implies, a cyst. However, it may become solid if
    - - It undergoes malignant degeneration, and becomes solid
    - - It may become with debris, and appear to be solid

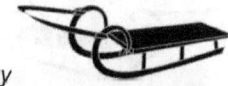

Mastering the Boards: Gastroenterology A.B.R. Thomson

Fibrovascular Polyp

➤ Clinical

- o Presentations
  - – Dysphagia
  - – Globus
  - – Asphyxiation
    - ▪ 2 cm (risk of tracheal obstruction → asphyxiation)

➤ Is the patient crazy – "Dr. Bob, I cough up a piece of tissue that disappears back into my mouth".

- o No, the patient is not making this up. This is likely a long fibrovascular polyp of the upper esophagus, near the cricoid.

➤ Treatment

- o Surgical resection
  - – Penetrating vessel
- o Endoscopic polyectomy
  - – No penetrating vessel: < 2 cm

A patient with dyspepsia has **nodules** in the esophagus. There is no esophagitis, no cobblestoning of the mucosa, and no whitish exudate.

- • Give the name of the likely diagnosis, and describe the histopathology.
  - o Large squamous cells
  - o Cytoplasm of these large squamous cells contains glycogen, and appear nodular.

Clinical curiosities: Cobblestoning of

- o Buccal mucosa
  - – Cowden syndrome
- o Tongue
  - – Crohn disease

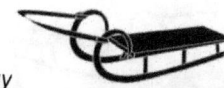

Mastering the Boards: Gastroenterology   A.B.R. Thomson

Esophageal Cancer

➤ Clinical

- Give presenting symptoms for **esophageal cancer**.
  - o Esophagus
    - – Dysphagia, odynophagia
    - – Back or chest pain with/without swallowing
    - – Halitosis
    - – Tracheoesophageal fistula
  - o Nerves
    - – Hoarseness from recurrent laryngeal nerve involvement
    - – Horner syndrome (miosis, ptosis, absence of sweating on ipsilateral face and neck)
    - – Phrenic nerve involvement from hiccups
  - o Nodes
    - – Supraclavicular adenopathy
  - o Systemic
    - – Weight loss
    - – Clubbing
    - – Signs/symptoms of metastases

➤ Clinical

- Give risk factors for esophageal squamous cancer and for adenocarcinoma.

	Squamous Cell Carcinoma	Adenocarcinoma
o Age	>60	>50
o Gender	M	M
o Alcohol	+	-
o Smoking	+	-
o GERD	-	+
o BE	-	+
o HIV	+	+

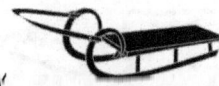

- o Previous head and neck squamous cell carcinoma
- o Radiation therapy
- o Lye ingestion
- o Plummer-Vinson (Paterson-Kelly) syndrome
- o Achalasia (33x ↑)
- o Nutritional deficiencies – Riboflavin, niacin; high starch diet without fruits and vegetables
- o Nitrosamines; "bush teas" (diterpene phorbol esters)
- o Gluten sensitive enteropathy (GSE)
- o Tylosis palmaris

Abbreviations: BE, Barrett epithelium; GERD, gastroesophageal reflux disease

➢ Classification

PRE-OPERATIVE CLASSIFICATIONS

o **Ultrasound** (US) TNM classification for esophageal cancers

uT1	Tumour invading the mucosa and the submucosa
uT2	Tumour invading the mucosa without going beyond
uT3	Tumour invading the tunica adventitia (or the serous membrane)
uT4	Tumour invading the adjacent structures
uN0	No lymph node invasion
uN1	Lymph nodes invaded around tumour; round, same echogenicity as the tumour
uN2	Lymph nodes invaded distant from the tumour (5 cm above or below the upper or lower pole of the tumour)

o **CT scan** (CT) TNM classification for thoracic esophageal cancers

ctT1	Non-visibility or mass <10 mm in diameter
ctT2	Mass 10-30 mm in diameter
ctT3	Mass >30 mm in diameter with no sign of invasion t mediastinal structures
ctT4	Idem + sign of spread to mediastinal structures

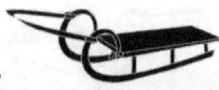

o Lymph nodes (N)*

ctN0   No detectable adenopathy

ctN1   Regional adenopathy (mediastinal and/or perigastric)

o Distant metastases

ctM0   No distant metastasis

ctM1   Presence of distant metastases (including celiac and cervical adenopathies)

o Definition of US and CT stages

US or CT   I TI N0 M0
stages
             IIa T2 N0 M0; T3 N0 M0

             IIb T1 T2 N1 M0

* lymph nodes >10 mm are considered to be high risk of being metastatic

POST-OPERATIVE CLASSIFICATIONS:

o TNM classification

T-Primary tumour

T0   No sign of primary tumour

Tis   Carcinoma in situ

T1   Tumour invading the lamina propria or the submucosa

T2   Tumour invading the muscularis

T3   Tumour invading the tunica adventitia

T4   Tumour invading the adjacent structures

o N-Regional adenopathy

Nx   Lymph nodes not evaluated

N0   No sign of regional lymph node involvement

N1   Regional lymph node metastases

o Cervical esophagus: cervical lymph nodes, internal jugular, peri-esophageal and supraclavicular nodes

Printed with permission: Veuillez V, et al. *Best Pract Res Clin Gastroenterol* 2007;21(6): 949.

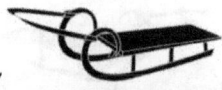

➢ Treatment

- Give **palliative treatments** for the care of the patient with esophageal carcinoma.
  - ○ Non-endoscopic techniques
    - – Surgery
    - – Radiation therapy
      - ▪ External beam radiotherapy
      - ▪ Intraluminal radiotherapy (brachytherapy)
    - – Chemotherapy
  - ○ Endoscopic techniques
    - – Laser therapy
      - ▪ Thermal (Nd:YAG)
      - ▪ Photodynamic therapy
    - – Dilation
    - – Electrocoagulation (BICAP probe)
    - – Chemical injection therapy
    - – Stent placement
  - ○ Nutritional support
    - – Nasoenteric feeding tube
    - – Percutaneous endoscopic gastrostomy (PEG)

Printed with permission: Siersema PD. *Nat Clin Pract Gastroenterol Hepatol* 2008;5(3): pg.143.

"The greatest joys in life are found not only in what we do and feel, but also in our quiet hopes and labors for others."

Bryant McGill

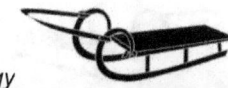

Submucosal Tumours

- o Muscle
  - – Leiomyomas
  - – Leiomyosarcomas
- o Nerve
  - – Schwannomas
- o Desmoid tumours

❖ **Lipoma**

- o EGD/C
  - – Single indentation of mucosa
  - – Yellowish
  - – Smooth
  - – Easily indented ("pillow" sign, aka "cushion" sign; sensitivity o 40%, specificity of 99%)
- o Easily tented (mucosa can be piled away from submucosal growth by gently tugging on mucosa biopsy forcep; known as "tenting" sign)
- o EUS
  - – Layer 1,3*,5 (hyperechoic – light)

❖ **Carcinoid tumour**

- o EGD/C commonest sites (in USA)
  - – Appendix ⎤
  - – Rectum   ⎬ usually are single

  - – Ileum   ⎤
  - – Stomach   ⎬ often are multiple
- o EUS
  - – Usually layer 2
  - – Hypoechoic
  - – Homogeneous

❖ **Granular cell tumours** (ECT)

- o Often in esophagus (mid and lower third)
- o EUS layer 2 or 3
- o Hypoechoic on EUS
- o Homogeneous
- o Usually benign unless > 4 cm
- o IHC (immunohistochemistry) – S -100 protein positive

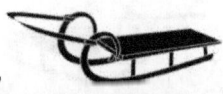

❖ **Duplication cysts**

o Usually in proximal small intestine

o May or may not communicate with the lumen

o Epithelium
  - Squamous
  - Columnar, or
  - Ciliated

o Contain mucoid fluid

o Usually benign

Gastrointestinal Stromal Tumours (GIST)

➢ Types
  o Leiomyomas
    - Commonest stromal tumour
      ▪ Endogastric (grow into the lumen)
      ▪ Mid or lower third of esophagus
    - Perform at least annual EUS for small tumours
  o Polypoid leiomyomas < 2 cm endoscopic snare resection

➢ Diagnosis
  o EUS plus FNA

➢ Laboratory
  o C-kit (a stem cell factor receptor) (~99%)
    - CD34 (a hematopoietic cell progenitor cell antigen) (70%)
    - Smooth muscle actin (20% to 30%)
    - S 100 protein (marker of neural differentiation)

➢ Pathology
  o Mutational activation of genes
    - KIT
    - PDGFRA
    - DC117
  o Site
    - Stomach   ~70%
    - Small bowel   ~25%
    - Colon/rectum   5%
  o Malignant potential
    - All GISTs > 10 m
  o Immunohistochemical (IHC) studies

99

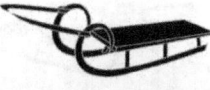

- Give how to distinguish GIST from leiomyomas (LM) and leiomyosarcomas (LMS).

IHC antibody	GIST	LM/LMS
o C-kit (CD117)	+	-
o Smooth muscle actin	-	+
o Desmin	-	+

Note: EUS/FNA rather than IHC will differentiate between leiomyoma and leiomyosarcomas.

- ➢ Treatment
  - o Medical
    - – TK (tyrosine kinase) inhibitors, e.g., imatimib, used as adjuvant or no adjuvant therapy (before surgical resection)
      - ▪ GISTs ≥ 3 cm
      - ▪ ↓ GIST recurrence is post-op yr 1
  - o Surgical
    - – Obtain negative tumour resection margins
    - – Laroscopic resection if possible
    - – Structural changes from previous EUSs
    - – Open en bloc esophagectomy for
      - ▪ Tumour ≥ 2 cm
      - ▪ Involvement of GE junction
  - o Leiomyosarcomas
    - – May require partial or total esophagectomy
  - o GCTs granular cell tumours, aka schwannomas submucosal, hypoechoic on EUS, layer 243, 5-100 protein positive on IHC

- ➢ Postsurgical follow-up (suggested, but not evidence-based)
  - o GIST
    - – Clinical (history & physical)
      - ▪ Every 3 month to 6 month for 5 years, then every year
    - – CT scan
      - ▪ Every 3 months to 6 months for 3 years to 5 years, then every year
  - o Leiomyosarcoma
    - – Clinical & CT
      - ▪ Every 3 months to 6 months for 2 years to 3 years, then every year
      - ▪ Consider regular imaging of the chest
    - – If margins of resected leiomyosarcoma are positive, perform follow-up as above, only more intense long-term:
      - ▪ Every 3 months to 6 months for 2 years to 3 years
      - ▪ Then every 6 months for 2 years, then every year

100

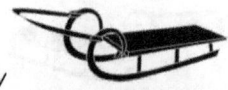

ESOPHAGEAL VARICEAL BLEEDING (EVB)

- Demography
  - Presence of varices at diagnosis of cirrhosis
    - Compensated
      - 30%
    - Decompensated
      - 60%
  - Risk of first EVB 12% per year
  - Risk of death from each EVB ~20%

- Risks
  - Frequency of EV
    - Cirrhosis 40%
    - Cirrhosis plus ascites 60%
  - Rates of development of EV
    - 2.5- 5% per year
  - Rate of progression of small to large EV
    - ~10% per year
  - Risk of new EV bleeding
    - Overall, ~25% in 2 years
    - Diameter < 5 mm, 7%
    - > 5 mm, 30%
  - EV bleeding stops spontaneously in ~ 50%
    - Within 5 days of initial bleeding, 40%
  - The mortality rate for each episode of variceal bleeding is 30%
  - Rebleeding of EV after initial EV bleeding
    - 50% per year
  - Occult infection from spontaneous bacterial peritonitis (SBP) may increase the rate of early rebleeding
  - Antibiotics are used on an empirical basis in cirrhotic patients with a variceal bleed or ascites
  - In person with hepatic cirrhosis, esophageal varices develop in 2.5% of persons per year
  - The risk of EV bleeding increase with:
    - longer varices
    - the presence of red wale marks on the varices
    - or in the person with more extensive liver dysfunction

Abbreviations: EVBL, endoscopic variceal band ligation; SBP, spontaneous bacterial peritonitis; TIPS, transjugular intrahepatic portosystemic shunt

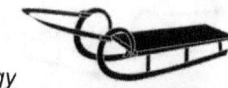

- Give factors in a person with liver disease and known esophageal varices which predict a high risk for the first variceal bleeding in the future.

  o Clinical
  – Child's class/ MELD score > 15
  – Previous variceal bleed
  – Alcohol consumption

  o Endoscopic
  – Large esophageal varices
  – Red colour sign
  – Presence of gastric or proximal esophageal varices
  – Presence of portal hypertensive gastropathy

  o Hemodynamic
  – Intra-esophageal variceal pressure
  – ↑ HVPG > 12 mm Hg

  o Blood tests
  – Platelets < 140-150 k
    ▪ Ratios spleen diameter/platelets
    ▪ Liver span/albumin
  – Collateral flow on Doppler ultrasound
  – Flow reversal in PV

  o Ultrasound
  – Congestion index of the portal vein
  – Portal vein size > 10-13 mm

Adapted from: Franchis de, R, and Dell'Era A. *Best Pract Res Clin Gastroenterol* 2007; 21(1): 11.

➢ Pathophysiology

- Give the pathogenesis of EV (esophageal varices).

When the pressure (P) in the esophageal varix rises (> 12 mm Hg), when the radius (r) of the varix increases (small → large varices), and when the thickness of the wall of the varix (w) becomes thin because of the enlarging and dilating vein, then according to the law of Laplace (T = Pr/w), the tension (t) on the wall of the varix becomes so great that a hole develops in the ruptured wall of the vein, and profuse bleeding occurs.

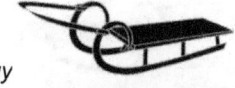

- Give the zones of venous drainage in EV.

  o Truncal zone
  - 10 cm in length, above perforating zone
  - 4 longitudinal veins in the lamina propria

  o Perforating zone
  - Above palsade zone
  - Network of esophageal submucosal veins anastomose with periesophageal external veins
  - Periesophageal veins drain into azygous system

  o Palisade zone
  - 2-3 cm above GE junction
  - 4 longitudinal veins anastomose with veins in the lamina propria
  - No anastomosis with periesophageal external (i.e., no perforating veins) veins
  - Limited soft tissue support high risk of bleeding

  o Gastric zone
  - 2-3 cm below GE junctions
  - Longitudinal veins in submucosal and lamina propria these longituding veins gather at the gastric cardia and drain into short gastric and left gastric veins

- Give the importance of portal pressure (PP) in EVD.

  o Portal vein (PV) pressure is normally 5 to 10 mm Hg

  o Cirrhosis → ↓ NO production → intrahepatic vasoconstriction (reversible) → splanchnic arteriolar vasodilation → ↑ PV (portal vein) blood flow → ↑ PP → hepatic sinusoids become distorted → ↑ resistance to outflow through HV (hepatic vein) → ↑ PP

  o HVPG = PV pressure (or WHVP) – HV pressure =

1 to 5 mm Hg	normally
>10 mm Hg	EV develop
> 12 mm Hg	EVB

  o The WHVP (wedge hepatic venous pressure) can be obtained from catheterization of HV, as also can the free HV pressure

- Hepatic Venous Pressure Gradient (HVPG)

  o WHVP approximates the value of PV pressure, so can be used to estimate HVPG.

  o Clinically useful to measure portal pressure
  - HVPG = WHVP – FHVP
  - Splenic pulp pressure gradient (SPPG)
  - In presinusoidal portal hypertension, HVPG is normal, but SPPG is increased

103

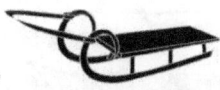

- HVPG cannot be obtained when the hepatic veins are blocked, e.g.,
  - BCS (Budd-Chiai syndrome)
  - Intrahepatic, presinusoidal causes of portal hypertension (e.g., idiopathic portal hypertension

- Endoscopic variceal pressure
  - Varices (miniature pneumatic pressure sensitive gauge on an endoscope
  - Endoscopic balloon
  - Represents the gradient between pressure in portal vein and the intra-abdominal inferior vena cava (IVC)
  - Not useful to measure presinusoidal causes portal hypertension (only good for sinusoidal and causes of PH)
  - Portal vein thrombosis (PVT) causes presinusoidal portal hypertension, which is not correctly assessed by HVPG (is normal in PVT)

Abbreviations: HVPG, hepatic venous pressure gradient; FHVP, free hepatic vein pressure; SPPG, splenic pulp pressure gradient; WHVP, wedge hepatic venous pressure

➢ Classification
  - F1
    - Small
    - Straight
    - Straight
    - Tortuous
    - < 1/3 of lumen of esophagus (< 5 mm diameter)
  - F2
    - Large, tortuous, fill < 1/3 of lumen
  - F3
    - Large, coil-shaped fill > 1/3 of lumen
    - Fill > 1/3 of lumen of esophagus (> 5 mm diameter)

➢ Terminology
  - Screening
    - Determine if there are EV (esophageal varices)
    - Screening for EV by EGD
      - Before 1st EVB in cirrhotic, compensated or decompensated
      - Consider: if ↑ ratio of platelet count/spleen size (standard deviation score) → EGD

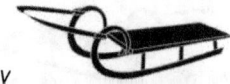

- o Pre-primary development of EV
- o Primary prophylaxis
    - Prevent the first EVB (esophageal variceal bleeding)
- o Secondary prophylaxis
    - Prevent recurrent EVB
- o Acute bleeding
    - Stop EVB

- ➢ Laboratory

- • Give the clinical, laboratory, and abdominal ultrasound imaging findings which increase the pretest probability of the cirrhotic patient having EV (a clue: HE, jaundice and ascites are not predictive for the presence of EV).
    - o Splenomegaly
    - o ↑ INR
    - o Platelets < 88,000/mL
    - o diameter of portal vein > 13 mm, shown on abdominal ultrasound

- ➢ Diagnostic imaging

- • Give findings seen on abdominal Doppler ultrasound which suggest the presence of portal hypertension.
    - o Portal vein
        - Reversed (hepatofungal) blood flow
        - Diameter > 13 mm
        - ↑ portal blood flow
    - o Splenic and mesenteric vein
        - Loss of changes on respiration
    - o Portosystemic collateral vessels
    - o Splenomegaly

- • Give advantages of MDCT (multidetector row CT) venous EUS in the evaluation of the patient with portal hypertension and possible esophageal varices.
    - o MDCT is useful to
        - Detect varices in the gastric fundus
        - Distinguish submucosal from perigastric varices

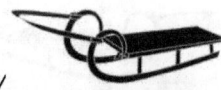

- Give two advantages of gadolinium-enhanced magnetic resonance imaging versus EUS in the evaluation of the patient with portal hypertension and possible varices.

  - MRI is useful to measure
    - Portal and azygous blood flow
    - Stiffness of spleen

- Give advantages of EUS in the evaluation of the patient with portal hypertension and possible varices.

  EUS is useful to measure:

  - Cross-sectional area of varices

  - Size and blood flow in
    - Left gastric vein
    - Azygous vein
    - Paraesophageal collaterals

  - Transmural pressure in the varix

  - Effectives of endoscopic therapy (including recurrence of varices after EVBL [esophageal variceal band ligation])

> **Prophylaxis of Bleeding from EV**

- Give the recommended times for repeated endoscopy (EGD) for screening for gastroesophageal varices (GEV) in a patient with cirrhosis.

Findings on Initial Endoscopy	Repeated EGD
o No GEV	q 2 to 3 yr
o Small GEV	q 1 to 2 yr
o Large GEV	q 1-3 months, with endoscopy varices obliterate, then every 2 to 3 years

o **Pre-primary** prophylaxis	– Before varices develop, to prevent future bleeding
	  ▪ Prophylactic treatment not proven
	  ▪ Repeat EGD in 2-3 years

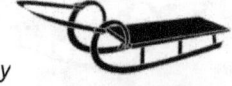

- o Low risk, primary prophylaxis
  - – NSBB (non-selective beta blockers)
    - ▪ Small, medium or large EV, plus
    - ▪ Red wale marks; or
    - ▪ Child B or C cirrhosis
    - ▪ Of no use for pre-primary prophylaxis
      - – ↓ progression of small to large EV
      - – ↓ cumulative probability of EVB

```
┌──────────────────────────────────────┐
│  CHILD Classs                          │
│                                        │
│  < 5 mm   A  - wait and see            │
│           C  - NSBB                    │
│                                        │
│  > 5 mm        NSBB or EVL             │
└──────────────────────────────────────┘
```

- o High risk
  - – NSBB (non-selective beta blockers)
    - ▪ ↓ MR (mortality rate) from EVB (5% versus 10% with placebo)
    - ▪ ↓ MR (trend) from all causes (21% versus 27% with placebo; or 0.7)
  - – EVL (endoscopic variceal ligation)
    - ▪ If NSBB fail to prevent enlargement of EV → EVL
    - ▪ EVL may be superior primary prophylaxis for large (F2 or F3) varices
  - – Risk of first bleed
    - ▪ No β-blocker   25%
    - ▪ With β-blocker   15%
    - ▪ ARR   10%
    - ▪ NNT   10%
  - – Mortality rate
    - ▪ No β-blocker, 28%
    - ▪ With β-blocker, 24%
    - ▪ ARR, 5%
    - ▪ NNT, 22
  - – Shortcoming!
    - ▪ Using HR or a ↓ HR as an indirect marker for the adequacy of NSBB
    - ▪ Only persons with better liver function (~1/3 of total group) respond to NSBB
    - ▪ Using HR / ↓ HR is not a good predictor of HVPG
    - ▪ When HVPG < 12 mm Hg, EV bleeding does not occur
    - ▪ When HVPG < 12 mm HG, EV bleeding does still occur

Abbreviation: ARR, absolute risk reduction; EV, esophageal varices; EVL, endoscopic variceal ligation; GV, gastric varices; NNT, numbered needed to treat; NSBB, non-selective beta blocker

- o Dosing of NSBB
  - – Starting dose of nadolol
    - ▪ MAP (mean arterial pressure)
      - – < 85 mm Hg   20 mg po per day
      - – > 85 mm Hg   40 mg po per day

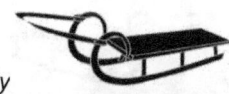

Mastering the Boards: Gastroenterology   A.B.R. Thomson

SO YOU WANT TO BE A GASTROENTEROLOGIST!

NSBB (non-selective beta blockers) reduce the beta adrenergic vasodilatory tone in the mesenteric arterioles, and this reduces portal vein in flow and portal pressure. However, NSBB leads to unopposed and therefore ↑ alpha adrenergic vasoconstriction and therefore ↑ portohepatic outflow resistance. The alpha 1 effect partially offsets the beneficial beta effect. Therefore, it may be reasonably postulated that nitrates, which decrease portal pressure, would be beneficial when added to NSBB to reduce the portal pressure and EVB.

- Give the reason why the combination of nitrates with NSBB is **not** recommended for primary prophylaxis for EVB.
  - The combination of nitrates plus NSBB do not achieve consistent
    - ↓ EVB (NNT ~ 10)
    - ↓ MR from EVB (perhaps is even increased by nitrates)

Nadolol and propranolol are non-selective beta blockers (NSBB) which reduce portal pressure mainly by ↓ WHVP (a surrogate for portal pressure). Carvedilol is a mixed adrenergic blocker, with beta blocking and alpha blocking activity.

- Give a comparison of the use of propranolol versus carvedilol for the primary prevention of EVB (i.e., give the advantages of carvedilol vs propranol)

Endpoint	Propranolol	Carvedilol
o Portal venous inflow	↓	↓
o Hepatic vascular tone	-	↓
o Reduction in portal pressure	13%	20%
– MAP		
– HVPG		
– HVG ≤ 12 mm Hg	14%	64%
– GFR	↓	-
– CO	↓	-
o Plasma volume	-	↑
o Rate of 1st EVB	23%	10%

Abbreviations: CO, cardiac output (a predictor of HRS [hepatorenal syndrome]); EVB, esophageal variceal bleeding; GFR, glomerular filtration rate; HVPG, hepatic venous pressure gradient; MAP, mean arterial pressure

108

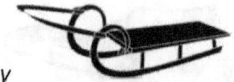

- Give the management strategy for esophageal varices after the initial screening endoscopy in patients with cirrhosis.

No Varices	o Repeat endoscopy in 3 years (sooner if decompensation occurs)		
Small varices	o CTP B/C patient or EV with red signs o CTP A patient, with no red signs	– NSBB optional – If no, ß-blockers given, repeat endoscopy in 2 yr (sooner if decompensation occurs)	▪ Start propranolol (20 mg bid) or nadolol (20 mg qd) ▪ Titrate to maximal tolerable dose or a heart rate of 55-60 bpm ▪ No need to repeat EGD ▪ Same as above
Medium/ large varices	o All patients independent of CTP class	– NSBB (propranolol, nadolol), or – EVL*	▪ Same as above ▪ Ligate q 1-2 wk EV ▪ First surveillance endoscopy 1-3 mon after obliteration, then q 6-12 mon indefinitely

109

*Choice depends on patient characteristics and preferences, local resources

Abbreviations: CTP, Child Turcotte Pugh ; EGD, esophagogastroduodenoscopy; EV, esophageal varices; EVL, endoscopic variceal ligation; NSS, non-selective beta blocker

Printed with permission: Garcia Tsao, et al. *Am J Gastroenterol* 2009; 104: 1806.

- o Endoscopic variceal ligation (EVL)

Outcome	No EVL RR
– Risk of first EVB	0.36
– EVB-related mortality	0.20
– All-cause mortality	0.50

- o EVL has comparable benefit as NVBB for primary prevention; except
  - – Possibly EVL being superior for large EV
  - – Cost effectiveness considering
    - ▪ QoL (quality of life) EVL > NSBB
    - ▪ Life-years gained EVL = NSBB
- o After first EVL for primary prophylaxis of EVB
  - – Repeat EGD
  - – Every 2 weeks until all EV are obliterated, then
  - – Check for recurrence of EV 1 to 3 mon later, then q 6 to q 12 mon
- o EVL is the endoscopic method of choice to treat esophageal varices.
- o No beneficial effects have been observed combining endoscopic sclerotherapy (EST) and EVL.
- o Proton pump inhibitors may enhance the safety of EVL
- o Variceal bleeding is markedly reduced when the HVPG decreases to < 12 mm Hg or by >20% from baseline
- o EVL may reduce variceal size until variceal obliteration
- o EVL has no effect on portal pressure
- o Variceal obliteration with tissue adhesives (e.g., cyanoacrylates) is effective in the treatment of gastric varices

Abbreviations: EVL, endoscopic variceal ligation; EST, endoscopic sclerotherapy; HVPG, hepatic venous pressure gradient

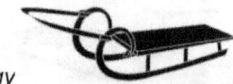

- Give the first and second line management strategy in the prevention of recurrent variceal hemorrhage (secondary prophylaxis).

o First line therapy	– Nonselective ß-blockers (propranolol, nadolol)	▪ Start propranolol (20 mg b.i.d) or nadolol (20 mg q.d) ▪ Titrate to maximum tolerable dosage or a heart rate of 55-60 b.p.m ▪ No need for repeat endoscopy
	– Endoscopic variceal ligation (EVL)	▪ Ligate every 1-2 weeks until variceal obliteration is achieved ▪ First surveillance endoscopy 1-3 months after variceal obliteration, then every 6-12 months
o Second line therapy (if combined pharmacologic + endoscopic treatment has failed)	– TIPS or – Shunt surgery (CTP class A patients, where available)	

Abbreviations: BID, twice daily; BPM, beats per minute; CTP, Child Turcotte Pugh; QD, once daily; TIPS, transjugular intrahepatic portosystemic shunt

Printed with permission: Macmillan Publishers Ltd: Garcia Tsao et al. *Am J Gastroenterol* 2009; 104:1802-1829, Table 3, page 1809.

➢ Secondary prophylaxis of EV prevention of rebleeding

- o Risk of rebleeding after first EV bleed 80% at 2 years

- o If CTP score ≥ 7, consider liver transplantation

- Give the endoscopic red colour signs seen on GEV at endoscopy, and indicated which sign are suggestive of recent bleeding (*) (aka "stigmata")
  - o "wale" marks*
    - Longitudinal, whip-like marks
  - o Cherry-red spots*
    - < 3 mm red spots
  - o Hematocystic spots ≥ 4 mm blood-filled blisters
  - o Diffuse redness

111

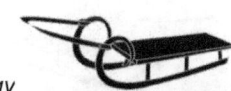

Approach for

- CHILD A
    - NSBB or NSBB plus EVL (endoscopic variceal ligation; [depends on whether measurements can be done to assess Δ HVPG])
- CHILD C
    - EVL
        - No rebleeding
            - EVL repeated
        - Rebleeding
            - EVL

Clinical Caution BARB Failure and EVL

"A patient who does not achieve a decrease in the HVPG to less than 12 mm Hg, or greater than 20%, on a beta blocker [β-adrenergic receptor blocker, a non-selective beta blocker (NSBB)] may not respond well to endoscopic variceal ligation [EVL] either" (Sleisenger and Fordtran's Gastrointestinal and Liver Disease. 10th Edition. Saunders/Elsevier, Philadelphia, 2016, page 1545).

- Primary (before the first bleeding episode) or secondary (after the first esophageal variceal bleed) prophylaxis with either non-selective beta-blockers or EVBL (endoscopic variceal band ligation) is recommended in Class A cirrhotic patients with medium or large varices, or Child Class B and C patients with varices of any size
- If EVBL cannot control the bleeding, the patient may benefit from a distal splenorenal shunt procedure or TIPS
- Repeat EGD
    - Cirrhosis
        - Compensated, q 2 to q 3 yr
        - Decompensated, q 1 yr

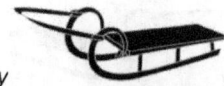

Mastering the Boards: Gastroenterology   A.B.R. Thomson

SO YOU WANT TO BE A HEPATOLOGIST!

- Give the factors which help the clinician to stratify the risk of failure to control EV bleeding at 5 days after the first EGD, (↑ likelihood of rebleeding* early after the initial EV bleed).

Risk factors for failure to control bleeding at 5 days	Risk factors for rebleeding after initial control for 24 hour*	Factors for risk of death from bleeding EV
○ Active EV bleeding at EGD	– Bleeding in ER – Bleeding gastric varices	▪ > 4 units PRBC ▪ Renal failure ▪ Alcoholic cirrhosis
○ ↓ Hct (hematocrit)	– ↓ albumin	▪ MELD > 18 ▪ HE
○ ↑ ALT or ↑ AST	– ↑ creatinine	▪ HCC
○ CHILD C > B > A	– Excessive transfusions	▪ ↑ bilirubin
○ Bacterial infection		▪ ↓ albumin ▪ Overall MR
○ PVT (portal vein thrombosis)		– 1 week, ~ 7%
○ HVPG > 20 mm Hg		– 6 weeks, 20%

Abbreviations: HCC, hepatocellular cancer; HE, hepatic encephalopathy; HVPG, hepatic venous pressure gradient; MR, mortality rate; PRBC, packed RBC

*Rebleeding is defined as "……recurrence of bleeding after initial control for 24 hours during which the vital signs and hemoglobin level are stable" (Feldman M., et al. Sleisenger and Fordtran's Gastrointestinal and Liver Disease. 10th Edition. Saunders/Elsevier, Philadelphia, 2016, page 1544).

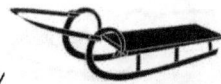

- Give a comparison of the outcomes of endoscopic band ligation (endoscopic variceal ligation, EVL) versus non-specific beta-blockers for primary prophylaxis of esophageal variceal bleeding.

Ligation Versus Beta-Blocker	RR
o Variceal bleeding	0.57
o Gastrointestinal bleeding (all types)	0.69
o Bleeding-related mortality	0.84
o All cause mortality	1.03
o Severe adverse event	0.34

Abbreviations: RR, relative risk

Source: Klebl, FH and Schölmerich J. *Best Pract Res Clin Gastroenterol* 2008; 22(2): 373-87; Villanueva, Candid., et al. *Best Pract Res Clin Gastroenterol* 2008;22(2): 263.

- Give the diagnosis and management strategy of patients with acute variceal hemorrhage.

o ***Diagnosis***	–	Any of the following findings on upper endoscopy performed within 12 hr of admission:
	–	Active bleeding from a varix or stigmata of variceal hemorrhage (white nipple sign) or
	–	Presence of gastroesophageal varices without another source of hemorrhage
o General management	–	Cautious transfusion of fluids and blood products, aiming to maintain a hemoglobin of ~8g/dL
	–	Antibiotic prophylaxis (3-7 days) with:

- Ciprofloxacin 500 mg b.i.d (p.o) or 400 mg b.i.d (i.v), or

- Ceftriaxone 1g/day (i.v) particularly in facilities with known quinolone resistance and in patients with two or more of the following: malnutrition, ascites, encephalopathy, serum bilirubin >3 mg/dL

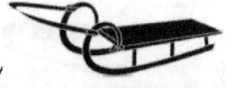

- o **Specific initial management**
  - – Pharmacological therapy initiated as soon as diagnosis is suspected; Octreotide 50 mcg i.v bolus, followed by continuous infusion 50 mcg/hr (3-5 days), and
  - – Endoscopic therapy (ligation preferable) performed at time of diagnostic endoscopy (performed within 12 hr of admission)
- o Rescue management
  - – Considered in patients with bleeding esophageal varices who have failed pharmacological and endoscopic therapy, or
  - – In patients with bleeding gastric fundal varices who have failed one endoscopic therapy: TIPS or Shunt therapy (CTP A patients where available)

Abbreviations: BID, twice a day; CTP, Child Turcotte Pugh; PO, orally.

Printed with permission: Garcia Tsao, et al. Am J Gastroenterol 2009; 104:1808.

Clinical Gem

- o NSBB (non-selective beta blockers) reduce the risk of development of ascites/SBP (spontaneous bacterial peritonitis) but

- o May not be safe to use in refractory ascites because of ↓ renal blood flow and ↓ GFR (glomerular filtration rate)

Clinical Tip: Esophageal Varices and Prophylaxis of Bleeding

- o "….prophylactic treatment to prevent variceal bleeding is recommended in all patients with large esophageal varice irrespective of the presence or absence of red colour signs…." (Sleisenger and Fordtran's Gastrointestinal and Liver Disease. 10th Edition. Saunders/Elsevier, Philadelphia, 2016, page 1544).

- EV/EVB and pregnancy

Non-selective beta blockers (NSBB) are efficacious to prevent primary and secondary bleeding from esophageal varices in persons with cirrhosis and portal hypertension.

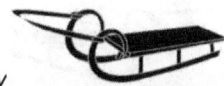

- Give the management of the NSBB of the cirrhotic woman who becomes pregnant.

  o Beta-blockers and FDA category

  Trimester 1   C

  Trimester 2 or 3   D
  - Bradycardia in the fetus
  - Intrauterine growth retardation

SO YOU WANT TO CONTINUE TO STUDY AND NOT HAVE A LIFE! OR BE A NERD?

- In the setting of hepatomegaly and ↑ AP, give the meaning of the Darrier sign.

  o Darrier sign is dermatographia, scratching the skin and urticarial develop
  o Caused by histamine release from macrophages, such as in systemic mastocytosis

---

Upper GI bleeding in Patient with Possible Esophageal/Gastric Varices

In the patient with UGIB (upper GI bleeding) and with signs of chronic liver disease, give the patient

o Octreotide sc
  - For NVUGIB (non-variceal upper GI bleeding)
    - Octreotide 50 mcg to 100 mcg bolus, then 25 mcg per hour for up to 3 days
  - For EVB (esophageal variceal bleed)
    - 50 mcg bolus, followed by 50 mcg per hr
  - If somatostatin to be used for NVUGIB
    - 250 mcg by bolus, then 250 mcg/hr, for 3 to 7 days

o Antibiotics (fluoroquinolone) before and 7 days after UGIB if EV is found

o Endoscopy
  - Diagnosis
    - Exclude EVB/GVB (esophageal or gastric variceal blood) if liver disease and varices
      - Prophylactic antibiotics
      - If EVB or GVB → EBL

o In fact, while recurrent EV bleeding is common, EGD must be performed with each presentation since just because EV are present does not mean they have bled.

116

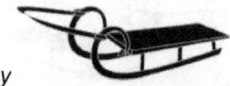

- o Characteristic signs on the varices and seen on EGD will establish whether the acute UBIB in the patient with liver disease or known EV arose from bleeding EV, from PUD, from a Mallory-Weiss tear of the gastroesophageal junction, from portal hypertensive gastropathy, GAVE (gastric antral vascular ectasia), or a Dieulafoy vascular lesion

- Give the reason why a person with isolated IgA deficiency should not be given a blood transfusion.

  - o The patient would have IgG and IgE antibodies (anti-IgA antibodies), which would react against the IgA in the transfused blood, just as would happen with IV immunoglobulins.

If a blood transfusion is contraindicated in a person with isolated IgA deficiency, give what is done if an urgent situation is faced and a blood transfusion would be lifesaving.

  - o The RBCs may be washed, removing most of the serum containing the IgA in the blood to be transfused. The washed and packed RBC may then be given safely.

- Compare and contrast the endoscopic findings and treatment of portal hypertensive gastropathy (PHG) and gastric antral vascular ectasia (GAVE).

	PHG	GAVE
➤ Feature findings		
o Site	Fundus	Antrum
o Mosaic pattern	Yes	No
o Red colour signs	Yes	Yes
o Findings on gastric mucosal biopsy		
- Thrombi	No	+++
- Spindle cell proliferation	Sparse	++
- Fibrohyalinosis	No	+++
➤ Management	o ↓ portal hypertension	o Estrogens
	o β adrenergic blockers	o Antrectomy
	o TIPS	o (TIPS doesn't help) Endoscopic laser therapy
	o Liver transplantation	o Liver transplantation

117

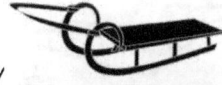

*Note: Gastric vascular ectasia (EVE) may occur anywhere in the stomach, not just in the asntrum, so do not distinguish GAVE/ EVE from PHG just on the site of localization

- Give the **SARIN** classification of gastroesophageal varices (GEV) or isolated gastric varices (IGV).

    - GEV1   – GV in continuity with EV
                        – Extend 2 to 5 cm below GE junction
                        – Easiest to obliterate with cyanoacrylate

    - GEV2   – GV in continuity with EV
                        – GV extend to cardia and fundus

    - IGV1   – No EV
                        – GV in fundus
                        – Most difficult to obliterate with cyanoacrylate

    - IGV2   – No EV
                        – GV in gastric body, antrum, and pylorus

    - Bleeding risk

        – GEV2/IGV1 > GEV1, IGV2 (unless patient is matched for CTP score, in which case the risk of bleeding is similar in each type of varix)

Transjugular Intrahepatic Portosystemic Shunt (TIPS)

With the TIPS (transjugular intrahepatic portosystemic stent) a coated stent is inserted between the hepatic vein (HV) and a branch of portal vein (PV) to form the equivalent of a portocaval shunt

- Give accepted indications for TIPS.

    - Varices
        – Bleeding esophageal [EV] or gastric [GV]) varice, MELD score < 114
        – Preventing rebleeding of EV

    - Ascites, refractory

    - Hepatorenal syndrome

    - Budd-Chiari syndrome (BCS)

    - Hepatic hydrothorax

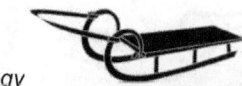

Making Sense: TIPS, MELD Score and Survival

- Give TIPS-associated complications.
    - Vessels
        - Carotid artery (unintential)
        - Jugular vein
        - Portal vein
            - Laceration in liver capsule
            - Intraperitoneal bleed
        - Hepatic artery
        - Pulmonary artery hypertension
    - Shunt
        - Thrombosis
        - Stenosis
        - Migration
        - Hepatic encephalopathy
        - Hepatic failure
    - Sepsis

- Give the reason why TIPS is still recommended in some patients with bleeding esophageal varices.
    - When MELD score < 14, the patient has an excellent prognosis, so that this prognosis may allow the exploitation of the benefits of TIPS.
    - When MELD score > 24, the mortality rate is very high (~30% in 3 months), so the TIPS will be of no value.
        - What the patient with a high MELD score needs is a liver transplantation

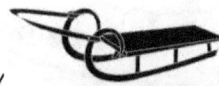

Clinical TIPS on TIPS

- o "when bleeding from varices cannot be controlled after two sessions of endoscopic therapy within a 24-hour period, TIPS placement is the usual salvage treatment"
- o "broad spectrum antibiotic coverage is recommended when TIPS placement is carried out as an emerging procedure….[or] in a patient with primary sclerosing cholangitis"
- o TIPS has no effect on survival (↓ variceal bleeding, ↑ hepatic encephalopathy)
- o Development of stent steatosis is at least 25% in TIPS

Ectopic Varices

➢ Definition
- o Varices which occur at site other than the esophagus or stomach

➢ Treatment
- Give the treatment options for bleeding ectopic varices.
  - o EVL
  - o NSBB
  - o Transhepatic embolization
  - o TIPS
  - o Surgical ligation
  - o Selective surgical shunt e.g., splenorenal shunt

Abbreviations: EVL, endoscopic variceal ligation, NSBB, non-selective beta blocker; TIPS, transjugular intrahepatic portosystemic shunt

Please see Sleisenger and Fordtran's Gastrointestinal and Liver Disease. 10th Edition. Saunders/Elsevier, Philadelphia, 2016, Figure 92-19, page 1514 for suggested "algorithm for the management of bleeding from ectopic varices in patients with portal hypertension".

SO YOU WANT TO CONTINUE TO STUDY AND NOT HAVE A LIFE! OR BE A NERD?
- In the setting of hepatomegaly and ↑ AP, give the meaning of the Darrier sign.
  - o Darrier sign is dermatographia, scratching the skin and urticarial develop
  - o Caused by histamine release from macrophages, such as in systemic mastocytosis

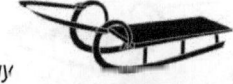

MANOMETRY CASES

Describe the manometric findings, and give a differential diagnosis.

Case 1: Clinical history: Presenting symptom of heartburn

➢ Describe the following esophageal motility studies; give the differential diagnosis, and state the most likely manometric diagnosis.

Lower Esophageal Sphincter (Normal values in brackets):	Esophageal Body (Normal values in brackets):
Resting pressure: 21 mmHg (16-30) Relaxation duration: 5.3 seconds (>2) % Relaxation: 93% (80-100%) Residual Pressure: 1.5 mmHg (<8)	Peristaltic contractions: 100% (>80%) Simultaneous contractions: 0% (<20%) Mean contraction amplitude: 73 mmHg (30-180) Mean contraction duration: 2.5 sec (<5.8) Lower amplitude contractions: 0% (<30%) Spontaneous activity between swallows: none

Acid infusion test: Not done

Pharyngo-esophageal sphincter (PE): Not done

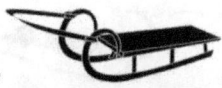

Case 2

Clinical history: Presenting with dysphagia

Lower Esophageal Sphincter (Normal values in brackets):	Esophageal Body (Normal values in brackets):
Resting pressure: 23 mmHg (16-30) Relaxation duration: 13 seconds (>2) % Relaxation: 92% (80-100%) Residual Pressure: 3.3 mmHg (<8)	Peristaltic contractions: 20% (>80%) Simultaneous contractions: 80% (<20%) Mean contraction amplitude: 128 mmHg (30-180) Mean contraction duration: 8.1 sec (<5.8) Lower amplitude contractions: 0% (<30%) Spontaneous activity between swallows: none

Acid infusion test: Not done

Pharyngo-esophageal sphincter (PE):

Resting Pressure: 26.5 mmHg (40-150)

Pharyngeal contraction pressure: 48.4 mmHg (40-150)

Coordination: Yes

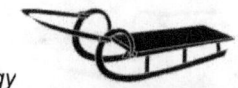

Case 3

Clinical history: Presenting with heartburn

Lower Esophageal Sphincter (Normal values in brackets):	Esophageal Body (Normal values in brackets):
Resting pressure: 34 mmHg (16-30) Relaxation duration: 10.3 seconds (>2) % Relaxation: 98% (80-100%) Residual Pressure: 0.5 mmHg (<8)	Peristaltic contractions: 100% (>80%) Simultaneous contractions: 0% (<20%) Mean contraction amplitude: 241 mmHg (30-180) Mean contraction duration: 6.1 sec (<5.8) Lower amplitude contractions: 0% (<30%) Spontaneous activity between swallows: none

Acid infusion test: Felt pharyngeal burning by two minutes of infusion, which became stronger by three minutes and radiated to epigastric area. With water, all symptoms gone by six minutes.

Pharyngo-esophageal sphincter (PE): Not done

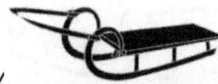

Case 4

Clinical history: Presenting with chest pain, heartburn, regurgitation and dysphagia

Lower Esophageal Sphincter (Normal values in brackets):	Esophageal Body (Normal values in brackets):
Resting pressure: 1 mmHg (16-30) Relaxation duration: ? seconds (>2) % Relaxation: ?% (80-100%) Residual Pressure: ? mmHg (<8) Difficult to assess relaxation due to low LES pressure	Peristaltic contractions: 0% (>80%) Simultaneous contractions: 0% (<20%) Mean contraction amplitude: ? mmHg (30-180) Mean contraction duration: ? sec (<5.8) Lower amplitude contractions: 0% (<30%) Spontaneous activity between swallows: none

Acid infusion test: Not done

Pharyngo- esophageal sphincter (PE):

Resting pressure: 44.8 mmHg (40-150)

Pharyngeal contraction pressure: 54.3 (40-150)

Coordination: Yes

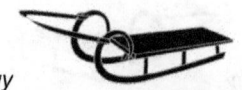

Case 5

Clinical history: Presenting with dysphagia, heartburn, regurgitation, chest pain, vomiting

Lower Esophageal Sphincter (Normal values in brackets):	Esophageal Body (Normal values in brackets):
Resting pressure: 23 mmHg (16-30) Relaxation duration: 6 seconds (>2) % Relaxation: 58.5% (80-100%) Residual Pressure: 9.3 mmHg (<8)	Peristaltic contractions: 0% (>80%) Simultaneous contractions: 100% (<20%) Mean contraction amplitude: 16 mmHg (30-180) Mean contraction duration: 2.7 sec (<5.8) Lower amplitude contractions: 100% (<30%) Spontaneous activity between swallows: none

Acid infusion Test: Not done

Pharyngo-esophageal sphincter (PE): Not done

"Don't worry about the neurobiological mechanisms of motivated learning – just provide a safe, stimulating and welcoming environment."

Grandad

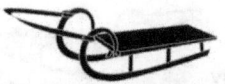

Cases 6 to 10 were kindly provided by Dr. Dan Sadowski (University of Alberta)

Case 6 – Channel water perfused esophageal manometry

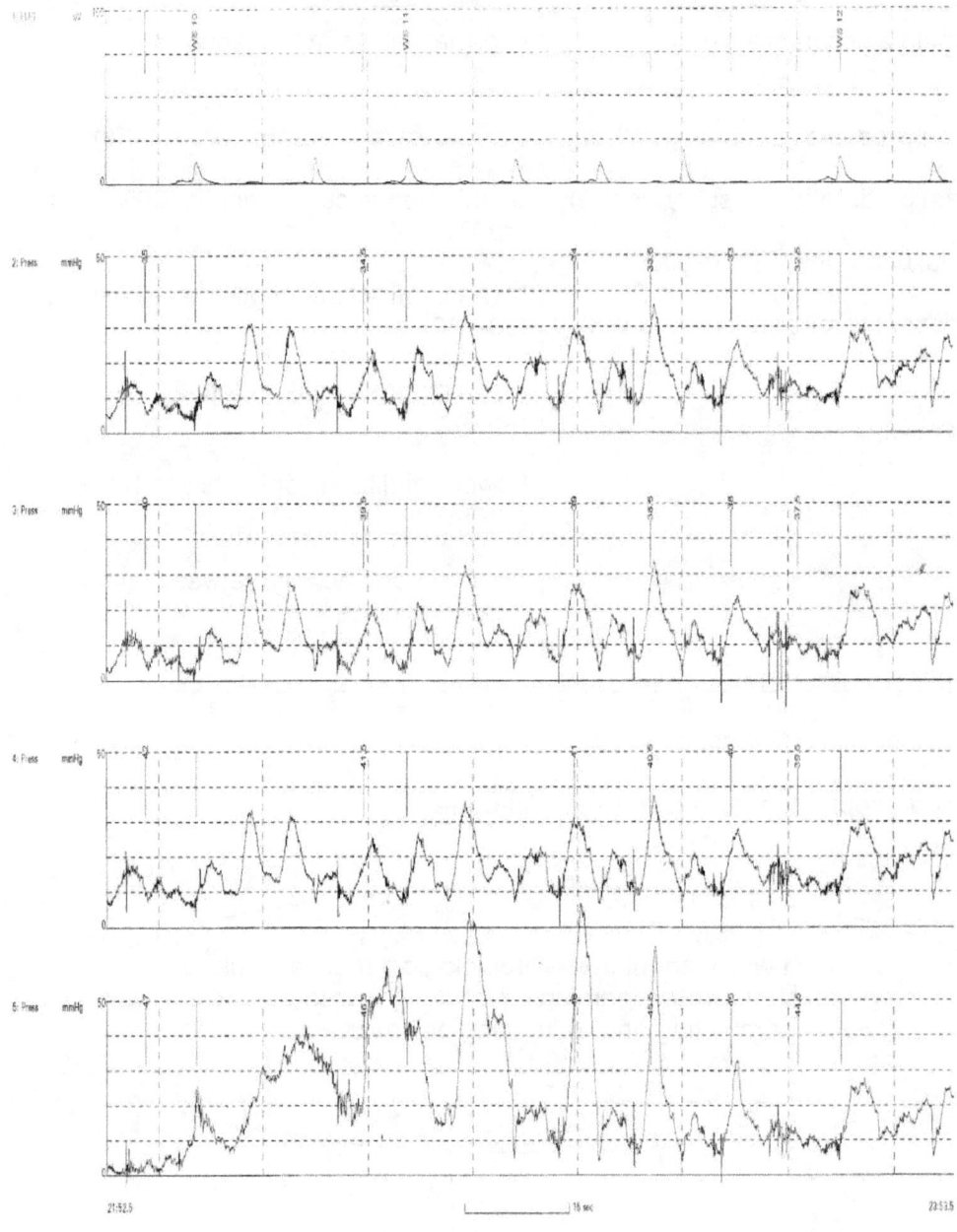

Case 7 – Channel water perfused esophageal manometry

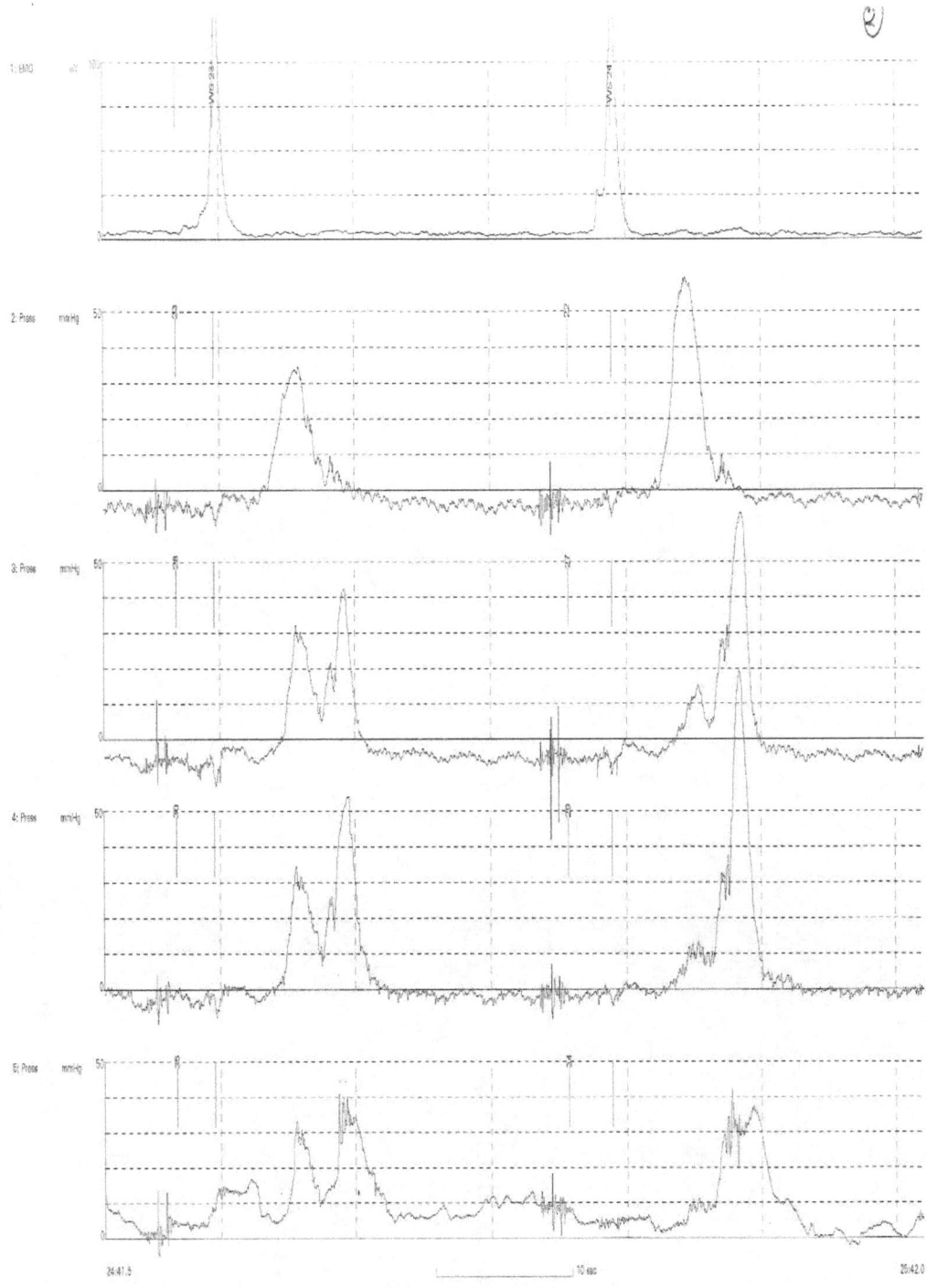

127

Case 8 – Channel water perfused esophageal manometry

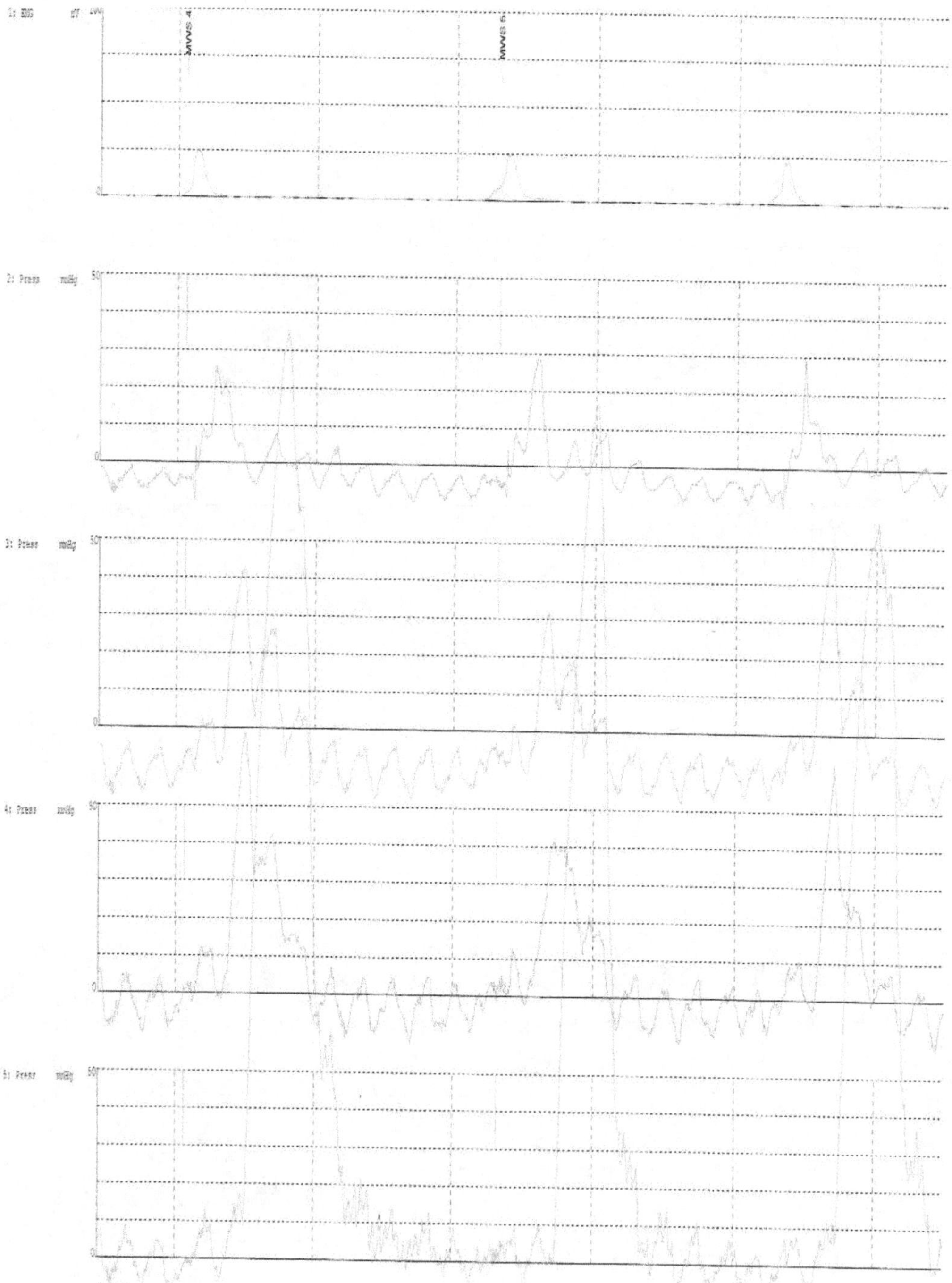

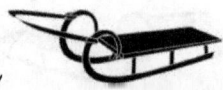

128

Case 9 – Channel water perfused esophageal manometry

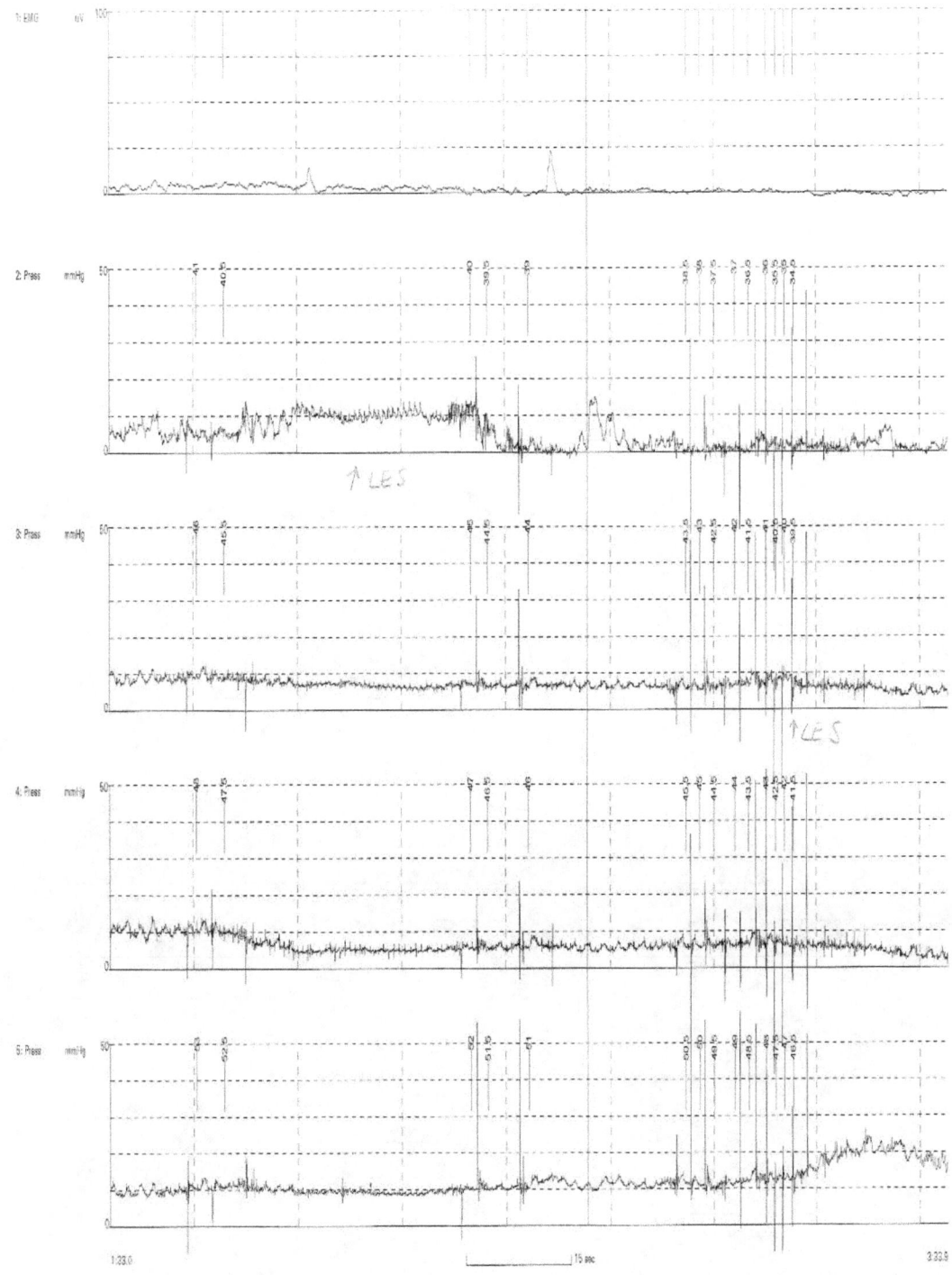

Case 10 – Channel water perfused esophageal manometry

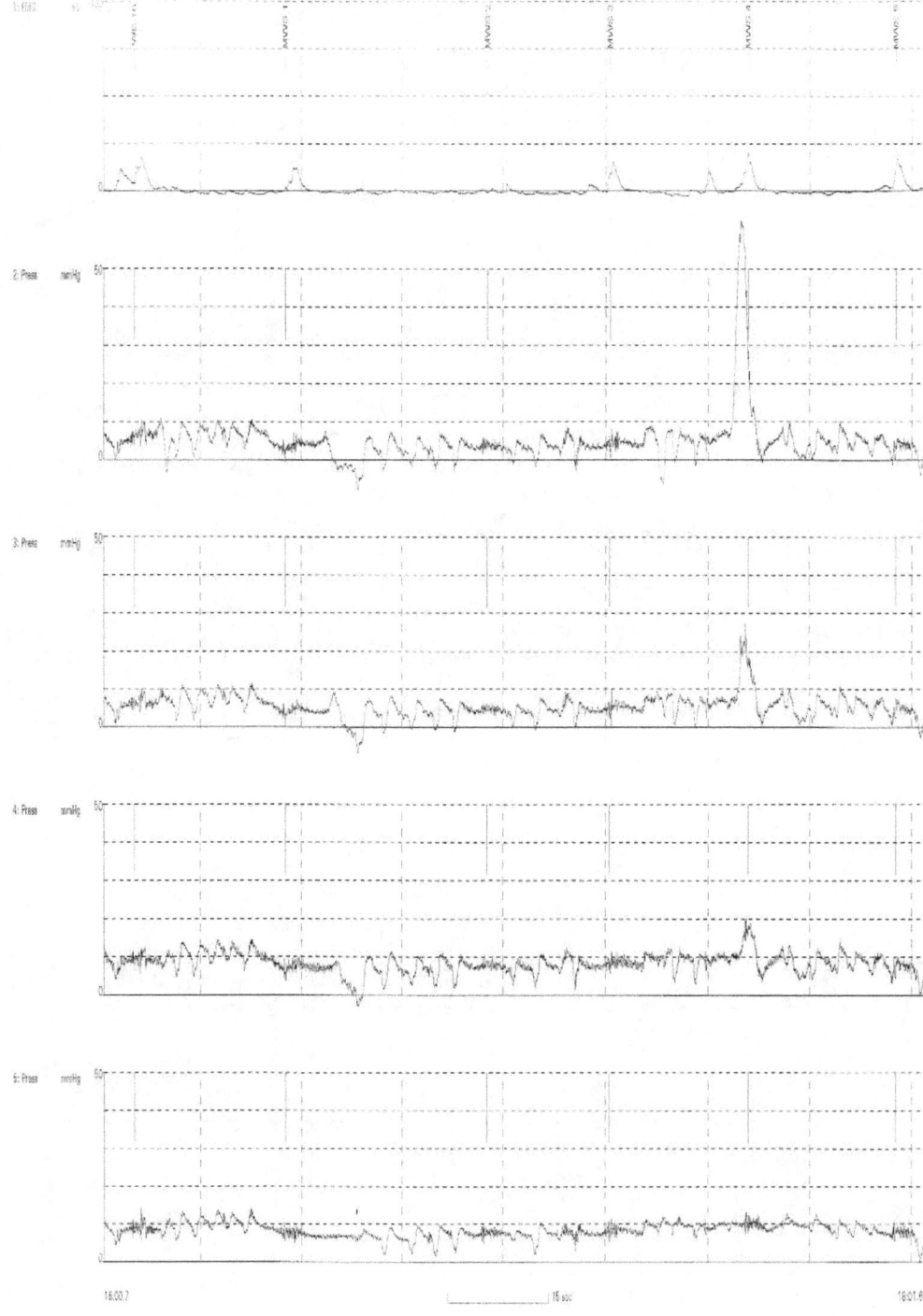

ABBREVIATIONS

5-ALA	5-aminolevulinic acid
ACE	Angiotensin-converting enzyme
Ach	Acetylcholine
ALS	Amptrophic lateral sclerosis
ANS	Autonomic nerve system
APC	Argon plasma coagulation
ARR	Absolute risk reduction
BARB	β-adrenergic receptor blocker (aka NSBB, non-selective β blocker
BE	Barrett epithelium
BID	Twice a day
BMI	Body mass index
BPM	Beats per minute
CAP	Community acquired pneumonia
CE	Chromendoscopy
CE	Capsule endoscopy
CIC	Computed interval chromendoscopy
CMV	Cytomegalovirus
CNS	Central nervous system
CPAP	Continuous positive airway pressure
CRP	C-reactive protein
CTP	Child Turcotte Pugh
DCI	Distal contractile index
DES	Diffuse esophageal spasm
DSRS	Distal splenerenal shunt
DU	Duodenal ulcer
EB	Evidence-based
EB	Esophageal body
EE	Eosinophilic esophagitis
EGD	Esophageal gastroduodenoscopy
EGJ	Esophagogastric junction

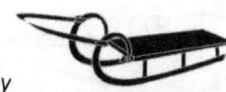

EGD	Esophagogastroduodenoscopy
EGID	Eosinophilic gastrointestinal diseases
EHT	Endoscopic hemostatic therapy
EIM	Esophageal pH impedence monitoring
EMC	Early mucosal cancer
EMD	Esophageal motility disorders
EMIIT	Esophageal multichannel intraluminal impedence testing
EMR	Endoscopic mucosal resection
ENT	Ear nose throat
EoE	Eosinophilic esophagitis
ER	Esophageal ring
ESR	Endoscopic submucosal resection
EST	Endoscopic sclerotherapy
EUS	Endoscopic ultrasound
EV	Esophageal varices
EVBL	Endoscopic variceal band ligation
EVL	Endoscopic variceal ligation
EW	Esophageal web
FE	Fluoresence endoscopy
FH	Functional heartburn
FHVP	Free hepatic vein pressure
FICE	Fuijnon intelligent chromendoscopy
FNA	Fine needle aspiration
GER	Gastroesophageal reflux
GERD	Gastroesophageal reflux disease
GFR	Glomerular filtration rate
GI	Gastrointestinal
GIST	Gastrointestinal stromal tumour
GSE	Gluten sensitive enteropathy
GU	Gastric ulcer
GV	Gastric varices

132

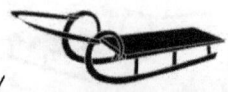

GVH	Graft-versus-host disease
H2RA	Histamine2-receptor antagonist
HCAP	Healthcare associated pneumonia
HCC	Hepatocellular cancer
HDGC	Hereditary diffuse gastric cancer
HE	Hepatic encephalopathy
HGD	High grade dysplasia
HGM	Heterotropic gastric mucosa
HREM	High resolution esophageal manometry
HREPT	High resolution esophageal pressure topography
HRHDME	White light high resolution endoscopy
HSV	Herpes simplex virus
HVPG	Hepatic venous pressure gradient
IBD	Inflammatory bowel disease
IBS	Irritable bowel syndrome
IEM	Ineffective esophageal motility
IPF	Interstitial pulmonary fibrosis
LES	Lower esophageal sphincter
LESP	Lower esophageal sphincter pressure
LGD	Low grade dysplasia
LIFE	Light induced fluorescence endoscopy [FE]
LES	Lower esophageal sphincter
LSC	Lifestyle changes
MAC	Mycobacterium avium complex
MC	Microscopic colitis
MCTD	Mixed connective tissue diseases
MG	Myasthenia gravis
MII	Multichannel intraluminal impedence
MMC	Migrating motor complex
MR	Mortality rate
MS	Multiple sclerosis

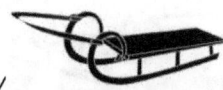

MSK	Musculoskeletal
NAB	Nocturnal acid breakthrough
NBI	Narrow band imaging
NCCP	Non-cardiac chest pain
NERD	Normal esophageal reflux disease
NG	Nasogastric tube
NR	Not reported
NNT	Numbered needed to treat
NSBB	Non-selective beta blocker
NSS	Non-selective beta blocker
NVUGIB	Non-variceal upper GI bleed
OCT	Optical coherence tomography
Od	Rx given once a day
PBC	Primary biliary cirrhosis
PDT	Photodynamic therapy
PEG	Percutaneous endoscopic gastrostomy
PNS	Peripheral nervous system
PO	Orally
POEM	Peroral endoscopic myotomy
PPI	Proton Pump Inhibitor
PRBC	Packed RBC
QD	Once daily
RF	Radiofrequency ablation
RR	Relative risk
SBP	Spontaneous bacterial peritonitis
SCD	Sudden cardiac death
SIBO	Small intestinal bacterial overgrowth
sLESR	Swallow-associated lower esophageal sphincter relaxations
SSIM	Subsquamous intestinal metaplasia
TG	Therapeutic gain
TIPS	Transjugular intrahepatic postoperative shunt

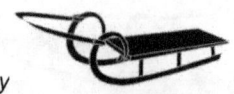

TK	Tyrosine kinase
tLESR	Transient LES relaxation
UC	Ulcerative colitis
UES	Upper esophageal sphincter
VFSA	Video fluoroscopy swallowing assessment
VFSS	Videofluroscopy swallowing study
WHVP	Wedge hepatic venous pressure
ZD	Zenker diverticulum
ZES	Zollinger-Ellison syndrome

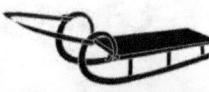

STOMACH

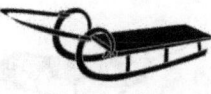

TABLE OF CONTENTS

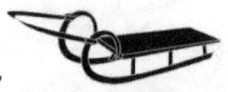

Mastering the Boards: Gastroenterology   A.B.R. Thomson

DYSPEPSIA

➤ Definition
- o Dyspepsia is pain or discomfort in the upper abdomen which may be associated with symptoms described as heartburn, indigestion, nausea, fullness, poor digestion some described as heartburn, e.g., Rome III
- o Epigastric pain or burning (termed "epigastric pain syndrome")
- o Postprandial fullness (termed "postprandial distress syndrome")
- o Early satiation (meaning "inability to finish a normal sized meal or postprandial fullness")
- o Uninvestigated dysplasia
  - – Blood work, ECG may be performed as needed, but the dyspeptic patient has not been investigated with an EGD (esophagogastro-duodenaoscopy)
- o There may also be "alarm symptoms" (suggesting possible esophageal or gastric malignancy):
  - – "VBAD"
    - ▪ Vomiting
    - ▪ Bleeding – hematemesis, melena
    - ▪ Anemia
    - ▪ Dysphagia, odynophagia
  - – "FWLMS"
    - ▪ Family history of upper GI cancer
    - ▪ Weight loss (non-intentional)
    - ▪ Liver disease jaundice, ascites
    - ▪ Mass in abdomen, or lymphadenopathy
    - ▪ Surgery on stomach in past

Note:
- o The PPV (positive predictive value) of alarm symptoms is low, but the NPV (negative predictive value) is 99%;
- o Thus, absence of "red flag" or "alarm" symptoms argues against upper GI malignancy being a cause of dyspepsia.

➤ Demography
- o Annual occurrence in general public ~25%

➤ Types
- o Using the Rome III classification, give subtypes of functional dyspepsia
  - – Post-prandial distress (PPD)
  - – Epigastric pain syndrome (EPS)
  - – Reflux-like
  - – Ulcer-like
  - – Dysmotility-like

139

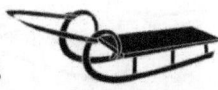

- There is so much overlap in symptoms that it is not possible to confidently distinguish between the usual causes of dyspepsia (i.e., poor specificity)
  - GERD (gastroesophageal reflux disease)
  - PUD (peptic ulcer disease, comprised of DU [duodenal ulcer] and GU [gastric ulcer])
    - DU classically
      - On an empty stomach
      - 2 to 3 hours pc, hen buffering acid of food has been lost, and HCl
      - Secretion is no longer high between 11 pm to 2 am
  - NERD (normal endoscopy reflux disease) and NUD (non-ulcer dyspepsia) describe the same condition of reflux-like dyspepsia and non-ulcer dyspepsia, in which the patient suffers from dyspepsia, but the EGD is normal (thus NERD and NUD are forms of "investigated dyspepsia" since an EGD has been performed).

- Warning: exceptions – although the absence of VBAD FWLML alarm symptoms is reassuring (NPV, 99%) in the dyspeptic person, the presence of upper GI tract malignancy must be excluded by EGD in several circumstances:
  - Age over a cut-off (guidelines vary from 45 to 55 years of age; suggestion – use age 50, or earlier if one of the following is present)
  - Family or personal history of cancer of esophagus or stomach
  - Personal origin from an ARGD of the world with a high incidence of GCa; e.g., Japan, South America
  - Personal origin from an area or group of persons with a high prevalence of H. pylori infection (because H. pylori infection may be a factor causing GCa)
  - The age cut-off is determined by the point at which the incidence of ECa/GCa begins to rise; e.g., 1% at age < 50 in N. Europe, USA, Canada
  - Middle aged Caucasian male with > 10 year history of moderately severe GERD occurring ≥ 3 times per week (risk of Barrett esophagus and ECa)

- Also call: the odds ratio (OR) of gallstones in a dyspeptic is low (OR, 2.0) and even if the patient is shown to have gallstones on abdominal ultrasound, that is not sufficient proof that the dyspepsia is not caused by GERD, PUD, NERD/NUD), or ECa/GCa.

- Overlap with IBS
  - Dyspepsia in persons with IBS, 14%
  - Reflux-like dyspepsia in IBS, 32%
  - IBS in persons with dyspepsia, 37%

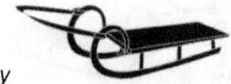

- ➢ Treatment approaches
  - ○ Clinical approach
    - – Age < 50 years, not in an "exception" group, no alarm symptoms → empiric anti-secretory, or
    - – T & T ("test and treat" for H. pylori) if in a high prevalence H. pylori area
    - – Age > 50 years, in an "exception" group, or with alarm symptom(s) → EGD
    - – There are pro's and con's for each approach
    - – If patient is in a low H. pylori risk area or group, then T&T is not the preferred approach
    - – For economic and availability reasons, the "scope (EGD) and treat" approach may not be viable, and there is some evidence that the anti-secretory pathway may not be the cheapest over the long run, and may not give the greatest improvement in the quality of life of the patient.
  - ○ Empirical therapy
    - – Empiric anti-secretory approach with OTC (over-the-counter) antacids, H2RA (H2 receptor antagonists), and half-dose
    - – PPIs may already have been by the patient before consulting a physician
    - – In guidelines, by "anti-secretory trial of therapy" is usually meant to be a standard dose of any PI, given po od ½ hour before breakfast, given for 4 to 8 weeks.

Tips on What's New A Word of Caution

  - ○ There is a poor correlation between dyspeptic symptoms and findings at EGD.

  - ○ Attempts to predict the pre-EGD probability of finding a serious lesion have included the patient's age, the presence of "red flags" (alarm symptoms), a family history of esophageal/gastric cancer, or belonging to a demographic group with such as high risk (e.g., in Canada, persons with a high risk of an H.pylori infection, e.g., "new Canadian" [immigrant] from a high endemic area), First Nations persons.

  - ○ Test-and-treat (for H. pylori)
    - – Prevalence of H. pylori in Northern Europe/Canada is about ~25% (~10% amongst locally born children)
    - – Distinguish between H. pylori infection and H. pylori disease, e.g., prevalence of H. pylori in Canadian adults, ~25% prevalence of GU/DU, ~5% (by EGD)

141

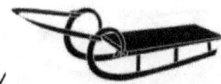

- Empiric treatment of H. pylori infection in investigated dyspeptics is higher, in part because DU and GU associated disease is being treated, rather than just H. pylori-associated gastritis, the associated symptoms from which generally respond poorly to the eradication of H. pylori.
- If using a biopsy-based test for H. pylori
  - Stop PI for at least 1 week before taking EGD biopsy
  - Take 2 EGD biopsies from gastric antrum, 2 from body, and 1 from angularis
- Positive serology for H. pylori only indicates previous exposure; a negative serology test excludes H. pylori-associated disease
  - Specificity is even lower with increasing age and in cirrhosis; determine presence of active infection with UBT or stool antigen test.

- Give the benefits and limitations associated with interventional/ diagnostic approaches to the patient with dyspepsia who is under 50 years of age and who has no alarm symptoms.

Diagnostic Approach	Benefits	Limitations
o "Watchful waiting" only	– Patients with mild and transient symptoms are not prescribed medication or investigated.	▪ No clinical studies
o Empirical Antisecretory therapy (PPI or H2RA)	– Addresses symptoms immediately – Documented effect on reflux symptoms and ulcer-related symptoms	▪ Recurrence after therapy is the rule; EGD is often only postponed, and may be false negative
o Treat based on clinical diagnosis	– Clinically meaningful. Low costs	▪ Unreliable.
o Treat based on subgrouping and computer-based algorithms	– Clinically attractive. Low costs	▪ Does not reliably predict EGD diagnosis or response to therapy
o H.*pylori* test-and-treat	– Infected patients with ulcer disease will have symptomatic benefits. Reduces endoscopy rates. Safe and cost-effective compared with endoscopy. Possible reduced risk of later ulcer development.	▪ Low benefit in those without peptic ulcer disease will not benefit. Continuing or recurrent symptoms may frustrate patients and clinician.

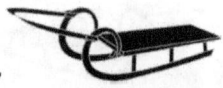

Diagnostic Approach	Benefits	Limitations
o H.*pylori* test-and-scope	– Potential to reduce upper EGD rates in H. pylori low-prevalence areas	▪ Only meaningful if a decision about eradication therapy in infected patients is influenced by endoscopy result. Increases endoscopy demands. Not applicable in H. pylori-high prevalence areas
o Early endoscopy	– Diagnostic "gold standard". Might lead to reduced medication in patients with normal findings. Increased patient satisfaction in some trials.	▪ Invasive. Costly. About half of EGDs will be normal. Long waiting lists may lead to false negative results. Not the preferred option for many patients. Does not diagnose non-erosive reflux disease (NERD).

Abbreviations: EGD, esophagogastroduodenoscopy; H2RA, H2 receptor antagonist; NERD, non-erosive reflux disease; PPI, proton pump inhibitor.

Adapted from: Bytzer P. *Best Pract Res Clin Gastroenterol* 2004; 18(4): pg.683.

CLINICAL SCENARIO
- o An MCQ is directed at the issue of the recommended follow-up of a dyspeptic < 55 years whose UBT is positive and they are given successful triple therapy for H. pylori. You are tempted to answer that the correct follow-up is to repeat the UBT to determine if the infection has been eradicated.
  - – Wrong. Successful triple therapy for H. pylori in this setting means the patient has lost her/his dyspepsia. The only circumstances were the UBT must be **repeated** is
    - ▪ Persistent dyspepsia despite treatment of H.pylori infection.
    - ▪ The patient with complicated H. pylori-associated peptic ulcer (e.g., hemorrhage) must be proven by repeat testing that the anti-H. pylori treatment has effectively eradicated the bug (expected cure rate for triple therapy is only 80%).
    - ▪ After endoscopic mucosal resection (EMR) for an early gastric cancer (EGCA) in a person who was previously positive for H. pylori

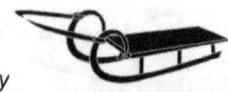

GASTRIC SECRETION OF HYDROCHLORIC ACID (HCl)

- Give the secretory cells of the stomach, and give one chemical/peptide/hormone which each cell secretes.

  o Goblet cell – mucus

  o Parietal cell – HCl, intrinsic factor

  o Chief cells – pepsinogen, gastric lipase

  o D cells – somatostatin

  o G cells – gastrin

  o Mast cells – histamine

  o Enterochromaffin-like cells (ECL) – histamine

An understanding of gastric parietal cell secretion of HCl and G cell secretion of stimulatory gastrin as well as D cell secretion of inhibitory somatostatin, is important to understand the pathophysiology of UD, as well as the gastric effects of hypergastrinemia, including the ZES of the sporatic or MEN-/types.

- Give the physiology of gastric secretion of acid, and its control.

There are redundant and overlapping pathways for acid secretion and inhibition.

❖ Parietal cell

  o Secretory vesicles are lined with membrane containing the H^+/K^+-ATPase acid-secreting pump.

  o With food stimulation the secretory vesicles traffic to and incorporated into the luminal membrane of parietal cells, forming the secretory canaliculi.

  o The pathway for K^+ to reach the H^+ - K^+ ATPase is in a short-circuited state in fasting state, but upon stimulation this pathway allows access of the K^+ to the H^+ - K^+ ATPase, exchange of H^+ for K^+ and thus HCl secretion.

  o The parietal cell is stimulated by the cephalic, gastric and intestinal components, with activation occurring through
    - ↑ Ca^{2+} (intracellular Ca^{2+})
    - ↑ cAMP → cAMP-dependent PK (protein kinase) cascade

  o When activation of the parietal cell causes, or inhibition increases, the H^+-K^+ ATPase moves back (reinternationalization) into the cytoplasmic side of the parietal cell.

  o Reinternalization of the H^+ - K^+ ATPase occurs by way of the cytoplasmic tail of the beta subunit of the enzyme.

144

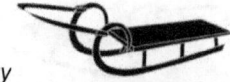

❖ Gastrin and Gastrin Receptors
  o Gastrin is released from G cells in the gastric antrum as a result of amino acids (AA) in the stomach (as well as protein and peptides), and from distention of the stomach.
  o Gastrin binds to the
    – CCK2 (aka CCK-B, or gastrin) receptors on
      ▪ Parietal cells
      ▪ ECL cells in body of stomach, adjacent to parietal cells
    – CCK1 (aka CCK-A) receptors on D cells, pancreas, gallbladder and brain
  o Physiology
    – Acutely
      ▪ ↑ histamine releases from ECL cells → histamine stimulates H2 receptor of parietal cells to secrete HCl
      ▪ Releases ↑ histamine synthesis in ECL cells
      ▪ Releases somatostatin (more from CCK rather than gastrin) → ↓ histamine release from ECL cells
      ▪ Stimulation of ECL cells to release histamine
        – Gastrin
        – PACAP (pituitary adenylate cyclase-activating polypeptide)
        – VIP (vasoactive intestinal peptides)
      ▪ Antigens stimulate gastric mucosal mast cells – release of histamine
    – Chronically
      ▪ Causes hypertrophy of parietal cells and ECL (enterochromaffin-like) cells
  o Note paradoxical effect of gastrin
    – ↑ histamine release from ECL cells
      ▪ ↑ HCl secretion
    – ↑ somatostatin release from D cells
      ▪ ↓ G release
      ▪ ↓ HCl secretion

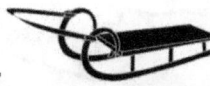

❖ Somatostatin

● Give factors responsible for increasing and/or decreasing the release of somatostatin from the D cells.

  ○ ↑ release – Gastric acidity (↑ H+ → somatostatin → ↓ H+ [feed-back loop])
  – Minor distention of stomach, acting through VIP neurons
  – ↑ gastrin
  – ↑ VIP activation
  – ↑ gastrin → ↑ somatostatin
    ▪ ↓ ECL secretion of histamine
    ▪ ↓ gastrin release
  – Major inhibitory mechanism of somatostatin
    ▪ Reduction of gastrin-stimulated release of histamine from ECL cells
  ○ ↓ release – Major distention of stomach
  – Ach

❖ Other GI peptides

  ○ Other peptides which inhibit acid secretion by way of ↓ ECL histamine release from ECL histamine release
  – CGRP (calcitonin gene-related peptide)
  – PYY (peptide YY)
  – Prostaglandins
  – Galanin
  – CCK2 and CCK2 receptors are G-protein-coupled receptors
  – Signaling by way of pertussis toxin-insensitive G-proteins
  – Agonist stimulation of receptors

❖ Prostaglandins

  ○ Produced and stored in gastric macrophages and capillary endothelial cells.

  ○ ↓ acid secretion by way of inhibiting
  – Gastrin-stimulated histamine release
  – Histamine-stimulated parietal cell acid secretion

146

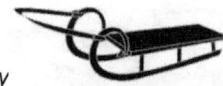

❖ Distention

    o Initially, little distention
        - VIP neurons are activated to release somatostatin
        - Somatostatin inhibits antral G cells

    o Then, more distention
        - Stimulation of release of acetylcholine (Ach; cholinergic)
            ■ Directly stimulates M3 receptors on parietal cell
            ■ ↑ gastrin
            ■ ↓ somatostatin

➢ AA in stomach

    o Direct effect of AA → G cells → ↑ gastrin

    o Indirect effect of AA
        - Activate Ach neurons
        - Activate GRP (gastrin related peptide) neurons → G cells → ↑ gastrin

---

SO YOU WANT TO BE A GASTROENTEROLOGIST!

Histamine released from ECL cells act on the H2-receptors on the basal membrane of gastric body parietal cells, increasing HCl secretion.

- Give the mechanism of action of the H3 receptors to alter gastric acid secretion.
    o Histamine stimulates H3 receptors → ↓ secretion of somatostatin from D-cells

    o The ↓ somatostatin → ↓ inhibition of parietal cell acid inhibition, and → ↑ HCl secretion (inhibition results in stimulation)

PYY (peptide YY) is contained in ECL cells in the terminal ileum and colon. Resection of the terminal colon (R. hemicolectomy) may be associated with increased gastric acid secretion, which sometimes results in diarrhea which responds to the use of a PPI.

- Give the mechanism of this surgically induced increased acid secretion.
    o PYY inhibits gastrin-stimulated histamine release → ↓ parietal cell secretion of HCl

    o This inhibition is lost with ileal resection and R. hemicolectomy

---

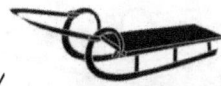

Acid Rebound

➢ Definition

  o An increase in acid secretion to above pretreatment values when an anti-secretory drug (e.g., PPI, H2RA) is suddenly discontinued. The amount and duration influence the magnitude of the acid rebound, which is usually ~15%, which may be sufficient to cause a post-treatment recurrence of symptoms.

• Give the pathophysiological mechanism(s) for the phenomenon of acid rebound which occurs when anti-secretory treatment is suddenly stopped.

  o Acid secretion inhibition → ↑ gastrin
    – Up-regulation (hypertrophy/hyperplasia) of
      ▪ Parietal and G cells (in antrum and on pancreatic islet cells), as well as other ECL cells
      ▪ Ach pathways
    – Down-regulation of D-cells
  o Suddenly stopping PPIs
    – A given stimulus causes more release of gastrin and Ach, more parietal cells to be stimulated by Ach and gastrin, and less down regulation of acid secretion from somatostatin inhibition of somatostatin (relative loss of inhibition and gain of secretion)

Gastric Secretion of Pepsin

The secretion of pepsinogen from gastric body chief cells is increased by
    – Ach
    – Gastrin/CCK
    – Secretin
    – VIP

• Give the explanation why secretion of pepsinogen is essential for normal secretion of gastric acid, and why secretion of gastric acid is essential for normal function of pepsinogens.

  o Pepsinogens are converted to pepsins, which begin the process of digestion of dietary proteins to amino acids (AA).
  o AA directly stimulate G cells to ↑ gastrin, and indirectly activated Ach neurons as well as GRP neurons.
  o This ↑ gastrin leads to ↑ histamine released from ECL cells, which in turn stimulates the H2 receptors on the parietal cell to stimulate secretion of H^+.
  o Pepsins become inactive at pH > 4, so the low intragastric pH (↑H+) maintains pepsins in an active form, which then maintains the AA-stimulation of release of gastrin from G cells, as well as release of Ach and GRP from neurons.

148

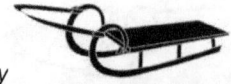

H. PYLORI (HP) INFECTION AND PEPTIC ULCER DISEASE (PUD)

➢ Demography

    o Note that while about 30% of Canadians have an Hp infection, less than 5% develop an Hp-associated disease.

➢ Pathophysiology of Hp-associated PUD

● Give bacterial factors and host factors which are important in the H. pylori-associated development of peptic ulcer, lymphoma and gastric cancer.

❖ The H. pylori organism

    o Adhesion/colonization

       – The genetically 'distinct strains'

       – Bacterial genes encoding proteins in the motility apparatus of H. pylori (movement of organism from lumen of stomach, into the mucus layer) and genes for urease (provides for 2 pH optimum values of 3.0 and 7.2).

       – Colonization occurs only in gastric epithelium or where there is gastric metaplasia.

       – O-glycans in deeper portions of the glandular mucosa present colonization

       – SLPI (secretory leucocyte protease inhibitor) produced by H. pylori reduces colonization.

       – F3 ab A, a bacterial gene product may be liquid for the host Lewis (Le) b receptor or MUC 5AC, enhancing colonization.

       – H. pylori urease binds to MHC (major histocompatibility) class II molecules to ↑ apoptosis.

       – TFF_1 (trefoil protein) on gastric epithelial cells and mucus bind H. pylori

       – TLRs (Toll-like receptors) in the PAMPS (pathogen-associated molecular receptors) family recognize H. pylori or their bacterial products which recognize LPS (lipopolysaccharide) or flagellin.

       – Cag PAI (cag pathogenicity island) is a segment of H. pylori DNA which provides cag E (type N secretion apparatus)

       – Cag PAI

          ■ Allow host gastric cellular membrane translocation

          ■ ↑ IL-8 expression

          ■ SRC kinase s phosphorylate tyrosine in Cag A protein

       – All H. pylori have the vac A gene, and half produce the protein, Vac A (vacuolating cytotoxin)

       – Vc A is a ligand for the cell membrane receptor, protein-tyrosine phosphatase.

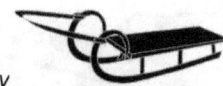

- ❖ The host

  - o Intensity of host inflammatory response
    - – OipA (outer inflammatory protein A)
    - – ↑ IL-8 → ↑ neutrophil infiltration
    - – Peptidoglycan, acting by type IV secretion system
    - – HP-NAP (H. pylori neutrophil-activating protein)
      - ▪ ↑ chemotaxis of neutrophils, monocytes
      - ▪ ↑ ROIs (reactive oxygen intermediates)
    - – ↑ recruitment of neutrophils and macrophages → ↑ iNOS (inducible nitric oxide synthase)

  - o Host immune response
    - – Polymorphism for IL-1β → ↑ IL-1 → intense mucosal inflammation (gastritis)
    - – IL-8, IL-10, TNF-α (tumour necrosis factor) also ↑ gastritis
    - – Morphological changes in gastric epithelial cells
      - ▪ TJ (tight junctions) complexes become broken
      - ▪ ↑ epithelial cell proliferation and apoptosis
    - – ↑ gene expression
    - – Inflammatory cytokine
      - ▪ ↑ signaling mechanism for gene expression
    - – ↑ MAP (mitogen-activated protein) kinases
    - – ↑ lost cell redox factor-1
    - – ↑ activity of NF-kB (nuclear factor kappa B)
    - – ↑ activity of AP-1 (activator protein-1)
    - – ↑ oxidative stress
      - ▪ ↑ oxidation of DNA
    - – NOD_1 (nucleotide-binding oligomerization domain-1) in host
      - ▪ Sense H. pylori
      - ▪ ↑ NF-kB
    - – GI physiology
      - ▪ SST (somatostatin), gastrin effects on secretion of gastric HCl and duodenal HCO_3^-
      - ▪ Mucus - ↓ volume
      - ▪ ↓ mucosal hydrophobicity
    - – TNF-α and IFN-γ (interferon-gamma)
      - ▪ ↑ effects of HP-NRP
      - ▪ Prime neutrophils
    - – ↑ phagocytosis of H. pylori infected gastric epithelial cells

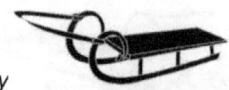

- – ↑ chemokines e.g., ENA-78 GRO-α activate neutrophils
- – ↑ cytokine induction
    - TNF-α
    - IL-6, IL-12, IL-17, IL-18
    - Heat shock protein 60
- – T cell
    - ↓ IL-4 activation of STAT6 → ↑ Th1 and ↓ Th2 response
    - ↑ Th1 response
    - ↑ apoptosis
    - ↑inflammation
    - ↑ atrophy
    - ↑ dysplasia
- – ↑ IL-1β, IFN-α, TNF-α
    - ↑ Fas antigen expression → Fas-FasL (ligand) interactions → ↑ gastric epithelial cell death by apoptosis
- – ↓ NFAT (↓ nuclear translocation of a transcription factor) → ↓ IL-2

- – Dysregulation of Treg (regulatory T cells)
- – ↑ IgA, IgA, IgM and complement
- – ↑ monoclonal antibodies to H. pylori cross-react with gastric epithelial cells
- – Innate host responses impaired by catalase, urease

> Transmission

- Give the modes of transmission of H. pylori (Hp), and the impact of one person in the family being positive for H. pylori on the rate of H. pylori infection by others in the family.

- ❖ Modes of transmission of Hp

    - o Gastro-oral vomitus-oral, fecal-oral

- ❖ Epidemiology

    - o About 50% of the world's population have an H. pylori infection, but only about 15% develop peptic (gastric or duodenal) when disease, and ~1% develop gastric cancer or MALT lymphoma. So, there a disconnect between H. pylori infection in the stomach, and H. pylori-associated diseases

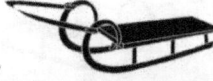

- Hp positive parent
  - Spouse 68% Hp⁺
  - Children 40% Hp⁺

- Hp negative parent
  - Spouse 9% Hp⁺
  - Children 3%Hp⁺

- Community Risk
  - Adults - approximately 25-30% (depends on person's age)
  - Higher (30%) in older persons
  - >50% First Nations Canadians, new Canadians from high Hp prevalence areas
  - New Canadians from high prevalence countries

❖ H. pylori-associated diseases

- H. pylori may be
  - Associated with, or causative of GU and DU, as well as gastritis, gastric cancer and gastric mucosa associated lymphoid tumour (MALT lymphoma)
  - Worsen chance of developing ASA/NSAID-associated GU/DU
  - Worsen effect of smoking on slow healing of peptic ulcer, and higher risk of relapse of ulcer

- Give how H. pylori causes DU.

  - Antrum D cells ↓ - ↓ S - ↓ inhibition of G cells - ↑ G - ↑HCl - ↑ metaplasia – H. pylori in metaplasia H. pylori infection develops in metaplasia of the duodenum.

MIND TEASER

- Give the reason why the rate of symptom relief with Hp-triple therapy higher for dyspepsia in functional dyspepsia in functional dyspepsia with an EGD, than in uninvestigated dyspepsia.

  - EGD shows an ulcer, so pretest probability for symptom relief is higher.

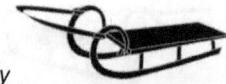

- ❖ Hp-associated diseases
  - ○ GI
    - – Non-investigated/investigated dyspepsia
    - – Non-ulcer dyspepsia
    - – Acute/chronic gastritis
    - – Atrophic gastritis (AG) – acceleration with PPI of AG-IM-Dys-GCa → intestinal metaplasia (IM) → dysplasia (Dys) → GCa (non-cardia gastric cancer)
    - – Duodenal and gastric ulcer (DU and GU) (only ~20% of Hp⁺ persons develop clinical disease)
    - – ↑ adverse effect of smoking on PUD
      - ▪ Once associated H. Pylori infection has been cured, smoking loses its adverse on ulcer healing and relapse.
    - – ↑ ASA/NSAID adverse effects on peptic PUD
    - – ↑ risk of ulcer relapse (80% for H. pylori +, 10% for H. pylori-)
    - – Maltoma
    - – Fundic gland polyps
    - – Hypertrophic gastric folds
    - – Protective against GERD (possible)
    - – Halitosis
    - – Carcinoid tumours
    - – Colorectal cancer (possible association, due to hypergastrinemia)
    - – Pancreatic cancer (possible association)
  - ○ Non-GI diseases
    - – Head – Otitis media, migraines, headaches
    - – CNS – Parkinsonism, CVA
    - – Heart – Atherosclerotic diseases
    - – Lung – Chronic bronchitis, COPD, SIDS
    - – Blood – ITP, iron deficiency; B12 deficiency
    - – Skin – Idiopathic chronic urticaria, acne, rosacea
    - – Growth retardation in children
    - – Vomiting in pregnancy

Abbreviations: COPD, chronic obstructive pulmonary disease; CVA, cerebrovascular accident; DU, duodenal ulcer; GCa, gastric cancer; GERD, gastroesophgeal reflux disease; GU, gastric ulcer; ITP, idiopathic thrombocytopenic purpura; PUD, peptic ulcer disease; SIDS, sudden infant death syndrome

Adapted from: Hunt R. *AGA Institute Post Graduate Course* 2006; pg. 333-342.; and adapted from Graham DY. and Sung JJY. *Sleisenger & Fordtran's gastrointestinal and liver disease: Pathophysiology/ Diagnosis/ Management* 2006. pg. 1054; and 2010, pg. 839.

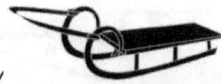

Helicobactor Pylori-Positive Peptic Ulcer Disease (PUD)

MCQ ALERT

- o A MCQ scenario speaks to the need for it to be proven that a previous H. pylori infection has been eradicated. Given the need to be certain the test is not falsely negative, watch out for
    - – UBT – falsely negative if patient has been on PPIs, H2RA or antibiotics in the week before the test.
    - – Biopsy (EGD necessary)-based techniques if the test will be falsely negative and the H. pylori may have migrated to the gastric body; biopsy need to be taken from mucosa of both gastric antrum and body before you may be confident that the pathology report of "no H. pylori seen" signifies that the infection has truly been cured, and that the H. pylori are not simply hiding in the mucus adjacent to the mucosa of the gastric body.

➢ Pathophysiology

SST (somatostatin) and gastrin are produced with the gastric antrum, and gastric acid is secreted by the parietal cells in the gastric body.

- Give the explanation why gastric acid secretion falls with acute or chronic H. pylori gastritis, yet why gastric acid secretion rises with antral gastritis.

❖ Acute or chronic H. pylori pangastritis
- o H. pylori
    - – Directly
        - ▪ ↓ gene expression of parietal cell H^+/K^+ -ATPase α-subunit
        - ▪ ↓ gastrin release
        - ▪ ↓ duodenal HCO_3^-
    - – Indirectly
        - ▪ Produces anti-secretory cytokines IL-1β and TNF-α
        - ▪ Activates CGRP sensory neurons → ↑ SST (somatostatin) → ↓ gastrin
        - ▪ ↓ HCl secretion for body parietal cells

❖ Chronic H. pylori antral gastritis
- o ↓ SST
    - – Proinflammatory/prosecretory cytokines
    - – Prosecretory H_3 agonist (N^3-methyl histamine)
- o ↑ gastrin (from ↑ SST, and from ↑ IL-8 and PAF
- o ↑ gastrin → ↑ ECL cells in fundus/body → ECL hyperplasia
- o ECL hyperplasia → ↑ HCL secretion from parietal cell antibodies

154

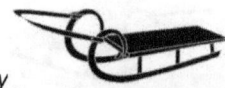

> Treatment

- Give recommended indications for *H. pylori* eradication therapy (ET) in the patient taking NSAIDs or ASA.
  - o Reduce PUD formation
  - o Reduce recurrent PUD
  - o Reduce recurrent PUD bleeding (in ASA or NSAID high risk users) (ET does not prevent further PUD bleeding in high risk ASA/NSAID users on PPI)

Abbreviation: ET, eradication therapy

Adapted from: Lai LH, and Sung JJY. *Best Pract Res Clin Gastroenterol* 2007; 21(2): pg. 270.

  - o Combine anti-H. pylori therapy with PPI to
    - − ↑ anti-H. pylori effect of antibiotics
    - − Accelerate improvement of ulcer healing and symptom relief
  - o Optimal pH for outcomes for different upper GI disorders (18 hours per day)

≥ 3	GU, DU
4	GERD
5	H. pylori eradication
6	Non-variceal upper GI bleeding

❖ Therapeutic options
  - o Uncomplicated peptic ulcer
    - − PPI of your po bid for 2 weeks with 2 antibiotics followed by PPI od for 2 weeks
    - − If patient experiences frequent recurrent recurrences
      - ▪ Perform UBT with patient off PPI for 1 week
      - ▪ If UBT positive, retreat H. pylori
      - ▪ If UBT negative, consider PI po od continuously as maintenance therapy
  - o Complicated peptic ulcer
    - − Complications of hemorrhage, obstruction, perforation
    - − Treat PUD plus H. pylori infection as above for uncomplicated ulcer
    - − Either repeat UBT off PPI therapy, and retreat and prove eradication of H. pylori, with no PPI maintenance therapy (PPI po od), or
    - − PPI maintenance therapy (PPI od), because of
      - ▪ Risk (low) of reinfection with H. pylori
      - ▪ Risk (low) of reulceration even without reinfection with H. pylori
      - ▪ Possibility that the original ulcer may have been caused by ASA/NSAIDs plus H. pylori infection

155

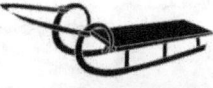

- o Non-ulcer
  dyspepsia
  - – In persons with H. pylori (Hp) associated non-ulcer dyspepsia, eradication of Hp results in longterm symptomatic relief in about 8% of patients (NNT, ~4)

- o Caution alert
  - – Every patient being considered for long-term use of ASA/NSAIDs/Coxibs should be tested (by UBT) and heated for H. pylori of positive
  - – Depending upon patient (host) and medication considerations, some persons on long-term on PPI po od, even after eradication of any associated H. pylori infection.

Helicobactor Pylori-Negative Peptic Ulcer Disease

- o The preparation of all peptic ulcers which are H. pylori-negative is increasing (~25%)
- o Ensure that if the diagnosis of H. pylori infection is based on UBT or gastric mucosal biopsies, anti-secretory therapy must be stopped at least 1 week before taking (mucosal gastric) biopsies and biopsies must be taken from antrum (2), body (2), and angularis (1).
- o Before deeming that the patient has H. pylori-negative peptic ulcer disease, care must be taken to exclude
  - – H. pylori infection, using 2 different types of standard tests
  - – Use of ASA, NSAIDs, Coxibs, bisphosphonates (check platelet aggregation or thromboxane B2 levels)
  - – Fasting hypergastrinemia (ensure patient not currently taking anti-secretory therapy)

- • Give factors which suggest that. H. pylori-negative (Hp-) peptic ulcers are more serious/severe than are H. pylori-positive peptic ulcers (Hp+).

	Clinical	Hp+	Hp-
o	Bleeding ulcer	4%	50%
o	Recurrent ulcer bleeding	11%	42%
o	ASA risk ≥ grade 3	18%	~50%
o	Mortality rate	37%	88%

Abbreviations: ASA, American Society of Anesthesiologist

156

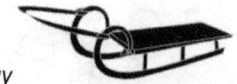

- Give theories why Hp-negative peptic ulcers are peptic ulcers are more serious than Hp-positive peptic ulcers (GU/DU).
  - H. pylori involving the gastric body may ↓ secretion of HCl from parietal cells.
  - H. pylori may have an anti-secretory effect, making PPI therapy more efficacious.

Dyspepsia and Pregnancy

  - Upper GI symptoms are common in pregnant women, and when EGD has been performed the findings are esophagitis (34%) and gastritis (25%).
  - Predictors of heartburn during pregnancy include young age of the mother, her parity, increasing gestational age, and the presence of heartburn before pregnancy (which occurs in 14% of mothers) (Marrero JM, et al. *Br J Obstet Gynaecol* 1992:731-4).
  - Only calcium-containing antacids should be used for GERD symptoms, since
    - Aluminum-containing antacids may cause fetal neurotoxicity,
    - Alginic acid (Gaviscon, sucralfate) may cause fetal distress
    - Magnesium-containing antacids may cause renal stones, respiratory distress and cardiovascular impairment, and hypotemia.
  - Nizatidine is not recommended for lactating mothers (FDA C, due to report of growth retardation of rodent pups)

- Give factors to carefully consider when performing endoscopy in pregnant women.
  - A strong indication is always needed, particularly in high-risk pregnancies
  - Whenever possible, endoscopy should be deferred until the second trimester
  - The lowest possible dose of sedative medication should be used (wherever possible FDA category A or B drugs)
  - Procedure time should be short
  - To avoid inferior venal cava or aortic compression, the patient should be positioned in the left pelvic tilt or left lateral position
  - Presence of fetal heart sounds should be confirmed before sedation and after the procedure
  - Obstetric support should be immediately available
  - No endoscopy should be performed in patients with obstetric complications (placental rupture, imminent delivery, ruptured membranes, or pre-eclampsia)

Printed with permission: Keller J, et al. *Nat Clin Pract Gastroenterol Hepatol* 2008; 5(8): 435.

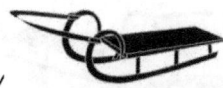

ZOLLINGER-ELLISON SYNDROME (ZES)

A Tricky Question

- In a patient with a known enterochromaffin-like cell (ECL) gastric "carcinoid" tumour, (term is now replaced by "ECL" tumour), what does the development of flushing and wheezing (carcinoid syndrome) tell the clinician?

  o Carcinoid syndrome does not occur unless there is hepatic involvement.

- Give the presenting clinical features of Zollinger-Ellison Syndrome (ZES).
  o Abdominal pain (75%-100%)
  o Diarrhea (35%--73%) (isolated presentation in up to 35%)
  o Pain and diarrhea (55%-60%)
  o Heartburn (44%-64%)
  o Duodenal and prepyloric ulcers (71%-91%)
  o Multiple ulcers in unusual places
  o Stomal ulcers
  o PUD refractory to treatment
  o Ulcer complications (bleeding, 1%-17%; perforation, 0%-5%, or obstruction, 0%-5%)
  o MEN-1 associated tumours (22%-24%)

Abbreviations: MEN, multiple endocrine neoplasia; PUD, peptic ulcer disease; ZES, Zollinger-Ellison syndrome

Adapted from: Metz DC, and Jensen RT. *Gastroenterology* 2008;135:. 1469.

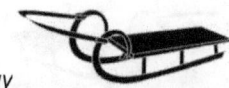

- Give the investigation of the patient with fasting hypergastrinemia, performed after a detailed history and physical examination.
  - ➢ Laboratory tests
    - o Confirm fasting state for gastrin measurement, and not on PPIs
    - o Calcium, PTH, TSH
    - o Creatinine (exclude renal failure)
    - o Chromogranin A
    - o Urinary metanephrins
    - o Schillings test, serum B12
  - ➢ Provocative tests
    - o Secretin infusion (increases gastrin paradoxically in ZES)
    - o Ca^{+2} infusion (marked increase in serum gastrin)
    - o Basal and pentagastrin stimulated acid secretion (↑↑ BAO), BAO/MAO>60% (ZES)
    - o Food-stimulated acid secretin (G-cell hyperplasia/hyperfunction)
  - ➢ Endoscopy
    - o EGD
      - – Multiple ulcers in unusual sites
      - – Biopsy antrum for G-cell number (to distinguish between G-cell hyperplasia [↑G-cell number] vs G-cell hyperfunction (normal G-cell number); H. pylori infection
      - – Thick gastric folds
      - – Fundic gland polyps
    - o EUS for possible tumour localization (especially wall of duodenum)
  - ➢ Diagnostic imaging
    - o Abdominal ultrasound
    - o CT/ MRI, head (pituitary fossa tumour in MEN I)
    - o Ostreotide scan
    - o MBIG scan
    - o Galium[68] scan
    - o CT scan of abdomen
    - o MRI of abdomen
    - o Parathyroid scan

Abbreviations: EUS, endoscopic ultrasound; ZES, Zollinger-Ellison syndrome

Hypergastrinemia and hypersecretion of gastric acid may occur with sporatic gastrinoma, or with a gastrinoma-associated with MEN-1 (multiple endocrine neoplasia type 1).

159

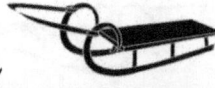

Mutiple Endocrine Neoplasia Type I (MEN-1) **Gastrinomas**

➢ Clinical

  o Parathyroid ~100% for
    – Symptomatic hypercalcemic patients
    – Parathyroid gland removal
    – Parathyroid autograft ± cervical thymectomy

  o Pancreas
    – ~80% of MEN-1 patients
    – 40% have asymptomatic ↑ gastrin (serum), or ZES

  o Pituitary adenomas, ~20% (usually a lactotroph adenoma)

➢ Types

- Give the tumours found in patients with multiple endocrine neoplasia-type I (MEN-1), and their approximate frequency % is shown.

Tumours	Approximate Frequency (%)
o Parathyroid	90 (78-97)
o Pancreatic endocrine tumour	80 (81-82)
- Gastrinoma	54
- Insulinoma	21
- Glucagonoma	3
- VIPoma	1

160

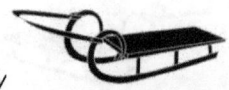

Tumours	Approximate Frequency (%)
o Pituitary tumours	40 (21-65)
- Prolactin-secreting	30 (15-46)
- Growth-hormone secreting	16 (6-20)
- Cushing syndrome	16
o Adrenal cortical adenoma	30 (27-36)
o Thyroid adenoma	20 (5-30)

- Give differences between **sporatic versus MEN-1-associated gastrinomas**.

Clinical	Sporatic	MEN-1 Associated
➤ Pathlogy		
o Carcinoid tumours	~1%	30%
o Number of tumours	Often single	Often multiple and in different sites
o Site, gastrinoma triangle	80%	Pancreas, duodenal wall
o Growth rate of metastases	Rapid	Slow
o Liver metastases at diagnosis	~24%	6%
➤ Prognosis		
o Survival overall		100% at 20 years
➤ Laboratory		
o Identification of source of excess gastrin	Yes	No – imaged tumours may not be source of ↑ gastrin
➤ Clinical		
o Family history	No	Yes
➤ Treatment		
o Consider exploratory laparotomy with curative intent when no evidence of metastatic disease	Yes	No
o Surgical cure (duodenotomy and subtotal pancreatectomy)	50%	No definitive evidence of benefit of surgery

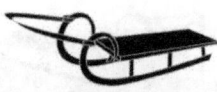

- ○ Optimal outcome is to reduce acid secretion to < 10 mEq/h, measured just before the next planned dose of PPI
  - – Control symptoms
  - – Reduce complications of peptic ulcers
  - – Control gastrin-producing tumour (gastrinoma)
- ○ In patients with metastatic gastrinoma, there may be some benefit from external beam radiotherapy, and some gastrinoma with somatostatin receptor-positive tumours benefit from octreotide or lanreotide-SR for control of symptoms.
- ○ Therapeutic options directed at the metastatic liver disease include
  - – Resection
  - – Embolization of the hepatic artery ± chemotherapy
  - – Radiofrequency ablation (RFA) or cryoablation ± surgical debulking
  - – Systemic chemotherapy
    - ▪ Streptozocin
    - ▪ Doxorubicin
    - ▪ Temozolomide
    - ▪ mToR (mammalian target of rapamycin)
    - ▪ TK (tyrosine kinase) inhibitors
    - ▪ Peptide receptor radioligand therapy

"Be an advocate, seek something good for everyone: seek justice and love."

Grandad

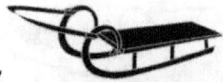

NON-STEROIDAL ANTI-INFLAMMATORY DRUGS (NSAIDs)

➢ Useful background

- o Dyspepsia may be associated with the use of NSAIDs, COXIBs, ASA
- o The relative increased risks of ulcer and ulcer bleeding is NSAIDs > COXIBs
- o Ulcers (DU, GU) occur in ~25% of persons on NSAIDs
- o NSAID-associated ulcers are often asymptomatic
- o The absolute risk of a bleeding GU/GU associated with the use of NSAIDs is ~25%
- o This risk of bleeding with NSAIDs and COXIBs is increased with
  - − The use of
    - ▪ ASA
    - ▪ Clopidogrel
  - − H. pylori infection
- o NSAIDs (excluding naproxen) and COXIBs increase the risk of
  - − Hypertension
  - − Renal dysfunction
  - − Fluid retention
  - − Coronary artery disease events
- o PPIs but not H₂RAs reduce (by ~50%) but do not eliminate the risk of endoscopic ulcer, ulcer symptoms and recurrent ulcer bleeding
- o Eradication of an H. pylori infection ↓risk of
  - − Endoscopic ulcer in persons starting on
    - ▪ NSAIDs
    - ▪ ASA
  - − Beneficial before starting NSAID therapy
  - − Ulcer bleeding in persons already on ASA (weak data)
  - − Mandatory in persons with a history of peptic ulcer disease
  - − In the patient with NVUGIB associated with H. pylori (Hp) infection start the Hp. treatment as soon as oral feeding is started
- o Maintenance therapy with PPIs is "…superior to H. pylori eradication alone in primary or secondary prevention of endoscopic ulcers among NSAID users" (Rostom et al., Aliment Pharmacol Ther 2009; 29: 481-496.

Adapted from Rostom, A. et al., Aliment. Pharmacol. Ther. 2009; 29: 481-496.

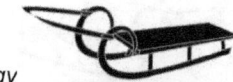

Mastering the Boards: Gastroenterology   A.B.R. Thomson

- ➢ Pharmacological consideration
  - o COXIBs
    - – COX-2 inhibitors are "…probably as effective as a combination of non-selective NSAIDs combined with PPI in patients at risk for ulcers".
    - – Considering celecoxib versus diclofenac plus PPI, "….neither treatment could eliminate the risk of recurrent bleeding in very-high-risk patients" (recent history of bleeding peptic ulcer, 6 month risk of ulcer 20% to 25%, risk of recurrent bleeding, 5%).
    - – "…..COX-2 inhibitors but also non-selective NSAIDs, with the exception of full-dose naproxen (1000 mg a day), increase cardiovascular risk" (risk ratio for most myocardial infarction, 1.42), and "…….. there was no significant difference in cardiovascular risk between COX-2 inhibitors and non-selective NSAIDs. Naproxen (500 mg twice daily) was the only exception" (Feldman M., et al. Sleisenger and Fordtran's Gastrointestinal and Liver Disease. 9th Edition. *Saunders/Elsevier*, Philadelphia, 2010, page 875).

  - o H. pylori
    - – H. pylori increases risk of ulcer bleeding 1.79 fold, NSAIDs 4.85-fold, and H. pylori plus NSAIDs ~ 6 folds.
    - – "Among patients who are about to start NSAIDs therapy, eradication of H. pylori reduces [by about 50% but does not prevent] the subsequent risk of ulcer development."
    - – Thus, "…..eradication of H. pylori infection alone is not sufficient for the prevention of ulcer bleeding in NSAID users with high ulcer risk.
    - – Although H. pylori increases the ulcer risk in patients receiving low-dose aspirin, "co-therapy with PPI after eradication of H. pylori was still required…."

Adapted from: Feldman M., et al. Sleisenger and Fordtran's Gastrointestinal and Liver Disease. 9th Edition. *Saunders/Elsevier*, Philadelphia, 2010, Table 53.2, page 876; and 10th Edition, 2016, page 890.

"The covers of the book are too far apart."

Anonymous

- o Anti-platelet drugs
  - – Low-dose aspirin alone slightly decreases all-cause mortality (relative risk, 0.93; 95% confidence interval, 0.87-0.99) but increases the risk for major GI bleeding (adds ratio, 1.55; 95% CI, 1.27-1.90).
  - – PPI use with aspirin decreased the likelihood of bleeding (OR, 0.34; 95% CI, 0.21-0.57).
  - – Low-dose aspirin negates the GI mucosa-sparing effect of COX-2 inhibitor.
  - – In combination of ASA with clopidogrel or anticoagulants, the risk for major bleeding is higher than with aspirin alone (OR, 1.86; 95% CI, 1.49-2.31 and OR, 1.93; 95% CI, 1.42-2.61, respectively).
  - – The major complication of these anti-ischemic therapies is gastrointestinal bleeding.
  - – Omeprazole can significantly reduce the risk of adverse upper gastrointestinal events in patients receiving clopidogrel alone.
  - – The patients with acute coronary syndrome or ST elevation myocardial infarction, esomeprazole is superior to famotidine in preventing upper gastrointestinal complications related to aspirin, clopidogrel, and enoxaparin or thrombolytics.

Source: Ng F-H, et al. Am J Gastroenterol 2012; 107: 389-391; Goldstein JL, et al. Aliment Phamacol Ther 2011; 34: 808.

165

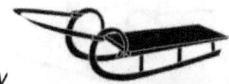

- Give the correlation between gastritis on biopsy, endoscopy and symptoms.

  o The correlation is poor between any two of these three factors.

- Give the finding on gastric mucosal biopsy which suggests that gastritis is due to NSAIDs/ASA.

  o Foveolar hyperplasia, a "corkscrew" appearance of the gastric foveolar, is suggestive of exogenous substance damage, such as from ASA/NSAIDs.

➢ Risk stratification
  o Because there is a poor association between NSAID-associated dyspepsia and peptic ulcer or peptic ulcer bleeding, there must be risk stratification for the development of peptic ulcer bleeding.
  o There are numerous patient-related risk factors associated with the used of NSAIDs, COXIBs, ASA, Clopidogrel. The magnitude of the relative risks should not be compared because various studies were used including different patient populations and risk factors.
  o Treatment algorithms often refer to low, moderate or high gastrointestinal (GI) risk, but actual values of relatives or absolute risk are not used to define these risk categories.
  o It is reasonable to accept that low GI risk comprises a group with no risk factors other than the intake of usual doses of a single agent (NSAID, COXIB, ASA, Clopidogrel).
  o An arbitrary definition of risk has been provided by Lanza et al. (Am J Gastroenterol 2009; 104: 728-738):
    - High risk
      ▪ History of a previously complicated ulcer, especially recently
      ▪ 3 or more risk factors
    - Moderate risk
      ▪ 1 or 2 risk factors
      ▪ > 65 years
      ▪ High dose NSAID therapy
      ▪ A previous history of uncomplicated (non-bleeding) ulcer
      ▪ Concurrent use of any dose of
        - ASA
        - Steroids
        - Anticoagulant

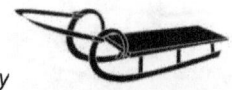

Mastering the Boards: Gastroenterology   A.B.R. Thomson

- Give the relative risk (RR) of clinical factors associated with upper gastrointestinal clinical events (bleeding, perforation, obstruction) in the person taking NSAIDs.

Clinical Features	Relative Risk*
o Age >60 – 75 years	2.5
o History of upper gastrointestinal symptoms	2.5
o History of peptic ulcer	2.5
o History of gastrointestinal bleeding	5
o *Helicobacter pylori* positive	2.0
o Severe rheumatoid arthritis disability	2.5
o History of cardiovascular disease	2.5
o Medications	
– High dose NSAIDs	7
– Multiple NSAIDs	10
– Concomitant low dose ASA	10
– Concomitant anticoagulants	10
– Concomitant corticosteroids	1.5
– Concomitant SSRIs	2.0

Abbreviations: ASA, acetylsalicylic acid; NSAID, nonsteroidal anti-inflammatory drug; SSRI, selective serotonin reuptake inhibitors

*RR, relative risks associated with various risk factors. Since these studies included differing patient populations and not all studies considered all risk factors, direct comparisons of the magnitudes of the risks (i.e., rows of the table) should be avoided.

Adapted from: Rostom et al. *Alim.Pharm.Therapeutics* 2009; 29:481-496.

"Life isn't a matter of milestones, but of moments."

Rose Kennedy

Gastroprotection

Useful background: Key points to consider regarding NSAIDs and gastroprotection

- o Concomitant PPI use reduces the risk of development of NSAID induced endoscopic lesions such as ulcers

- o Concomitant PPI use is strongly recommended for high risk NSAID users

- o It is not known whether concomitant PPI use reduces the risk of clinically significant GI events such as hemorrhage and perforation

- o PPI co therapy in high risk NSAID users is equivalent to COX-2 therapy in preventing NSID induced endoscopic lesions

- o PPI use is effective as secondary prevention of ulcer complications in patients needing antithrombotic therapy with aspirin or clopidogrel

- o As alternatives to PPIs, misoprostol and H_2RAs can be used in the prevention of NSAID related ulcers and their complications, and their use is cost effective

168

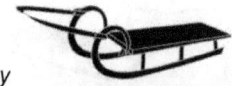

- PPI co therapy is effective in the healing and prevention of recurrence of ulcers in patients maintained on long term NSAID therapy.
- Persons with cardiovascular disease (CV) may be on aspirin (ASA) when they develop a NVUGIB.
- The reflex action may be to stop the ASA to reduce the risk of recurrent ASA-associated bleeding.
- This is successful from the GI perspective (recurrent bleeding is higher in patients on rather than off ASA, 10.3% vs 5.4%).
- However, this discontinuation of ASA in the high CV-risk patient leads to a higher CV mortality rate (12.9% vs 1.3%) (Sung et al., Ann. Int. Med.; 2010 152: 1-9).
- This person with both high CV and GI risk be kept on ASA and that gastroprotective therapy with a PPI be used.

Adapted from: Arora et al. *Clin Gastroenterol Hepatol* 2009;7: 725-735

Printed with permission: Lanza FL, et al. *AM J Gastroenterology* 2009; 104: 734.

- Give the recommendations for avoiding peptic ulcers (gastric or duodenal; GU, DU) associated with the use of nonsteroidal anti-inflammatory drugs (NSAIDs) as a function of low, moderate and high gastrointestinal, as well as low and significant cardiovascular risk (CV) (e.g., required use of ASA plus NSAID).

	Low GI Risk	Moderate GI Risk	High GI Risk
❖ Low CV Risk (no ASA)	o An NSAID with a low ulcerogenic potential at the lowest effective dose o Consider testing/ treating for H. pylori if starting NSAIDs o Avoid multiple or high dose NSAIDs	– NSAID plus – Misoprostol – COXIB	▪ COXIB plus PPI ▪ Misoprostol
❖ Significant CV Risk (requires ASA)	o NSAID plus a PPI	– NSAID and a PPI	▪ Avoid NSAIDs and COXIB, if at all possible

Abbreviations: COXIB, COX-2 inhibitor; CV, cardiovascular risk; NSAIDs, nonsteroidal anti-inflammatory drugs; PPI, proton pump inhibitor.

*these recommendations did not embrace the patients who required antiplatelet therapy, but the same principle is likely to apply.

Printed with permission: Lanza FL, et al. *Am J Gastroenterol* 2009; 104: 728-38.

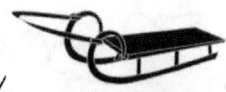

BARIATRIC SURGERY

➢ Indications

• In a sentence, give the indications for bariatric surgery
  o BMI > 40 kg/m², or
  o BMI > 35 kg/m² plus comorbid complications

➢ Benefits

• Give the benefits of bariatric surgery
  o ↓ all cause mortality rate (CV, CRC), as well as and other obesity-related cancers
  o ↓ diabetes
  o ↓ NAFLD histology score in > 80% (↓ fibrosis in 60%)
  o ↑ quality of life for patient

➢ Types of bariatric surgery
  o Restriction procedures
    – VBG (vertical banded gastroplasty)
    – LAGB (laparoscopic adjustable gastric banding)
    – SE (sleeve gastrectomy)
  o Malabsorption-producing procedures
    – BPD (biliopancreatic diversion)
    – BPD/DS (BPD plus duodenal switch)
  o Mixed procedures
    – RYGB (Roux-en-Y gastric bypass)
  o The post-operative complications of bariatric surgery are often subdivided into 3 phases
    1. 1 to 6 weeks
    2. 7 to 12 weeks
    3. 13 to 52 weeks

Gems & Pearls

  o Ursodeoxycholic acid (UDCA) ↓ risk of gallstones by 40% after R-en-Y gastric bypass

  o Vertical banded gastroscopy (VBG) → pseudoachalasia

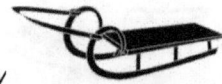

➤ Endoscopy in the Bariatric Surgery Patient

  o Be smart: review the operative notes and any relevant post-operative imaging studies to be aware of the "lay of the land".

  o Visualization may require the use of a narrower pediatric gastroscopy or colonoscopy.

  o ERCP of the biliopancreatic limb and retrograde evaluation of the bypassed stomach is especially difficult after RYGB (Roux-en-Y gastric bypass).

  o This difficult is increasing with more use of "distal bypass", with anastomosis of the biliopancreatic limb only 150 cm proximal to the ileocecal value.

  o Retrograde evaluation may be made easier with use of
    – Shapelock™ enteroscopy guide
    – Deep small bowel enteroscope
      ▪ Double balloon
      ▪ Spiral enteroscopy

  o Common Endoscopic finding after RYGB Bariatric Surgery
    – "gastritis" is common, but clinical significance is unclear
    – ~1/3 of symptomatic RYGB have a normal EGD
    – ~1/4 will have stenosis of stoma, usually 1 month after surgery

➤ Complications

• Give complications common to all bariatric surgical procedure.

  o CNS
    – Psychiatric disturbance

  o Lung
    – Atelectasis and pneumonia
    – Deep vein thrombosis
    – Pulmonary embolism

  o GI
    – Anemia
    – Diarrhea
    – Ulceration
    – GI bleeding
    – Stenosis
    – Gallstones

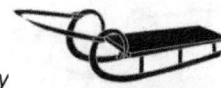

- o Metabolic
  - – Bone disease
  - – Too rapid weight loss
- o Surgical
  - – Wound infection
  - – Failure to lose weight
  - – Mortality (0.5-1%)

Abbreviation: CNS, central nervous system

Adapted from: Klein S. *2006 AGA Institute Post Graduate Course*: pg. 175.

- • Givethe name of bariatric surgical procedures, and list complications for each.
  - o Gastric bypass (Roux-en-Y)
    - – Anastomotic leak with peritonitis
    - – Stomal stenosis
    - – Marginal ulcers (ischemia)
    - – Staple line disruption
    - – Internal and incisional hernias
    - – Nutrient deficiencies (usually iron, calcium, folic acid, vitamin B12)
    - – Dumping syndrome
  - o Gastroplasty
    - – GERD
    - – Stomal stenosis
    - – Staple line disruption
    - – Band erosion
  - o Gastric banding
    - – Band slippage
    - – Erosion
    - – Esophageal dilation
    - – Band infections
  - o Biliopancreatic diversion
    - – Anastomotic leak with peritonitis
    - – Protein-energy malnutrition
    - – Vitamin and mineral deficiencies
    - – Dehydration

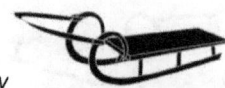

- Give the endoscopic treatment of complications after bariatric surgery.

❖ Stoma
  o Narrowing (symptomatic stomal stenosis)
    – Bougie dilators or balloons, using guide wire TTS (through-the-scope placement)
    – Optimal aperture diameter 10 mm to 15 mm
    – If multiple dilators needed, dilate slowly (up to 3 mm [3 French sizes] at each session, every 1 to 2 weeks until symptoms resolve
  o Reduction in size of enlarged stomas and pouches
    – Aim for stomal diameter ~ 12 mm
    – Objective is to reduce/eliminate symptoms e.g., slowing of expected weight loss from surgery; during syndrome)
    – Use sclerosants, suturing device, clips

❖ Marginal ulcer (MU) bleeding
  o Usually on jejunal side of gastrojejunal anastomosis
  o Early MU in 10%, late in 1%
  o Risk of MU associated with smoking, H. pylori infection, NSAIDs use
  o If bleeding occurs early after surgery, perform EGD in OR

❖ Leaks
  o Fistulae, dehiscence of staple line, gastric leaks
    – Tissue apposition
      ▪ Fibrin glue
      ▪ Biomaterial (from pig intestine)
      ▪ Clipping
    – Stents
      ▪ SEPS (self-expanding plastic stents)
      ▪ SEMS (self-expanding esophageal metal stents)

❖ Band erosion
  o Nd:YAG laser
  o Scissors
  o Cutters (endoscopic)

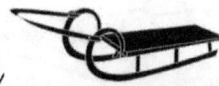

➤ Treatment

- Give the Phase 2 and 3 post-operative medical care of the patient with bariatric surgery (the gastroenterologist is often involved in the phases).
    - Nutrition
        - Eat slowly (< 1 oz per 10 minutes)
        - Eat solids, wait 30 min, then take beverage
        - Be aware of possible new food intolerance, e.g., red meat
        - Avoid snacks and high calorie fluid drinks, e.g., Coal "pop"
        - Identify and correct any vitamin D deficiency
        - Beware alcohol use disorder (10% in second post-op year)
        - Anticipate, possible deficiencies of
            - Thiamine
            - Copper 2 mg/day
            - Zinc 8 mg/day
            - Calcium (use calcium citrate po, which does not need gastric acidity for dissolution)
    - Medications
        - Medicals need to be crushable, or liquid
        - If anti-diabetic therapy, use metformin po (only small changes in blood sugar)
        - Reassess need for treatment of GERD (GERD symptoms may improve with weight loss)
        - Reassess need for contraception
            - ↑ fertility as weight is lost
            - Menses may return
            - Consider use of non-oral hormonal
        - Reassess need for drugs for obesity-associated arthralgias
            - ↓ need or NSAIDs is possible
            - Use acetaminophen if arthralgias persist
            - Return of post psychiatric issues
    - Be on lookout for
        - Psychiatric disorders
            - Emotional liability
            - Self-destructive behaviour
            - Bulimia
            - Somatization (nausea, vomiting)
        - GI disorders
            - Dyspepsia from development of stomal (aka marginal)
            - Nausea/vomiting

174

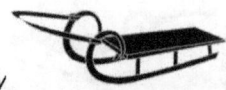

- Cholelithiasis
  - 22% at 6 months post-op
  - Consider UCDA (ursodeoxycholic acid, ursodiol) 300 mg bid for 6 months
- Dumping syndrome
  - Avoid foods which are associated with causing symptoms (e.g., sugar, pop)
  - Eat slowly, "by the clock"
  - Take liquids at end of rather than during a meal
- Prolonged vomiting
  - Only slowly advance intake to solid foods
  - Stomal stricture
  - Marginal ulcers
  - Small bowel obstruction, such as from internal hernia
  - Food intolerances
  - Somatization
  - Overrating
- New onset of heartburn, regurgitation, dysphagia
  - Gastric outlet obstruction from slippage of band, such as may occur if the patient had
  - An unrecognized or unrepaired hiatus hernia
- Hematemesis
  - Marginal ulcer
  - Mallory Weiss tear from vomiting
  - Severe esophagitis from partial gastric outlet obstruction
  - Band erosion through the wall of the stomach
- Slowing of initially satisfactory weight loss
  - Recidivism
  - Development of new and poor eating habits
  - Development of gastrogastric fistula
- Expected weight loss
  - RYGB
    - First 6 months 10 lbs to 15 lbs per month
    - 2 years
      - 65% of excess body weight, or
      - 35% of initial body weight
  - LAGB
    - 2 years
      - 45% of excess body weight, or
      - 25% of initial body weight

o Cosmetic and body image issue

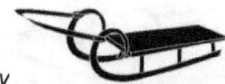

Nutrient Deficiencies After Gastric Surgery

- Give mechanisms or causes of iron- and B12-deficiency associated anemia, diarrhea, metabolic bone disease, and recurrent gastric ulceration in a patient having had a Billroth II partial gastrectomy for peptic ulcer disease (PUD), gastric cancer (GCa) or morbid obesity (bariatric surgery) and Roux-en-Y.

- ❖ Iron

  o Pre-surgery iron deficiency

  o ↓ intake from post-op symptoms (anorexia, early satiety)

  o ↓ acid → ↓ pepsin and ↓ meat digestion and release of iron

  o ↓ acid-mediated solubilizing and reducing of inorganic dietary iron (Fe^{3+} .[ferric] .. Fe^{2+}) ferrous])

  o ↓ absorption of Fe^{2+}, Ca^{2+}, BII, bypassing site of maximal absorption (duodenum)

  o Can be slow bleeding at surgical site

  o Bile gastritis

  o Gastric stump cancer

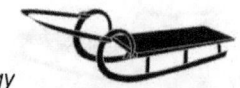

- ❖ Vitamin B12 (cobalamine)
  - ○ Pre-surgery deficiency
  - ○ Decreased intake
  - ○ Loss of stimulated and co-ordinated release of "R" factor
  - ○ Decreased intrinsic factor
  - ○ Loss of HCl/pepsinogen to liberate food B12
  - ○ Bacterial overgrowth syndrome

- ❖ Metabolic bone disease
  - ○ Pre-existing osteoporosis ↓ Ca^{2+} solubilization
  - ○ ↓ vitamin D or Ca^{2+} intake
  - ○ ↓ absoption due to ↓ solubility of Ca^{2+}
  - ○ Bypass of site of maximal absorption of Ca^{2+} (duodenum)
  - ○ Binding Ca^{+2} (unabsorbed fatty acids)

- ❖ Diarrhea
  - ○ Medications
    - – Magnesium-containing antacids, PPI's
  - ○ Stomach
    - – Early dumping syndrome
    - – Retained antrum (↑ gastrin)
    - – Hypergastrinemia → HCL hypersecretion (↑ volume, mucosal damage); loss of PPY from ileum, loss of inhibition of gastrin → ↑s. gastrin
  - ○ Small bowel
    - – Bypassed duodenum
    - – Bacterial overgrowth syndrome (BOS - aka small intestinal bacterial overgrowth {SIBO})
  - ○ Colon
    - – PPI-associated collagenous colitis
  - ○ Unmasked conditions
    - – Unmasked celiac disease
    - – Unmasked lactose intolerance
    - – Unmasked bile acid wastage
    - – Unmasked monosaccharide transporter defect
    - – Primary or secondary (unmasked) pancreatic insufficiency

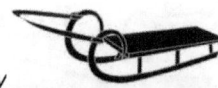

- ❖ Peptic ulceration (stomal/marginal ulcer, previous peptic ulcer disease [PUD])
  - ○ ↑ gastrin - ZES, incomplete vagotomy, gastric retention, afferent loop syndrome
  - ○ H. pylori infection
  - ○ NSAIDs, ASA use
  - ○ "Stump" Cancer
  - ○ Ischemia at anastomosis
  - ○ Bile gastritis

- ❖ Presentations of ZES (Zollinger Ellison Syndrome)
  - ○ PUD – severe, multiple, unusual sites; GERD-like symptoms
  - ○ Diarrhea
  - ○ Recurrent ulceration (with or without gastric surgery)
  - ○ Associated MEN I syndrome
  - ○ Thick gastric folds
  - ○ Fundic gland polyps

Abbreviations: BOS, bacterial overgrowth syndrome; GCa, gastric cancer; MEN, multiple endocrine neoplasia ; PPIs, proton pump inhibitor; PUD, peptic ulcer disease; ZES, Zollinger-Ellison syndrome

"Play a crucial role in finding your own humility and humanity."

Grandad

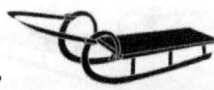

GASTRIC EMPTYING

- o Duodenal mucosal receptors for FA (fatty acids), AA (amino acids) and carbohydrates limit the rate of gastric emptying to ~ 150 kcal/hr.

- o Fat in the ileum slows small bowel emptying through the release of GLP-1 and -2, as well as PYY (peptide YY).

SO YOU WANT TO BE A WHAT - GASTROENTEROLOGIST!

It is widely taught that CCK stimulates pancreatic acinar cells to secrete enzymes, but in humans these acinar cells have no CKK receptors.

- Give the mechanism by which CCK stimulates pancreatic acinar cell secretion of enzymes.

  - o CCK acts on the cholinergic vagal afferent pathway, and its action (as well as that of secretin) is increased synergistically by 5-HT.

➢ Physiology

- Give the neuromuscular function of the stomach/or accommodation, grinding and mixing as well as emptying.

❖ Smooth muscle cells

- o Receptors in the excitable membrane of the smooth muscle cells

- o These receptors bind to amines and peptides which reach the smooth muscle cells from neurocrine, paracrine and endocrine pathways

- o The excitable membrane of the smooth muscle cells fires spontaneously, causing action potentials that cause the muscle cell to contract

- o The muscle cells are joined as a syncytium, which provides electrical coupling of neighbouring muscle cells

- o The contraction resulting from the spontaneous depolarization, action potential and syncytial coupling cause contraction in the circumferential and longitudinal axes.

179

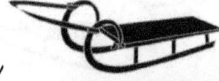

o Electrophysiology of smooth muscle

Site	RMP, mV	PP/SP
– Fundus	-50	-
▪ Effect of inhibitory vagal input	Receptive relaxation ($\downarrow$ fundic tone)	
– Corpus/antrum ▪ Effect of Ach or stretch	-60/-70	$\uparrow$ amplitude and duration of PP, occurrence of PP, occurrence of AP $\rightarrow$ low or high-amplitude contractions

    – Pylorus
       ▪ Electrical barrier between slow wave of distal antrum (3 cpm) and duodenum (12 cpm), i.e., the duodenal slow wave is 12 cpm (contractions per minute).

Abbreviations: AP, action potential; PP, plateau potential; RMP, Resting membrane potential

❖ PNS (parasympathetic nervous system) and SNS (sympathetic nervous system)

  o PNS
    – Stimulatory vagal nerves
    – $\uparrow$ gastric contraction
    – $\uparrow$ gastric secretion

  o SNS
    – Inhibitory

❖ ENS (enteric nervous system)

  o Main networks
    – SM submucosal
    – Myenteric
    – Deep muscular
       ▪ Interstitial cells of Cajal (ICC)
       ▪ Plexi involved in pacemaking
       ▪ Muscle propulsion (MMC)
          – Sensation
          – Secretion

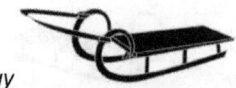

- o "Stimulation of excitatory enteric neurons leads to depolarization of IM-ICCs".
- o "The depolarization [of IM-ICCs]......causes positive chronotropic effects on the frequency of gastric slow waves", and also........increases the contractile response of smooth muscle to slow wave depolarizations........" (Feldman M., et al. Sleisenger and Fordtran's Gastrointestinal and Liver Disease. 9th Edition. Saunders/Elsevier, Philadelphia, 2010, page 793).
- o Thus, the ICC networks provide the control of frequency and propagation velocity for the circular muscle contractions that comprise gastric peristalsis waves" (Feldman M., et al. Sleisenger and Fordtran's Gastrointestinal and Liver Disease. 9th Edition. Saunders/Elsevier, Philadelphia, 2010, page 792).

❖ Autonomic nervous system (ANS)
- o Parasympathetic pathways from
    - – DMN (dorsal motor nucleus)
    - – NA (nucleus ambiguous)
    - – TS (tractus solitarius)
- o Vagus efferents pass to MP (myenteric plexus) in wall of stomach
- o Sympathetic pathways
    - – From IML (intermediolateral columns) in T5 to T10 levels of spinal cord from
        - ▪ Celiac ganglia to splanchnic efferents
            - – Myenteric ganglia   norepinephrine
        - ▪ Splanchnic efferents to
            - – Submucous ganglia ⎫ norepinephrine and somatostatin
            - – Circular muscle ⎭
            - – Blood vessels   norepinephrine and NPY
            - – Pyloric sphincter
            - – Non-sphincteric muscle

Abbreviation: NPY, neuropeptide Y; MMC (aka IMMC), interdigestive migrating motor complex

❖ ICC (interstitial cells of Cajal, aka pacemaker cells) → plateau or action potentials → slow waves/cysclic contractile activity
- o ICCs arise from c-kit-positive mesenchymal cell precursors
- o ICCs present in multiple layers of stomach wall
    - – Myenteric (MY-ICCs)
    - – Intramuscular (IM-ICCs)
    - – Submuscular
    - – Subserosal

181

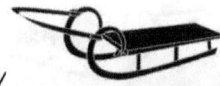

- o Types
  - – Phase 1
    - ▪ Quite; little contractile activity
  - – Phase 2
    - ▪ Random, irregular contractions
    - ▪ Peristaltic reflex
- o ICCs at the junction of the gastric fundus and body at the proximal part of the greater curve of the stomach have innate activity and spontaneously produce a slow wave (aka pacesetter potential, gastric myoelectrical activity)
- o Slow waves from occur at 3 cpm (cycles per minute) move circumferentially and distally at 14 mm/sec towards the antrum.
- o MY-ICCs (ICCs in the myenteric plexus between the circular and longitudinal muscle layers) general the slow waving.
- o The slow wave of the gastric myoelectrical activity has an uptake.
- o When this uptake of the slow wave depolarizes, there is a reduction in the threshold for the circular smooth muscle to contract.
- o When the membrane potential reaches the threshold potential, the force of contraction quickly increases (steep slope of the voltage-contraction curve)
- o The slow wave becomes linked with the plateau or action potentials.
- o "Action potential are superimposed on the plateau potentials in the terminal antrum and pyrolus" (Feldman M., et al. Sleisenger and Fordtran's Gastrointestinal and Liver Disease. 9th Edition. Saunders/Elsevier, Philadelphia, 2010, page 792; 10th edition, 2016, page 812).
- o The action potentials are associated with increased amplitude of the contraction of the smooth muscle.
- o This increased activity of the plateau or action potentials causes the gastric peristaltic contractions.
- o The fundus does not have MY-ICCs or a slow wave, so the fundus does not participate in the linking of slow wave to the plateau or action potentials, and therefore has no role in producing peristaltic contractions.
- o The IM-ICCs in the fundus
  - – Sensory cells for mechanoreception
  - – Innervated by inhibitory vagal neurons which regular tone and receptive relaxation in the fundus

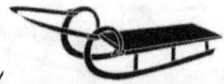

- o Electrode placed on the anterior wall may be used to detect the myoelectrical activity of the slow waves arising from the pacemaker region.
- o This recording of the gastric myoelectrical activity is employed clinically as the EGG (electrogastrogram).
- o The MY-ICCs produce the slow waves which depolarize the smooth muscle membrane depolarization by the MY-ICCs slow wave activates the voltage-dependent L-type calcium channels in the smooth muscle cell membrane
  - The depolarization which occurs during the upstroke of the slow wave redepolarizes to the value of the RMP, and the contraction ends.
  - Neurons of the ENS (enteric nervous system) are close to MY-ICCs and IM-ICCs.
  - Excitatory neurotransmitters include Ach (acetylcholine) and substance P.
  - Inhibitory neurotransmitters include NO (nitric oxide) and VIP (vasoactive intestinal polypeptide).
  - The spread of the slow wave and the smooth muscle contraction is integrated by IM-ICCs.
  - IM-ICCs are electrically coupled by way of gap junctions to the smooth muscle cells.
  - MY-ICCs initiate, and IM-ICCs mediate neurotransmission: they [integrate slow wave activity and smooth muscle activity] carry and coordinate the spread of slow waves.
    - MMC (migrating myoelectrical [motor] complex)

- ❖ Peristaltic reflex
  - o Responsible for the "law of the intestine"
  - o Ascending contraction: stimulus in the lumen, usually from distention by food
    - Transmitters of excitation of smooth muscle
      - Acetylcholine
      - Serotonin acting on 5HT4 receptors on cholinergic interneurons
      - Tachykinins
        - SP (substance P)
        - SK (substance K)
  - o Descending contraction: inhibition of smooth muscle below area of stimulation causes descending inhibition
    - Resistance to the movements of the food bolus which is being pulsed distally into the relaxed area by the ascending contraction and the proximal smooth muscle excitation.

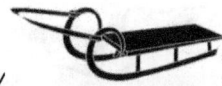

- Transmitters of inhibition of smooth muscle
  - NO (nitric oxide)
  - VIP (vasoactive intestinal peptide)
  - Somatostatin
  - GABA (gamma-aminobutyric acid)
  - Endogenous opiates
- Pylorus (antroduodenal junction)
  - 0.6 cm to 1.6 cm long, and maintains an area of high resting pressure
  - 3 times per minute phasic contractions sweep across this antroduodenal junction, emptying particles which are 1 mm to 2 mm in size
  - These phasic pyloric contractions are mediatedly NO, Ach and opiates.

- o Muscle activity: circular, oblique and longitudinal muscle layers of stomach, which leads to
  - Relaxation of fundus (accommodation)
  - Contraction of antrum (chemical digestion, shearing and pulverization, propulsion, rates pulsion, sieving, emptying of 1 mm to 2 mm particles)

- o Phase 3
  - Bursts of "regular, high – amplitude phasic contractions ["activity front"] that last from 5 to 10 min….and migrate from the antrum to the ileum (Feldman M., et al. Sleisenger and Fordtran's Gastrointestinal and Liver Disease. 9th Edition. Saunders/Elsevier, Philadelphia, 2010, page 794) in 90 to 120 min.
  - Motilin is of importance to Phase 3 contractions
  - Cyclical contractile activity beginning in phase 3 of MMC seen in stomach and small bowel, as well as,
    - LES (lower esophageal sphincter)
    - SOD (sphincter of Oddi)
    - Gallbladder

- ❖ GI peptides
  - o Released by food (see fasting and fed neuromuscular activity)
  - o Act on
    - ICCs
    - Smooth muscle
    - ENS
    - Vagal function
      - Afferent
      - Efferent

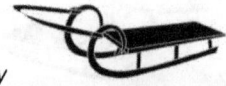

- Give GI peptides involved in gastric emptying.

  - CCK
    - Released from enteroendocrine cells in duodenal mucosa in response to fatty acids (from digested triglycerides) in the duodenum.
    - Activation of CCK receptors → sensation of fullness → ↓ food intake

  - PYY (polypeptide-YY)
    - Released from enteroendocrine cells in ileocolonic mucosa
    - ↓ gastric emptying and small bowel rate of transit ("ileal brake")
    - ↓ appetite, ↓ food intake

  - CRF (corticotropin-releasing factor)
    - Acts through central pathways in periventricular nucleus
      - Central dopamine 1 and 2
      - Vasopressin (AVP) pathways
    - Responds to emotional stress

  - SCF (stem cell factor)
    - ↓ SCF with ↑ BS (increased blood sugar), i.e., hyperglycemia)
    - ↓ SCF → ↓ ICCs and ↓ contraction of smooth muscle

- Give the process and mechanisms of gastric emptying of food and fluids.

  - The intake of food
    - Begins the processes of fundic receptive relaxation
    - Body grinding and mixing ("trituration")
    - Antral peristalsis
    - Antropyloroduodenal coordination
    - Emptying of 2 to 4 ml of chime, containing particles < 4 mm, by varying resistance of pylorus and antrum
    - The ICCs in the deep muscular plexus junction act in conjugation with the ENS (enteric nervous system)
    - The ICCs in the myenteric plexus do not depend on the ENS
    - ICCs in the pylorus are associated with inhibitory neural activity in this region, and thereby are important in the context of the rate of gastric emptying

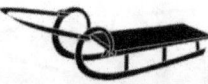

- o Receptive
  relaxation
  – Vagus and NO
  - Ingested food and fluid stretch the fundus and stimulate mechanoreceptors and chemoreceptors.
  - Secretin is released from enterochromaffin cells.
  - IPANs (intrinsic primary afferent neurons) in the submucosa or myenteric plexus of the stomach.
  - Activated mechano-/chemo-receptors stimulate IM-ICCs.
  - The IM-ICCs activate vagal efferent and vago-vagal reflexes.
  - The nucleus of the tractus solitaries, periventricular nucleus and dorsal motor nucleus of the vagus are stimulated.
  - There is inhibition of the vagal excitatory neurons.
  - NO (nitric oxide) and VIP (vasoactive intestinal peptide) are released.
  - NO and VIP are also inhibitory to the normal tone of smooth muscle of the fundus.
  - The end result is for filling of the fundus to result in receptive relaxation.
  - This process begins before mixing and grinding in the gastric body.

- o Other
  factors
  – Distension
  - Antrum
    - Capsaicin-sensitive afferent vagal nerves mediated by
      - 5-HT_3 (5-hydroxytryptamine)
      - GRP (gastrin-releasing peptide)
  - Duodenal CCK_A receptors
  - Duodenum
  - Colon
  – Perfusion of duodenum
  - Acid
  - Lipid
  - Protein

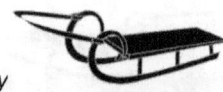

- o Body
  contractions
  - Relaxation of the fundus and proximal portion of the gastric body is replaced by contractions of the fundus and proximal corpus.
  - This pushes food into the rest of the body and antrum, where mixing and grinding occur.
  - This initial postprandial interval of receptive relaxation, mixing and grinding, is called the "lag phase".
  - The lag phase duration depends on the composition of the meal (usually about 45 to 60 min).

- o Emptying
  - Trituration of solid food into particles 1 to 2 mm in size begins the linear phase of gastric emptying.
  - The gastric peristaltic waves arise from the electrical activity of ICC, the plateau and, action potentials.
  - These peristaltic waves sweep waves through the body of the stomach at 3 cpm (cycles per min).
  - The clearance of the pyloric sphincter and the contraction of the duodenum present the emptying of the particles > 2 mm.
  - The antral contraction waves pump, pulsatile "squirts" of food and fluid into duodenum.
  - Depending on the strength of contraction (10 to 40 mm Hg) and duration of antral peristaltic wave, and the resistance provided by pyloric sphincter and duodenal contraction, usually 3 to 4 kcal/min is emptied into the duodenum.
  - About 50% of a meal will be emptied in 90 min ($T_{1/2}$ of gastric empting), and 95% has been emptied by 4 hours.
  - Non-caloric and then caloric liquids are emptied first without a lag phase and in a "mono-exponential emptying", pattern, then digestible material during the linear phase as a result of lower amplitude pressure waves.

- o Effect of
  food/fluids
  - The rate of gastric emptying may be modified by the amount and composition of the ingested food and fluids.
    - Volume
    - Viscosity
    - Osmolarity
    - Nutrient density
    - Fats
  - For further details, please refer to Feldman M., et al. Sleisenger and Fordtran's Gastrointestinal and Liver Disease. 10th Edition. Saunders/Elsevier, Philadephia, 2016, Table 49.1, page 882.

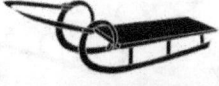

Modulation of Rate of Gastric Emptying

- Give the key factors involved in the **modulation of rate** of gastric emptying.

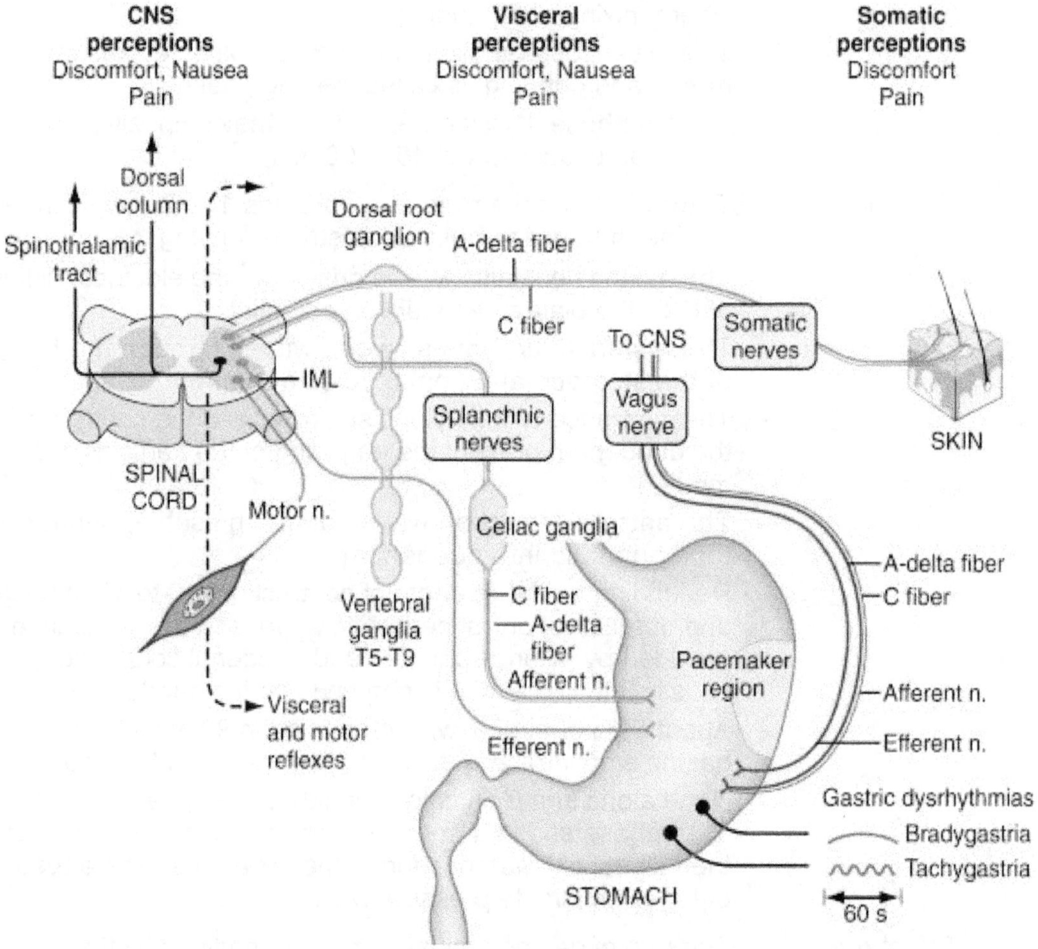

CNS perceptions
Discomfort, Nausea
Pain

Visceral perceptions
Discomfort, Nausea
Pain

Somatic perceptions
Discomfort
Pain

Dorsal column

Spinothalamic tract

Dorsal root ganglion

A-delta fiber

C fiber

To CNS

Somatic nerves

IML

Splanchnic nerves

Vagus nerve

SKIN

SPINAL CORD

Motor n.

Celiac ganglia

A-delta fiber

C fiber

Visceral and motor reflexes

Vertebral ganglia T5-T9

C fiber
A-delta fiber
Afferent n.

Efferent n.

Pacemaker region

Afferent n.

Efferent n.

Gastric dysrhythmias
Bradygastria
Tachygastria

STOMACH

60 s

- o Vagal and splanchnic nerve activity modulate the neuromuscular activities of the stomach.
- o The balance between excitatory and inhibitory nerves to the stomach leads to slower or faster gastric emptying.
- o There is slow wave gastric myoelectrical activity during fasting.
- o In the postprandial period there is summation of the slow wave activity linked to plateau and action potential activity.

188

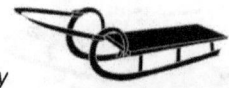

- Only a large meal, hypoglycemia and reduced fundic accommodation (relaxation) speed to emptying to the stomach (reduced $T_{1/2}$ of emptying).

- All other gastroduodenal, ileal and colonic neuromuscular factors, as well as meal-related factors delay gastric emptying (longer $T_{1/2}$).

- Gastric emptying may be slowed by either bradygastria (1 cpm [cycle per minute]) of low- or high- amplitude or by tachygastria (6 cpm), where the gastric dysrhythmia is not coordinated with opening of the pylorus.

- The vagus nerve contains afferent nerves with A-delta and C pain fibres with cell bodies in the nodose ganglia with connections to the nucleus tractus solitarius (not shown).

- Low threshold mechano- and chemoreceptors stimulate visceral sensations such as stomach emptiness or fullness and symptoms such as nausea and discomfort.

- These stimuli are mediated through vagal pathways and become conscious perceptions of visceral sensations if sensory inputs reach the cortex.

- The splanchnic nerves also contain afferent nerves with A-delta and C fibres that synapse in the celiac ganglia with some cells bodies in the vertebral ganglia (T5-T9).

- Interneurons in the white rami in the dorsal horn of the spinal cord cross to the dorsal columns and spinothalamic tracts and ascend to sensory areas of the medulla oblongata.

- These splanchnic afferent fibres are thought to mediate high-threshold stimuli for visceral pain.

- In contrast to visceral sensations, somatic nerves such as from the skin carry sensory information via A-delta and C fibres through the dorsal root ganglia and into the dorsal horn and then through dorsal columns and spinothalamic tracts to cortical areas of somatic representation.

- Changes in gastric electrical rhythm, excess amplitude contractions, or stretch on the gastric wall are peripheral mechanisms that elicit changes in afferent neural activity (via vagal and/or splanchnic nerves) that may reach consciousness to be perceived as visceral perceptions (symptoms) emanating from the stomach.

Abbreviations: IML, intermediolateral nucleus; n., nerve

Printed with permission: Feldman M., et al. Sleisenger and Fordtran's Gastrointestinal and Liver Disease. 9th Edition. Saunders/Elsevier, Philadephia, 2010 Figure 48-17, Page 801.

189

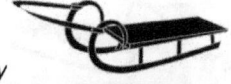

➢ Diagnosis

- • Give the best test to diagnose gastroparesis.
    - o A gastric emptying study performed with a solid and a liquid test meal will correctly establish whether the gastric emptying was slow at the time of testing.
    - o However, there is usually a poor correlation between the patient's symptoms, the T1/2 of emptying provided by the emptying study, or their response to prokinetic medications.

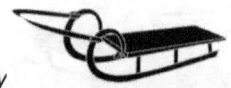

➢ Treatment

• Give the treatment of delayed gastric emptying.
  o Meal Factors
    – Small, frequent, fluid, neutral pH and temperature, isotonic, low energy density, low fat meals
    – Certain amino acids (e.g., L-tryptophan – [cheese])
    – Avoid offending foods and beverages
    – Vitamin B6 (thiamine) (FDA A)
    – Ginger
    – Soda crackers (unproven benefit!)

  o "prokinetics"
    – Metoclopramide
    – Domperidione
    – Cisapride
      ▪ Metabolized by CYP450 3A4:AEs
    – Antibiotics
      ▪ Macrolide
      ▪ Antifungals
      ▪ Phenothiazine
    – Long QT (QTc > 0.45 sec) syndrome
    – Erythromycin: 250 mg po tid, as needed, or maintenance induces high amplitude gastric propulsive contractions
    – Azithromycin
      ▪ AEs: ototoxicity
      ▪ Long QT syndrome → SCD (sudden cardiac death)
    – Antiametics
      ▪ Phenothiazines (do not give with cisapride →↑ risk of QTc > 0.45 sec → SCD)
      ▪ Antihistamine
      ▪ 5-HT3 antagonists e.g., ondansetron

  o PPIs to volume of gastric secretions
    – Botulinum toxin-injection into pylorus
      ▪ Unproven value

  o Treat complications
    – GERD, esophagitis
    – Dehydration, electrolyte disturbances
    – Malnutrition
    – Hypokalemia
    – Metabolic alkalosis
    – Hyperglycemia (in a diabetic)

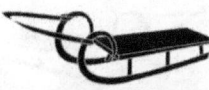

- o Gastric pacing
  - GES (gastric electrical stimulation)
    - High-frequency (12 cpm)
    - Short duration (300 <u>micro</u>sec)
  - Gastric pacing (to "entrain" the normal gastric slow wave rhythm)
    - Low-frequency (3 cpm)
    - Long duration (300 <u>milli</u>sec)
  - Sequential
    - Sequential pacing using a microprocessor
    - Activation of electrodes in a series around the distal 2/3 of the stomach

- o Treat associated disorders
  - Underlying disease/condition causing/ aggravating gastroparesis
  - Rectal/colonic distention
  - Pregnancy
  - Ascites
  - Hyperglycemia
  - Avoid circular vectoral motion
  - Avoid medications which may relax smooth muscle and thereby aggravate gastroparesis

- o Surgery
  - Decompression
    - Venting gastrostomy
    - Jejunostomy
  - Conversion
    - Previous partial gastrectomy → subtotal gastrectomy or near-total gastrectomy and Roux-en-Y gastrojejunostomy

- o Acupuncture
  - Stmulation of P6 acupuncture point
    - Acupuncture with electrical stimulation (acustimulation) represents one of the alternate forms of electrical therapy for gastroparesis.

- o Endoscopic therapy
  - Decompression with enterostomy tube

- o Gastric electrical stimulation ("humanitarian use device")

Adapted from: Quigley EMM. *Sleisenger & Fordtran's gastrointestinal and liver disease: Pathophysiology/Diagnosis/Management* 2006: pg. 1007.

192

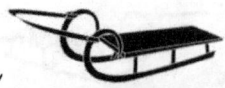

- Give the mechanism (s) of action of prokinetic drugs used for the treatment of symptoms of gastroparesis.

Drug	Receptor
o Metoclopramide	– Central/peripheral dopamine receptor antagonist (D_2) – 5-HT3 receptor antagonist – 5-HT4 receptor agonist
o Domperidone	– Peripheral D_2 antagonist
o Cisapride	– Muscarinic (acetylcholine) receptor agonist – -5-HT3 receptor antagonist – -5-HT4 receptor agonist
o Ondansetron	– -5-HT3 receptor antagonist
o Erythromycin	– Motilin receptor agonist
o Tegaserod	– 5-HT4 partial agonist
o Bethanechol	– Muscarinic receptor agonist
o Anticholinergic (buscopan, for tachygastria)	
o α-adrenergic antagonists	– α-adrenergic antagonist
o Botulism toxin injection	– Acetycholine esterase inhibitor
o Octreotide injection	– Somatostatin receptor agonist
o Viagra®	– Phosphodiesterase inhibitors (NO, nitric oxide)

Adapted from: Quigley EMM. *Sleisenger & Fordtran's gastrointestinal and liver disease: Pathophysiology/Diagnosis/Management* 2006: pg. 1007; and 2010, pg. 813.

- Give the smooth muscle receptors and examples of drugs which act on these receptors to treat GERD.
  - o D2
    - – Peripheral
      - ▪ Domperisone
    - – Peripheral and central
      - ▪ Metoclopramide

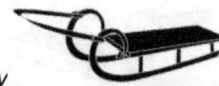

- 5HT
  - 5HT3 receptor antagonist
    - Metoclopramide
    - Cisapride
    - Ondansetron
  - 5HT4 receptor agonist
    - Metoclopramide
    - Cisapride
    - Tegaserol
- Ach
  - Muscarinic
    - Cisapride
    - Bethanecol
  - Anticholinesterase
    - Buscopan
    - Botilinum toxin
- Motilin — Erythromycin
- Phosphodiesterase — Viagara
- Somatostatin — Octreotide
- α-adrenergic antagonists — Clonidine

Diabetic Gastroparesis

➢ Definition

- o Some persons with severe, intractable gastroparesis, such as may occur with severe type I diabetes, may improve with near-total gastrectomy and Roux-en-Y anastomosis.

- o Usual causes related to impaired motility (gastroparesis) and mechanical obstruction.

- o Sometimes the term "gastroparesis" will be used interchangeably with delayed gastric emptying, and then implies a process rather than mechanism.

194

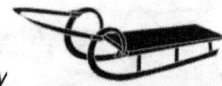

- ➢ Demography
  - o Diabetes is one of the most common etiologies of gastroparesis.
  - o 30-50% of outpatients with long-standing type 1 or type 2 diabetes mellitus (DM) have slow gastric emptying.
  - o The risk of developing gastroparesis among subjects with type 1 DM was elevated over 30-fold, whereas the risk in subjects with type 2 DM was increased almost 8-fold, relative to age- and sex-matched controls.
  - o Subjects with type 1 DM were four times more likely to develop gastroparesis than those with type 2 DM.
  - o The incidence of gastroparesis among those with diabetes is still rare.

Source: Chong RS, et al. Am J Gastroenterol 2012; 107: 82-88.

- ➢ Pathophysiology

- • Give pathophysiological processes involved in the gastroparesis associated with type 1 diabetes.
  - o Episodes of hyperglycemia (from poor control of blood sugars) → ↓ SCF (stem cell factor) → ↓ ICCs (interstitial cell of Cajal)
  - o Metabolic products
    - – ↑ glycosylation end products
    - – ↓ neural function
    - – ↓ smooth muscle function
  - o Vagal dysfunction, e.g., autonomic neuropathy, hyperglycemia in type 1 diabetes
  - o ↓ ICC in deep muscle plexus, e.g., in diabetes possible due to ↓ insulin and IGF-1 → smooth muscle cell produces ↓ stem cell factor
  - o ↑ oxidative stress (as in diabetes)
  - o ↓ inhibitory nitric oxide containing neurosis
  - o ↑ phosphodiesterase -5 activity
  - o Associated neuropathic or myopathic abnormalities of small bowel motility
  - o Abnormal electrical slow wave rhythms, possible from ↑ prostaglandins
    - – Brachygastria
    - – Tachygastria
    - – Mixture of brachygastria and tachygastria

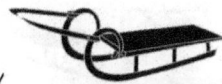

- ○ Abnormal function of
  - – Fundus
    - ▪ Abnormal distribution of food
    - ▪ ↓ relaxation
    - ▪ In response to distention of fundus phasic contraction → ↓ accommodation due to failure of recovery of ↓ tone of fundus during the fasting (postprandial) period; possibly due to a defect in the NO pathway ↓ (50%) of IMMC during fasting associated with antral contraction and the clearance of undigested solids > 1 mm to 2 mm.
    - ▪ Possibly due to neuropathy of the vagus nerve
  - – Body
    - ▪ ↑ dysrhythmias
  - – Antrum
    - ▪ ↓ MMC
    - ▪ ↓ postprandial motility
    - ▪ ↑ dysrhythmias
    - ▪ ↓ phase 3 contractions → ↓ emptying of nondigestible food (e.g., fibre)
    - ▪ ↓ motility (contractions)
    - ▪ ↑ lag time for emptying of stomach
    - ▪ ↓ frequency of distal antral contractions (< 1 per minute), causing hypomotility
    - ▪ ↑ IPPN (isolated pyloric pressure waves "pylorospams")
    - ▪ ↓ proximal gastric contraction, with failure of food still in stomach to be redistributed, again entering the antrum for trituration and emptying.
  - – Pylorus
    - ▪ ↑ motility (pylorospasm, leading to non-coordinated antral contraction and pyloric sphincter relaxation)

"Go as far as you can see; when you get there, you'll be able to see farther."

J. P. Morgan

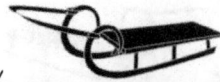

NAUSEA AND VOMITING

➢ Causes/associations

    o The vomiting centre is on the blood side of the blood-brain barrier

Please see Malagelada JR, and Malagelada C. Nausea and vomiting. *Sleisenger & Fordtran's Gastrointestinal and Liver Disease: Pathophysiology/ Diagnosis/ Management* 2006:pg.145.

➢ Mechanisms

• Give mechanisms for the development of **post-operative** nausea and vomiting (PONV).

    o Release of serotonin from bowel handling stimulates $5HT_3$ receptors on afferent serotonergic pathways that stimulate the brainstem

    o Reduced blood flow to brainstem during surgery

    o Activated cerebral cortical pathways

➢ Risk factors

• Give risk factors and methods to reduce PONV.

    o Risk factors
        – Post Puberty females
        – Non-smokers
        – Previous PONV
        – Use of volatile anesthetics
        – Intra-operative use of opiates
        – High dose neostigmine
        – Prolonged surgery
        – Intra-abdominal surgery
        – Major gynecological surgery

    o Anaesthetic methods to reduce the risk of PONV
        – Avoid opioids
        – Avoid nitrous oxide
        – Avoid high-dose reversal agent
        – Adequate hydration
        – High oxygen concentration
        – Propofol anesthetic

Abbreviation: PONV, post-operative nausea & vomiting

Printed with permission: Gan TJ, et al. *Anesth Analg* 2003;97(1):62-71.; and Williams KS. *Surg Clin North Am* 2005;85(6):1229-41.

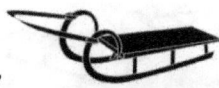

> Treatment

- Give the smooth muscle as well as the CNS receptors which are responsible for the mechanism(s) of action for drugs used for the treatment of **refractory nausea and vomiting**.
  - GI receptors
  - Central
    - H-1 receptor antagonists (inner ear) – diphenhydramine, promethazine
    - Cannabinoids – dronabinol, nabilone
    - Neurokinin (NK)-1-antagonist – aprepitant, talnetant, osanetant
    - Neuroleptic – chlorpromazine, haloperidol
    - Benzodiazepines
    - 5 HT3 antagonist – Ondansetron
    - Metocloprimide
      - D2 antagonist
      - 5HT3/ 5HT4
    - Tricyclic antidepressants (TCA)
    - Steroids (e.g., dexamethasone and Mannitol) (nausea and vomiting due to increased intracranial pressure)

- Give non-prescription drug, dietary and lifestyle modifications therapeutic options for the treatment of nausea and vomiting during **pregnancy**, including dietary and lifestyle modifications, and medical therapy.
  - Avoidance of precipitating factors
  - Frequent, small meals high in carbohydrate and low in fat
  - Stimulation of P6 acupuncture point
  - Ginger
  - Vitamin B6

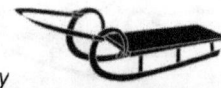

- Give drugs that may be used for nausea and vomiting in pregnancy and give the FDA pregnancy use category.

Drug	FDA Category	Usual Dosage
○ Vitamin B$_6$ (thiamine)	A	10-25 mg three times daily
○ Doxylamine	B	12.5 mg twice daily
○ Prochlorperazine	C	5-10 mg tid
○ Metoclopramide	B	10-20 mg four times daily (qid)
○ Domperidone, cisapride	C	1-20 mg tid or qid
○ Ondansetron	B	4-8 mg tid
○ Promethazine	C	12.5-25.0 mg qid

Adapted from: Thukral C, and Wolf JL. *Nat Clin Pract Gastroenterol Hepatol* 2006; 3(5): pg. 258; and Printed with permission: Keller J, et al. *Nat Clin Pract Gastroenterol Hepatol* 2008; 5(8): pg. 433.

SO YOU WANT TO BE A GASTROENTEROLOGIST!

Patients with a partial gastrectomy and Roux-en-Y anastomosis may develop nausea, vomiting, bloating and early satiety. These symptoms are due to the stasis of food in the gastric remnant as well as the distal Roux jejunal limb, especially, if the Roux limb is > 45 cm. This is called the "**Roux-en-Y stasis syndrome**".

- Give the pathophysiology and non-surgical treatment of the Roux-en-Y stasis syndrome.

  ○ The transection of the jejunum prevents the pacemaker wave generated in the duodenum from passing distal to the level of the transection

  ○ Ectopic pacemakers in the Roux limb cause retrograde contractions leading to ↑ filling of gastric remnant and the Roux limb

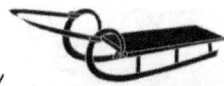

Mastering the Boards: Gastroenterology

A.B.R. Thomson

ACUTE NON-VARICEAL UPPER GI BLEEDING (NVUGIB; UGIB)

➢ Demography

- The overall incidence of hospitalization for UGIB is ~130/10^5 population; incidence is higher among men than women (153 vs 117/10^5).

- UGIB incidence, but not mortality was associated with lower socio-economic status.

- Overall case fatality rates at 30 days after hospital admission was 10.0%; fatality rates rose with age and were higher for men than women and for those with (vs without) comorbid illnesses.

- Adjusted fatality rates are 13% higher for patients admitted on weekends than on weekdays, and 41% higher for patients admitted on holidays than on weekdays (this difference in mortality could be attributed to reduced staffing and lack of availability of endoscopy on weekends and holidays in some hospitals).

- Patients admitted on weekends or holidays suffered higher mortality than those admitted on weekdays (13% higher on weekends, and 41% higher on holidays).

- Fatality rates decreased from 11.4% to 8.6% during the study period.

➢ Clinical

- A negative NG aspirate in the patient who presents with melanoma or hematoschezia reduces the likelihood of an upper GI source of the bleeding, but because of curling of the tube or duodenal bleeding which does not reflux into the stomach, 15-18% of persons with an upper GI source for bleeding will have a non-bloody aspirate.

- The distribution of the endoscopic type of bleeding ulcers is: clear-based, 55%; a flat pigmented spot, 16%; a clot, 8%; a visible vessel, 8%; and active bleeding, 12%.

- RCTs show that adding bolus plus infusion of PPI to endoscopic hemostatic therapy (EHT) significantly decreased bleeding (NNT, 12) surgery (NNT, 28) and death (NNT, 45).

Abbreviations: NG, nasogastric; NNT, number needed to treat

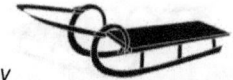

➤ Risk Stratification

• Initial bleeding

• Give patient-related adverse prognostic variables in persons with acute NVUGIB.

  o Increasing age

  o Increasing number of comorbid conditions (especially renal failure, liver failure, heart failure, cardiovascular disease, disseminated malignancy)

  o Shock – hypotension, tachycardia, tachypnea, oliguria on presentation

  o Red blood in the emesis or stool

  o Increasing number of units of blood transfused

  o Onset of bleeding in the hospital

  o Need for emergency surgery

  o Anticoagulant use, glucocorticosteroids

Abbreviations: NVUGIB, non-variceal upper GI bleeding

• Give the performance characteristics of the vital signs and acute blood loss.

Physical Finding	Sensitivity (%)		Specificity (%)
	Moderate Blood Loss	Large Blood Loss	
o Postural pulse increment ≥30/min, or severe postural dizziness*	7-57	98	99
o Supine tachycardia (pulse >100/min)	1	10	99
o Postural hypotension (≥ 20 mm Hg ↓ in SBP)	9	...	90-98
o Supine hypotension (SBP <95 mm Hg)	13	31	98

* best sensitivity and specificity for moderate and large blood loss

Adapted from: McGee S. R. Evidence-Based Physical Diagnosis. 2nd Edition. *Saunders/Elsevier,* St.Louis, Missouri, 2007, Table 15.2 pg. 167

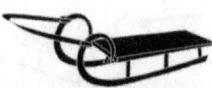

- Give a clinical method to estimate volume depletion.

Clinical	Class I	Class II	Class III	Class IV
o Blood loss (mL)	<750	750-1500	1500-2000	>2000
o Blood loss (% blood volume)	<15	15-30	30-40	>40
o Heart (beats/min)	<100	>100	>120	>140
o Blood pressure	Normal	Normal	Decreased	Decreased
o Pulse pressure	Normal or increased	Decreased	Decreased	Decreased
o Ventilatory rate (breaths/min)	14-20	20-30	30-40	>35
o Urine output (mL/hr)	>30	20-30	5-15	Negligible
o Mental status	Slightly anxious	Mildly anxious	Anxious and confused	Confused and lethargic
o Fluid replacement	Crystalloid	Crystalloid	Crystalloid and blood	Crystalloid and blood

Printed with permission: Atkinson RJ and Hurlston DP. *Best Pract Res Clin Gastroenterol* 2008; 22(2): pg. 234.

- Give the performance characteristics of hypotension and its prognosis.

Finding	PLR
o Systolic blood pressure <90 mm Hg	
– Predicting mortality in intensive care unit	4.0
– Predicting mortality in patients with bacteremia	4.9
– Predicting mortality in patients with pneumonia	10.0
o Systolic blood pressure ≤ 80 mm Hg	
– Predicting mortality in patients with acute myocardial infarction	15.5

Abbreviation: PLR, positive likelihood ratio

Source: McGee S. R. Evidence-Based Physical Diagnosis. 2nd Edition. *Saunders/Elsevier*, St.Louis, Missouri, 2007, Box 15.1 page 161.

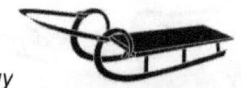

- Give the **Rockall Risk Score Scheme** for assessing prognosis in patients with NVUGIB (PUD), using clinical and endoscopic considerations.

Variable	0	1	2	3
○ Age (years)	< 60	60-79	≥ 80	≥ 80
○ Shock	SBP ≥ 100, PR < 100/min	SBP ≥ 100, PR ≥ 100	SBP < 100 mm, PR ≥ 100	SBP < 100, PR ≥ 100
○ Comorbidity	None	None	Cardiac failure, ischemic heart disease, any major comorbidity	Renal failure, liver failure, disseminated malignancy
○ Diagnosis at time of endoscopy	Mallory-Weiss tear, or no lesion identified and no stigmata of recent hemorrhage	All diagnoses except malignancy	Malignancy of the upper GI tract	-
○ Stigmata of recent hemorrhage	None, or dark spot only		-Blood in upper GI tract -Adherent clot -Visible or spurting vessel	-

Maximum score prior to endoscopic diagnosis=7, maximum score following diagnosis=11

Abbreviations: GI, gastrointestinal; NVUGIB, non-variceal upper GI bleeding; PUD, peptic ulcer disease; PR, pulse rate

➤ Prognosis

- Give factors which are predictive of a poor prognosis after hemorrhage from peptic ulcer.
  - ○ Clinical
    - – Age > 60 years
    - – Bleeding onset in hospital
    - – Comorbid medical illness
    - – Shock or orthostatic hypotension
    - – Multiple transfusions required

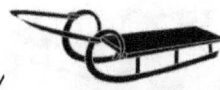

- o Laboratory
  - Coagulopathy
  - Multiple transfusions required
- o Endoscopy
  - Higher lesser curve gastric ulcer (adjacent to left gastric artery)
  - Posterior duodenal bulb ulcer (adjacent to gastroduodenal artery)
  - Endoscopic finding of active bleeding or visible vessel

Printed with permission: Barkun A, et al. Consensus recommendations for managing patients with non-variceal upper gastrointestinal bleed. *Ann Intern Med* 2003; 139: 843-57, Table 19-4.

- Give the **Forrest endoscopic classification** of bleeding gastroduodenal ulcers.
  - o 1a, spurting
  - o 1b, ouzing
  - o IIa, non bleeding visible vessel (VV)
  - o IIb, adherent clot
  - o IIc, flat pigment spot
  - o III, clean ulcer base
    - No scoring system has been validated to predict when rebleeding will occur after endoscopic hemostatic therapy (El munzer et al., 2008).
      - Thus it is not recommended to routinely perform a "second-look EGD".
    - Individualize such practice based on the unproven endpoints of clinically apparent recurrent bleeding, unexplained low level of hemoglobin concentration after appropriate transfusion, hemodynamic instability, multiple patient morbidities, or a high risk bleeding lesion seen at the index of EGD.

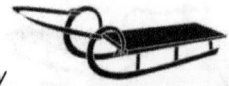

- Give the rates (%) of rebleeding, surgery and mortality, without and with **endoscopic hemostatic therapy** (ET), using the **Forrest classification** of bleeding peptic ulcers.

EGD Appearance	Prevalence	Rebleeding Rate (%) No EHT EHT(~70%↓)		Surgery Rate (%) No EHT EHT (~80%↓)		Mortality rate (%) No EHT EHT (~50%↓)	
		EHT°	EHT⁺	EHT°	EHT⁺	EHT°	EHT⁺
o Active Bleeding (Ib, ouzing)*	18	55	20	35	7	11	<5
o Visible vessel (IIa); not bleeding	17	43	15	34	6	11	<5
o Adherent clot (IIb)	15	22	5	10	2	7	<3
o Flat pigmented spot (IIc)	15	10	<1	6	<1	3	<1
o Clean ulcer base (III)	35	<5	<1	<1	<1	<1	<1

*Forrest 1a, active bleeding (spurting)

Abbreviation: EHT, endoscopic hemostatic therapy

Printed with permission: Atkinson RJ and Hurlstone DP. *Best Pract Res Clin Gastroenterol* 2008; 22(2): pg. 235.

Recurrent/Persistent Ulcer Bleeding

There are additional factors which increase the patient's risk for persistent or recurrent NVUGIB.

- o Rochwall score at index EGD
- o Active bleeding (Forrest Ia, Ib)
- o DU, lesser curve of stomach
- o Large GU/DU > 1 to 2 cm
- o End-stage renal disease on dialysis, OR, 3

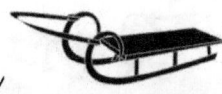

- Give clinical endpoints which suggest recurrent NVUGIB.
  - If you see blood: NG tube bloody, hematemesis, melena
  - Blood counts ↓ hemoglobin ≥ 2 g/dL after 2 consecutive stable hemoglobins taken 3 hrs apart
  - Vital signs
    - 1 hr of hemodynamic stability: HR ≥ 110 bpm, SB ≤ 90 mm Hg (in the absence of sepsis, cardiogenic shock) or ↑ HR / ↓ SBP within 8 hr post index EGD despite
      No other explanation e.g., sepsis, cardiogenic shock
      - Continued melena, hematochezia

- Give risk factors for persistent or recurrent gastrointestinal tract bleeding, as well as their approximate odds ratio (OR) for ↑ risk.

Risk Factors	OR
o Clinical Factors	
– Age ≥ 70 yr	2.2
– Age > 65	1.3
– Health status (ASA class 1 vs 2-5)	1.9-7.6
– Comorbid illness	1.6-7.6
– Erratic mental status	3.2
– Shock (systolic blood pressure < 100 mm Hg)	1.2-3.7
o Presentation of Bleeding	
– Hematemesis	1.2-5.7
– Red blood on rectal examination	3.8
– Melena	1.6
– Transfusion requirement	NA
o Laboratory Factors	
– Coagulopathy	2.0
– Initial hemoglobin ≤ 10 g/dL	0.8-3.0
o Endoscopic Factors	
– Ulcer location high on lesser curve	2.8
– Diagnosis of gastric or duodenal ulcer	2.7
– Ulcer location on superior wall of duodenum	13.9
– Ulcer location on posterior wall of duodenum	9.2
– Active bleeding	2.5-6.5
– High-risk stigma	1.9-4.8
– Clot over ulcer	1.7-1.9
– Ulcer size ≥ 2 cm	2.3-3.5

Printed with permission: Barkun A, Bardou M, Marshall JK. *Ann Intern Med* 2003; 139: 843-57, Table 19-5.

206

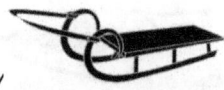

- Give risk factors for peptic ulcer rebleeding after successful endoscopic hemodynamic therapy.
    - Hemodynamic instability
    - Active bleeding at endoscopy (spurting more than oozing)
    - The large ulcers (either > 1 cm or > 2cm as the threshold)
    - Posterior duodenal ulcer or high lesser curve gastric ulcer
    - Need for red blood transfusion

- Give the clinical features of upper gastrointestinal bleeding elderly versus younger patients.
    - Similarities
        - Presenting manifestations of bleeding: hematemesis (50%); melena (30%); hematemesis and melena (20%)
        - Peptic ulcer disease most common etiology
        - Safety and efficacy of endoscopic therapy
    - Differences (elderly vs younger patients)
        - Fewer antecedent symptoms (abdominal pain, dyspepsia, heartburn)
        - Prior aspirin and NSAID use
        - Presence of comorbid conditions
        - Higher rates of hospitalization
        - Higher rates of rebleeding Higher mortality rate

Adapted from: Farrell JJ, and Friedman LS. *Gastroenterol Clin North Am.* 2001;30(2):377-407, viii.

CLINICAL TIP

- Give the reason why a person with isolated IgA deficiency should not be given a blood transfusion.

    - The patient would have IgG and IgE antibodies (anti-IgA antibodies), which would react against the IgA in the transfused blood, just as would happen with IV immunoglobulins.

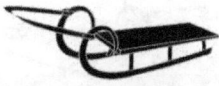

➢ Treatment

❖ UGIB inpatient with no suspected/known liver disease
- o Stabilize ABC's
- o IV fluids
- o Transfuse PRBC to maintain hemoglobin concentration at 70 g/L (90
  g/L for patient with angina/ischemic heart disease)
- o O$_2$ by nasal probes/mask, as indicated
- o ECG if clinically indicated
- o Routine blood work, including CBC, electrolytes, Cr/BUN, LEs, LFTs
- o Monitor renal function and adequacy of fluid replacement
- o Risk stratification
  - – Without/before EGD   ▪ Blatchford score
  - – With/after EGD   ▪ Rockall score
                             ▪ Forrest score
- o Acid inhibition
  - – Continuous IV PPI or bid PPI infusion may be given after EGD, to
    determine duration of PPI infusion
  - – IV PPI may be given before EGD to "down grade" Rockall risk
    score: 80 mg IV bolus over 30 min, then 8 mg/hr
    - ▪ High stigma lesion, continuous 72 hr IV infusion, followed by
      PPI po, duration depending upon lesion
    - ▪ Low risk lesion d/c IV infusion after EGD; switch to PPI o, for
      duration dependent upon diagnosis of cause

Abbreviations: EGD, esophagogastroduodenoscopy; LEs, liver enzymes;
LFTs, liver function tests; PRBC, packed red blood cells

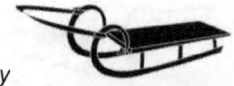

208

- Give the benefits of empiric PPI infusion before EGD is recommended in the care of patients with non-variceal UGIB.
  - Downgrade the severity of the lesion and the risk of it rebleeding or requiring surgery (i.e., changing Forrest Ib → IIa)
  - ↓ activation of platelets
  - ↓ peptic digestion of clot ↑ cost effectiveness
  - Downgrading of Rockall risk when giving IV PPIs to EGD /EHT

	IV PPI Infusion	Placebo
– Active bleeding on EGD	6%	15%
– Need for EHT	19%	28%

  - Oral PPIs
    - Use high dose oral PPI to approximate IV PPI infusion e.g., lansoprazole 30 mg tabs 4, then 30 mg (tabs 1) p q 30 min
  - Octreotide and somatostatin
    - Potential explanation for clinical benefit
      - ↓ splanchnic blood flow
      - ↓ gastric acid secretion
      - ↑ gastric cytoprotection
    - When to use
      - When EGD/EHT is not available, and PPI infusion or high-dose po has not been effective
  - Endoscopic hemostatic therapy (EHT)
    - Two modalities
      - Injection
      - Cautery
      - Clipping

      ] ~66% ↓ risk of rebleeding, need for surgery, and death
  - Assess for H. pylori infection
    - By standard methods
    - Beware that blood in the stomach may render the biopsy-based tests and the urea breath test negative
    - If a benign appearing gastric ulcer, take 6 gastric mucosal biopsies from the rim of the ulcer at the time of the initial EGD, or shortly after the bleeding has stopped, then repeat EGD after 8-12 wk of PPI treatment to confirm complete healing of the gastric ulcer.
    - Caution
      - If H. pylori infection diagnosed, tract with appropriate antibiotic and PPI combinations, and confirm eradication of H. pylori

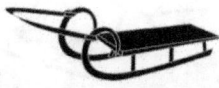

- Overall benefit of EHT, 2/3 ↓ in risk of rebleeding, surgery, death
  - OR for use of EHT in high-risk lesions
    - Recurrent bleeding, 0.46
    - Need for surgery, 0.59
- Overall benefit of PPI infusion after EHT, ~ ½ further ↓ in risk of rebleeding, surgery, death
- Timing
  - Usually with 24 hrs of index bleed
  - Earlier may be necessary in some patients
  - Best done with full GI bleeding term of experience endoscopy nurses, staff, trainees, and available anaesthesiologists and general surgeons
- Adherent clots
  - Gently wash to visualize nature of underlying lesion
- Use two modalities of endoscopic hemostatic treatment, e.g., injection of epinephrine plus thermal coagulation or hemostatic clips
  - Epinephrine 1:10,000 dilution, 0.5 to 2.0 mL aliquots given into 4 quadrants, within 3 mm of bleeding site

---

Clinical Heads-Ups

Hemospray®, a nanopowder which promotes hemostasis, has been shown in preliminary studies to be 95% effective in achieving acute hemostasis in persons with ouzing peptic ulcers.

- Planned and unplanned
  - A planned second-look EGD within 24 hrs of the index EGD may be justified, if there is
    - Poor visualization in the initial EGD
    - Possible poor EHT in the initial EGD
  - An unplanned second-look EGD or recurrent bleeding
    - Persistent
- Interventional Angiography: TAE (transarterial embolization)
  - Success of TAE for index bleed 52% to 88%
  - Risk of rebleeding 10% to 20%
  - After failure EHT – consider TAE for high surgical risk
    - Hematobilia or bleeding into pancreatic duct
- Surgery in NVUGIB
  - Mortality rate
    - Urgent ~25%
    - Elective ~5%
  - Recurrent (post-op) bleeding ~5%

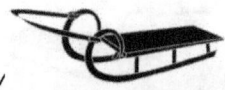

Guidelines Non-Variceal Upper Gastrointestinal Bleeding (NVUGIB)

ICUGBCG. Barkan AN, et al. Ann Intern Med 2010; 152: 101-113.

○ Resuscitation
  – ABC's 2 large bore IVs   – Crystalloid infusion

○ Risk Assessment
  – Blatchford score (predicts low score   – APACHE II
    for EGD)   – Barkan et al. predictors
  – Rockall preendoscopy score (low   – High risk of rebleeding or mortality
    score predicts low mortality)
    ▪ Patient   – > 65
               – Alcoholism, chronic   ▪ Lesion   – Active (Forrest Ia/b)
               – Cancer, active   bleeding or NBVV
               – Comorbidities   (Forrest IIa)
               – Chronic liver disease   – GU, posterior lesser
               – Heart failure   – DU, posterior wall
               – Poor socio-familial conditions

    ▪ Clinical   – FRBPR   ▪ Laboratory   – ↑ BUN / ↑ Cr$_s$
               – Shock   – ALT/AST
               – Syncope

NG tube in-out for melena/uncertain whether U-/LGIB

  – Correct coagulopathy   – Blood transfusions
    preendoscopy PPI therapy   – To maintain Hb 70 g/L

○ Endoscopy   – IIb (remove clot thermal   ○ Feed
  – Institutional protocol   coagulation)   – Low risk 24 hr
  – 24 hr GI bleeding team   – EHT   – High risk 2-3 d
  – Forrest Ia, b; IIa (EHT)   ▪ Injection coagulation
                                      ▪ Clipping

○ PPI therapy
  – Infusion, injection for 3 d for for Ia/b, then po for 4-12 wk
  – PPI po for 4 wk for DU, 12 wk for GU → repeat EGD
                                          Rebleeding

> **Note by Author**
> ○ PPI administration before EHT is recommended to downstage the Forrest Classification of a bleeding ulcer

○ Failed EHT   ○ Repeat   ○ Discharge
                      EHT   – PPI po for 4-12 wk test and treat for Hp
                                        ▪ Confirm eradication of Hp (because of high risk of
  – Therapeutic radiology   – Surgery   recurrent ulcer and bleeding if Hp eradication not
    ▪ Percutaneous   successful
      embolization   – If GU not biopsied at original EGD, then repeat EGD
                                   with 6 biopsies from edge of GU
                                – Confirm healing of GU after 8-12 wk PPI

Abbreviations: ALT/AST, aminotransferases; BUN, blood urea nitrogen; ASA, acetylsalicylic acid ("aspirin"); COX2, cyclooxygenase-2; Cr$_s$, serum creatinine; DU, duodenal ulcer; EGD, esophago-gastroduodenoscopy; EHT, endoscopic hemostatic therapy; FRBPR, fresh red blood per rectum; GU, gastric ulcer; Hb, hemoglobin concentration; Hp, *Helicobacter pylori* infection; ICUGBCG, International Consensus Upper Gastrointestinal Bleeding Conference Group; LGIB, lower gastrointestinal bleeding; NBVV, non-bleeding visible vessel; NG, nasogastric; PPI, proton pump inhibitor

❖ Upper GI bleeding in patient with suspected/known liver disease

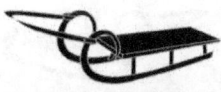

Mastering the Boards: Gastroenterology   A.B.R. Thomson

In the patient with UGIB (upper GI bleeding) and with signs of chronic liver disease, give the patient

- o Stabilize ABC's
- o IV fluids
- o Transfuse PRBC to maintain hemoglobin concentration at 70 g/L (90 g/L for patient with angina/ischemic heart disease)
- o O_2 by nasal probes/mask, as indicated
- o ECG if clinically indicated
- o Routine blood work, including CBC, electrolytes, Cr/BUN, LEs, LFTs
- o Monitor renal function and adequacy of fluid replacement
- o Octreotide sc
  - – For NVUGIB (non-variceal upper GI bleeding)
    - ▪ Octreotide 50 mcg to 100 mcg bolus, then 25 mcg per hour for up to 3 days
  - – For EVB (esophageal variceal bleed)
    - ▪ 50 mcg bolus, followed by 50 mcg per hr
  - – If somatostatin to be used for NVUGIB
    - ▪ 250 mcg by bolus, then 250 mcg/hr, for 3 to 7 days
- o Antibiotics (fluoroquinolone) before and 7 days after UGIB
- o Endoscopy (EGD)
  - – Diagnosis
    - ▪ Exclude EVB/GVB (esophageal or gastric variceal blood) if liver disease and varices
      - – Prophylactic antibiotics
      - – If EVB or GVB → EBL
  - – In fact, while recurrent EV bleeding is common, EGD must be performed with each presentation since just because EV are present does not mean they have bled (e.g., peptic ulcers are common in patients with cirrhosis)
  - – Characteristic signs on the varices and seen on EGD will establish whether the acute UBIB in the patient with liver disease or known EV arose from bleeding EV, from PUD, from a Mallory-Weiss tear of the gastroesophageal junction, from portal hypertensive gastropathy, GAVE (gastric antral vascular ectasia), or a Dieulafoy vascular lesion
- o Co-morbidities to be treated

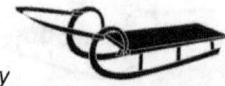

- For NVUGIB (non-variceal upper GI bleeding)
  - Octreotide 50 mcg to 100 mcg bolus, then 25 mcg per hour for up to 3 days
- For EVB (esophageal variceal bleed)
  - 50 mcg bolus, followed by 50 mcg per hr
- If somatostatin to be used for NVUGIB
  - 250 mcg by bolus, then 250 mcg/hr, for 3 to 7 days
- Exclude risks for future rebleeding
  - ASA/NSAIDs
    - Use preventive maintenance co-therapy
  - H. pylori
    - Test and treat, then repeat UBT ± EGD biopsies when off PPI for > 7 days
  - H. pylori-negative, NSAID-negative ulcer
    - Maintenance PPI po, in standard dose, ½ hr before breakfast

Abbreviations: ABC's, airway breathing circulation; EVB, esophageal variceal bleed; GVB, gastric variceal bleed; UBT, urea breath test (for H. pylori infection); EHT, endoscopic hemostatic therapy

- Give the **SARIN** classification of gastroesophageal varices (GEV) or isolated gastric varices (IGV).

  - GEV1   – GV in continuity with EV
    - Extend 2 to 5 cm below GE junction
    - Easiest to obliterate with cyanoacrylate

  - GEV2   – GV in continuity with EV
    - GV extend to cardia and fundus

  - IGV1   – No EV
    - GV in fundus
    - Most difficult to obliterate with cyanoacrylate

  - IGV2   – No EV
    - GV in gastric body, antrum, and pylorus

  - Bleeding risk
    - GEV2/IGV1 > GEV1, IGV2 (unless patient is matched for CTP score, in which case the risk of bleeding is similar in each type of varix)

213

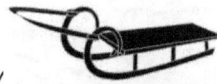

Clinical Tips: To glue or to band gastric varices (GV)

- o Cyanoacrylate injection of GV is superior to EVL or sclerotherapy
- o "Band Ligation of EV greater than 10 mm in diameter usually is unsafe" (Feldman M., et al. Sleisenger and Fordtran's Gastrointestinal and Liver Disease. 9th Edition. Saunders/Elsevier, Philadelphia, 2010, page 1512)
- o EVL of GV in cardia of stomach is safest
- o If bleeding occurs from IGV1 after TIPS, consider transhepatic embolization of fundal GV

➤ Primary prophylaxis
- o EGD surveillance 1 to 2 years
- o Npn-selective beta blocker (NSBB)
  - – Start when
    - ▪ ↑ EV size
    - ▪ Development of red wales
- o Possibly (one study) cyanoacrylate ("glue") injection for large GV

Outcome	"Glue"	NSBB or Placebo
– Probability of first bleed from GV	28%	45%
– Actuarial probability of survival	90%	72%

- o Do not use sclerotherapy, TIPS, or shunt of primary prophylaxis of GV.

"An alcoholic is a person who drinks more than his physician! Don't believe it. TRUST, BUT VERIFY."

Grandad

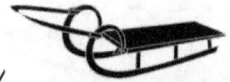

Mastering the Boards: Gastroenterology

A.B.R. Thomson

GASTRIC VARICES (GV)

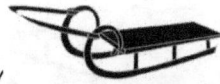

Mastering the Boards: Gastroenterology A.B.R. Thomson

GASTRITIS AND GASTROPATHIES

➤ Terminology

- o AMAG, autoimmune metaplastic atrophic gastritis

- o Carditis, inflammation of gastric cardia

- o DCAG, diffuse corporal atrophic gastritis (aka autoimmune metaplastic atrophic gastritis [AMAG], or type A gastritis)

- o EMAG, environmental multifocal atrophic gastritis

- o GCP, gastritis cystica profunda

- o Multifocal atrophic gastritis (MAG; aka metaplastic atrophic gastritis)
  - Patchy
  - Gastric body and antral mucosa
  - Often associated with
    - H. pylori infection
    - Hyperplastic, hypersecretory gastropathy (HHG; aka Ménétrier disease)

- o APG, H. pylori gastritis

- o PG, phlegmonas gastritis

➤ Causes/associations

- Give causes of histologically diagnosed gastritis.
  - o Drugs, chemicals, radiation
    - Medications
      - Aspirin, NSAIDs, COXIBs
      - Bisphosphonates, K⁺ tablets
    - Drugs, chemicals
      - Alcohol, bile, cocaine, chemotherapy, radiotherapy, red peppers, pickles
  - o Infection
    - Bacterial - H. pylori, Mycobacteria
    - Viral-CMV, HSV
    - Fungal
    - Parasitic
  - o Graft-versus-host disease (GVHD)
  - o Autoimmune gastritis (pernicious anemia)

216

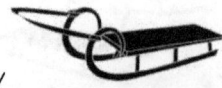

- o Ischemia
  - – Atherosclerosis
  - – Sepsis
  - – Burns
  - – Shock
  - – Mechanical ventilation
- o Associated with liver disease
  - – GAVE
  - – PHG
- o Trauma/foreign body
  - – Nasogastric or gastrostomy tubes
  - – Bezoar
  - – Prolapse/sliding hiatal hernia/paraesophageal hernia
  - – Cameron ulcer (ulcer in hiatus hernia)
- o Infiltration/tumour
  - – Lymphocytic/collagenous
  - – Granulomatous
  - – Eosinophilic
  - – Tumour
- o Miscellaneous'
  - – Gastritis cystica profunda
  - – Ménétrier disease (hyperplastic, hypersecretory gastropathy [HHG])

Abbreviations: CMV, cytomegalovirus; GAVE, gastric antral vascular ectasia; GVHD, graft-versus-host disease; HSV,herpes simplex virus; PHG, portal hypertensive gastropathy

Adapted from: Lee EL, and Feldman M. *Sleisenger & Fordtran's gastrointestinal and liver disease: Pathophysiology/Diagnosis/Management* 2006: pg. 1068.; and Printed with permission: Francis DL. *Mayo Clinic Gastroenterology and Hepatology Board Review*; 2008:67.

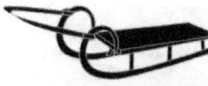

Mastering the Boards: Gastroenterology   A.B.R. Thomson

➤ Pathological types

- Give the characteristics of **distinctive gastritides**.
  - HPG (H. pylori gastritis)
    - Active gastritis (aka acute gastritis)
      - Neutrophils, lymphocytes, plasma calls in mucosa and submucosa
    - Epithelial damage
      - ↓ surface mucin
      - Nuclear changes
      - Lymphoid follicles
    - May be associated with
      - EMAG (environment multifocal atrophic gastritis)
      - Lymphocytic gastritis (> 5 lymphocytes per 100 cells)

  - EMAG (environmental multifocal atrophic gastritis)
    - 85% of EMAG caused by H. pylori
    - Body
      - Atrophic gastritis
      - Pseudopyloric metaplasia (stains positive for PG1 [pepsinogen 1])
    - Body/antrum
      - Atrophy
      - Intestinal metaplasia

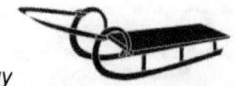

Mastering the Boards: Gastroenterology   A.B.R. Thomson

- AMAG/DCAG) (autoimmune metaplastic atrophic gastritis, aka diffuse corporal atrophic gastritis), or type A gastritis
  - Parietal cell antibodies to H^+, K^+ - ATPase
  - Thin fundic/body mucosa
  - Flat gastric folds
  - ↑ gastrin
    - ↓ HCl
    - Antral G-cells (secrete antibacterial HD-5 [human defensin-5)
    - Progression of metaplasia to dysplasia/GCA: ↑ CDX_2 (type III)

SO YOU WANT TO BE A GASTROENTEROLOGIST!

- AMAG (autoimmune metaplastic atrophic gastritis)/DMAG (diffuse corporal atrophic gastritis) results in increased antibodies to parietal cell antigens
- The parietal cell antibodies to H^+, K^+ ATPase lead to increased CD_4^+ lymphocytes.

- Give the consequences of the increased CD_4^+ lymphocytes in AMAG/AMAG.

  The increased CD_4^+ lymphocytes in the inflammation of AMAG/DMAG leads to

  - ↑ Th1 cytokines → ↑ secretion of immunoglobulins by B lymphocytes
  - ↑ cytotoxicity mediated by performin
  - ↑ FAS ligand-mediated apoptosis

- Phlegmonous gastritis (PG)
  - PG is also known as suppurative gastritis (SG).
  - PG/SG may progress to
    - ANG (acute necrotizing gastritis), which represents gangrene of the stomach
    - Emphysematous gastritis, as the result of the necrotic gastric wall becoming infected with a gas-forming organism (e.g., Clostridium welchii)

219

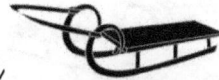

- Collagenous gastritis
  - Chronic gastritis
    - Superficial
    - Patchy
  - Atrophy
    - Focal
  - Collagen
    - Focal deposits
    - Subepithelial thickening of the collagen band (20 to 75 μm thick)

- Gastritis cystica profunda (GCP)
  - Rare
  - Unknown cause
  - May be associated with
    - Gastric surgery (Bilroth II)
    - Atrophic gastritis
    - Inverted hyperplastic gastric polyp
  - Histology
    - Foveolar hyperplasia
    - Cystic glands extending into muscularis mucosae, submucosa, muscularis propria

- Give the reason why do we need to know about it
  - GCP may be associated with
    - Synchronous or metachronous gastric adenocarcinoma (GCa)
    - GCa of postoperative gastric stump

  - Reactive gastropathies (aka acute erosive gastritis)
    - Necrosis of superficial lamina propria in area of erosion
    - Foveolar hyperplasia
    - Gastric pits
      - Elongated
      - Corkscrew
    - Hemorrhage
      - From > 25% of biopsy samples
      - Atypical nuclei
  - Hyperplastic Gastropathies may be confused with or miscalled Ménétrier disease (aka [hyperplastic, hypersecretory gastropathy])

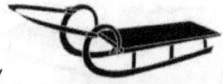

- o Carditis
  - – "Inflammation of the small rim of the cardiac glands at the proximal portion of the stomach" (Feldman M., et al. Sleisenger and Fordtran's Gastrointestinal and Liver Disease. 9th Edition. *Saunders/Elsevier*, Philadelphia, 2010, page 848).

- Give common causes/associations of **carditis**.
  - o GERD (gastroesophageal reflux disease)
  - o H. pylori infection
  - o EMAG (environmental multifocal atrophic gastritis)
  - o AMAG (autoimmune metaplastic atrophic gastritis)

×××

SO YOU WANT TO BE A GASTROENTEROLOGIST!

- Give the differences between Ménétrier disease and hyperplastic, hypersecretory gastropathy (HHG), both of which may show foveolar hyperplasia and cystic dilation on mucosal biopsy.

	Ménétrier Disease	Hyperplastic, Hypersecretory Gastropathy
o Protein losing gastropathy	+	+/-
o Acid secretion	↓	N/↑
o Parietal and chief cells	N/↓	↑
o Inflammation	+/-	-
o Mucus secretion	N/↑	-
o Associated with lymphocytic gastritis	+	-
o Carcinoid-like syndrome (↑ PGE_2)	+	-

Abbreviations: N, normal; PGE_2, prostaglandin E_2

Even in the absence of a decrease in parietal cells in Ménétrierr disease (MD), there is reduced acid secretion (hypochlorhydria) or achlorhydria.

- Give the explanation for the change in acid secretion in MD.

Acid secretion may be reduced or absent in MD even in the absence of a reduction in parietal cells, because of

  - o ↑ TGF-α (transforming growth factor-alpha)
  - o ↑ TGF-α → ↑ EGFR (epidermal growth factor receptor)
  - o EGFR is a receptor for tyrosine kinase (TK)
  - o ↑ EGFR and ↑ TK → ↓ HCl

×××

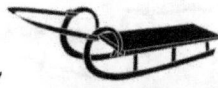

Mastering the Boards: Gastroenterology   A.B.R. Thomson

GASTRIC NEOPLASM

Gastric Polyps

Endoscopic alert
  - Thick gastric folds may be confused with gastric polyps.

- Give causes of thick gastric folds seen on an upper GI series or EGD.
  - Folds not actually thickened (e.g., barium study is wrong – i.e., varices)
  - Malignant – adenocarcinoma, lymphoma
  - Benign infiltration –granulomas (e.g., sarcoidosis, TB, Crohn disease)
    - Severe gastritis (ethanol, H. pylori)
    - Menetrier disease (hyperplasia)
    - Eosinophilic gastritis
  - Multiple gastric polyps (HNPCC, FAP, fundic gland polyps)
  - Hypersecretion (Zollinger-Ellison Syndrome)
  - Fundic varices
  - Worms

Abbreviations: EGD, esophagogastroduodenoscopy; FAP, familial adenomatous polyposis; GI, gastrointestinal; TB, tuberculosis

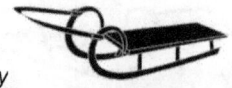

- Give the EGD characteristics and pathological features for types of benign gastric polyps.

Polyp Type	Location	Size	EGD	Pathological Features	Comments
o Fundic gland (75%)	– Fundus and upper body	<1 cm	o Smooth, glassy, transparent; usually multiple polyps are found	– *Helicobacter pylori*-associated gastritis is rare	▪ Associated with PPI use, may regress ▪ Dysplasia found in patients with FAP ▪ Fundic gland polyp: distorted glands and microcysts lined by parietal and chief cells; no or minimal inflammation
o Hyper-plastic (20%)	– Random, adjacent to ulcers or stoma sites, or the cardia if related to acid reflux	Generally <1 cm	o Small polyps have a smooth dome o Large polyps are lobulated, and erosions are common	– Atrophic gastritis with intestinal metaplasia – *Helicobacter pylori*-associated gastritis (25%) – Dysplasia is rare (<3%) and found in polyps <2 cm	▪ Hyperplastic elongated, cystic, and distorted foveolar epithelium ▪ Marked regeneration ▪ Stroma with inflammation, edema, and smooth muscle hyperplasia
o Adenoma	– *Incisura angularis*, found in the antrum than fundus	<2 cm	o Velvety, lobular surface; exophytic, sessile or pedunculated; usually solitary (82%)	– Atrophic gastritis with intestinal metaplasia – May be accompanied by coexistent carcinoma	▪ Dysplastic intestinal- or gastric-type epithelium ▪ Variable architecture

Polyp Type	Location	Size	EGD	Pathological Features	Comments
o Inflammatory fibroid	– Submucosal – Near the pyloric sphincter	Median 1.5 cm; generally <3 cm	o Single, firm, sessiole o Well-circumscribe o Uceration is common	– Pernicious anemia commonly found; atrophic gastritis – Genetic mutations are common	▪ CD34+ spindled stromal cells ▪ Inflammatory cells ▪ Thin-walled vessels in a myxoid stroma
o Peutz-Jeghers	– Random	<1 cm	o Pedunculated with a velvety or papillary surface	– Risk of adenocarcinoma rare in gastric polyps	
o Juvenile	– Found more in the body than in the antrum	Variable	o More rounded than hyperplastic polyps o Superficial erosion o Multiple	– Polyps may exclusively involve stomach – Risk of adenocarcinoma rare in gastric polyps	
o Xanthoma	– Antrum, lesser curvature, prepyloric	<3 mm	o Can be multiple in group o Sessile o Pale-yellow o Nodule or plaque	– Chronic gastritis – No association with hyperlipidemia	▪ Xanthoma aggregates of lipid-laden macrophages in the lamina propria
o Pancreatic heterotopias	– Antrum, prepyloric	0.2-4.0 cm	o Solitary o Dome-shaped with central dimple o Smooth surface	– Normal – Very rare instances of associated pancreatitis, islet-cell tumours, adenocarcinom	▪ Normal components of pancreatic parenchyma
o Gastrointestinal stromal tumour	– Random, submucosal	Variable (median 6 cm)	o Well-circumscribed o Overlying mucosa may be ulcerated	– Normal – 25% are malignant – Risk of aggressive behaviour depends on size and mitotic count	▪ CD117+, CD34+ spindle cell or epitheliod cell tumour ▪ Variable pattern, mitoses, and stroma

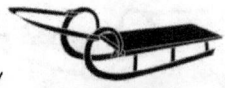

Polyp Type	Location	Size	EGD	Pathological Features	Comments

o Carcinoid	– Body and fundus	<2 cm, larger if sporadic	o Hypergastri-nemic lesions
			o Firm
			o Yellow, broad-based
			o Multiple
			o Sporadic lesions: large and single
				– Autoimmune atrophic gastritis with intestinal metaplasia
				– Parietal cell hyperplasia in ZES
				– Normal mucosa if lesion is sporadic
				– Associated with
				  ▪ Hypergastri-nemia
				  ▪ Autoimmune
				  ▪ Atrophic gastritis
				  ▪ ZES or MEN I
					▪ Nodular proliferation of neuro-endocrine cells >500 μm in diameter

Abbreviations: EGD, esophagogastroduodenoscopy; FAP, familial adenomatous polyposis; MEN, multiple endocrine neoplasia; ZES, Zollinger-Ellison syndrome

Adapted from: Carmack SW, et al. *Am J Gastroenterol* 2009;104(6): 524-532.; and Carmack SW, et al. *Nat Rev Gastroenterol Hepatol* 2009;6(6): 331-341.

Fundic Gland Polyps

➢ Clarification

    o The term "fundic gland polyp" needs to be understood in its context: when the endoscopist reports fundic gland polyps, strictly speaking this means that there are polyps in the fundus or fundic gland area of the stomach.

    o However, the term "fundic gland polyps" is sometimes used interchangeably with the term "fundic gland polyposis", which is defined by their characteristic histpathology.

➢ Causes/associations

    o Idiopathic (sporatic)

    o Hypergastrinemia

    o PPI use

    o H. Pylori infection (possible)

    o Familial adenomatous polyposis (FAP)

    o Cowden syndrome

225

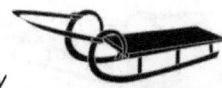

➢ Types

• Give the features which distinguish between sporatic versus familial fundic gland polyposis (FAP), as defined by the above histopathology.

Feature	Sporatic	Familial (FAP)
o Associated with mutations in		
– Beta-catenin gene	+	-
– APC gene (chromosome)	-	+
o Dysplasia	3%	25%

Stromal (Mesenchymal) **Tumours** (aka GIST, gastrointestinal stromal tumours)

➢ Pathology

  o Fat
    – Lipoma
    – Liposarcoma

  o Muscle
    – Leiomyomas
      ▪ Multiple in ~ 25%
    – Leiomyosarcomas
      ▪ Usually exogastric

  o Nerve
    – Schwannomas

  o Desmoid tumours

  o GIST (gastrointestinal stromal tumour) commonest stromal tumour in stomach
    – Usually in gastric fundus or small intestine
    – Endo- (into) or exogastric (away from lumen), given a dumbbell shape
    – Site
      ▪ Stomach   ~70%
      ▪ Small bowel ~25%
      ▪ Colon/rectum 5%
    – Malignant potential
      ▪ All GISTs > 10 mm

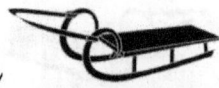

- ➢ Genetic mutations
  - ○ Mutational activation of genes
    - – KIT
    - – PDGFRA
    - – DC117

- ➢ Endoscopic diagnosis
  - ○ EUS plus FNA (fine needle aspiration)

- ➢ Markers for GIST
  - ○ C-kit (a stem cell factor receptor) (~99%)
  - ○ CD34 (a hematopoietic cell progenitor cell antigen) (70%)
  - ○ Smooth muscle actin (20% to 30%)
  - ○ S 100 protein (marker of neural differentiation)

- ➢ Treatment
  - ○ Medical
    - – TK (tyrosine kinase) inhibitors, e.g., imatimib
    - – TK inihibitors control GIST tumour growth in ~80% of patients

---

×××

SO YOU WANT TO BE AN ONCOLOGIST!

- • Give indications for imatinib neoadjuvant therapy prior to resection of a GIST.

  - ○ Unresectable/borderline resectable locally advanced GIST

  - ○ Potentially resectable locally advanced GIST, with extensive organ destruction

  - ○ Source of GIST
    - – Esophagus
    - – EG (esophagogastric junction)
    - – Duodenum
    - – Distal rectum

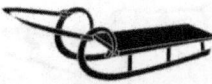

- o Surgical
  - For < 2 cm, resect if EUS shows
    - Irregular borders
      - Cysts
      - Ulceration
      - Echogenic foci
      - Heterogeneity (lack of homogeneity suggests area of necrosis)
    - \> 2 mitoses per 10 hpf
  - for ≥ 2 cm
    - Segmental resection; leaving the tumour pseudocapsule intact
    - Obtain negative tumour resection margins
    - Laparoscopic resection is possible
  - Neoadjuvant TKIs (tyrosine kinase inihibitors) for 6 months, with imaging and reassessment for consideration if possible suitable for resection surgery ("downstaging")
    - GISTs ≥ 3 cm
    - ↓ GIST recurrence post-op
- o Leiomyosarcomas
  - Adjacent structures
    - No invasion   Need a nodal resection), with TFM (tumour-free margins)
    - Invasion   En bloc segmental resection, with TFM

228

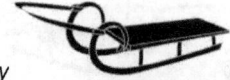

- Survival rates
  - 3 years   53%
  - 5 years   22%
- After ~ 2 years of TKI therapy, tumour may develop new KIT mutations, and tumour grows
  - Options
    - Continue imatinib
    - Switch from imatinib to sunitinib
    - Resection of residual disease, while continuing TKI to prolong progress-free survival
- Metastatic disease
  - Limited progression
    - Continue TKIs, plus surgery
  - Generalized progression
    - TKIs
  - Liver metastases
    - Isolated
      - Hepatic resection plus TKI for non-multifocal bilobar disease (resectable disease)
    - For non-resectable (multi-focal bilobar disease)
      - Hepatic arterial embolization with or without TCI (imatinib or sunitinib [a multi-targeted TKI for imatunib-resistant disease])

"Your present circumstances don't determine where you can go; they merely determine where you start."

Nido Qubein

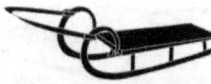

GASTRIC ADENOCARCINOMA (GAC)

- ➢ Incidence
  - o $8/10^5$ in North America
  - o Higher in Japan, some parts of China, Chile, Peru
  - o Lower incidence in Caucasians and in females.

SO YOU WANT TO BE A GASTROENTEROLOGIST!

- o Canadian guidelines recommend that a person with dyspepsia at age 50 or over, or dyspepsia at any age with alarm symptoms (vomiting, bleeding, anemia, dysphagia, weight loss) should have an EGD to diagnose the cause of dyspepsia.

- o Unfortunately, the waiting time for an EGD may be very long (~ 6 months), by which time an early gastric cancer (definition: "a cancer that does not invade beyond the submucosa regardless of lymph node involvement" (Sleisenger and Fordtran's Gastrointestinal and Liver Disease. 10th Edition. *Saunders/Elsevier*, Philadelphia, 2016, page 915) may possibly have advanced.

- • Give the reason why an upper GI (UGI) barium study is not recommended for investigation of dyspepsia, but is still understandably used in the at-risk dyspeptic patient waiting for EGD.

  - o It has all to do with performance characteristics: the sensitivity and specificity of an UGI to detect advanced gastric cancer (GCA) is about 65%, and 90%, respectively. So, a negative UGI does not exclude a serious lesion, and certainly does not exclude EGCA (early gastric cancer), because the sensitivity is disappointingly low.

  - o However, if the UGI shows a suspicious lesion thought to possibly be EGCa, with a specificity of ~ 90%, this information would be forwarded to the consultant and should inspire a prompt endoscopy (EGD).

  - o For staging an GCa, the TNM system is used.

  - o EUS (endoscopic ultrasound) is recommended to stage GAC, including GCA (early gastric cancer).

  - o This is because EUS has 90% accuracy to differentiate between mucosal and submucosal tumour invasion (note that accuracy for restaging T and N after neoadjuvant chemotherapy is lower, ~50%).

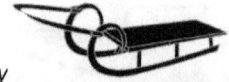

Mastering the Boards: Gastroenterology

A.B.R. Thomson

➢ Causes/associations

• Give reversible and non-reversible risk factors associated with the development of gastric adenocarcinoma (GAC).

- o Reversible – *H.pylori* infection (note: diffuse gastric cancer [linitus plastic] is not associated with H. pylori infection)
  - *Gastric atrophy*
    - Pernicious anemia
    - Chronic atrophic gastritis
    - Subtotal surgical resection with vagotomy for benign gastric ulcer disease
  - Diet
    - Salted, pickled or smoked foods
    - Low intake of fruits and vegetables
  - Life Style
    - Smoking (EtOH is not an independent risk factor)
    - Obesity
  - Esophageal --Barrett esophagus (cancer of gastric cardia)

  Abbreviation: HNPCC, hereditary nonpolyposis colon cancer

  Adapted from: *Sleisenger & Fordtran's Gastrointestinal and Liver Disease: Pathophysiology/ Diagnosis/ Management* 2016: pg 909.

- o Non-reversible
  - Genetic
    - First degree relative with gastric cancer (hereditary diffuse gastric cancer; 2-3 fold ↑ risk with mutations in E-cadherin CDH1 gene)
    - Predisposition for diffuse >> intestinal-type GCa
    - Familial clustering (in 10%)
    - Twins: monozygotic HR (hazard ratio), 9.9; dizygotic HR, 6.6
  - Molecular factors
    - ↑IL-1β → ↑ gastric MDSCs (myeloid-derived suppressor cells)
    - Polymorphisms
      - TNF-α
      - IL-10
      - TNF-α plus IL-10
  - TLRs (toll-like receptors, 27x ↑ risk of GCa i.e., pattern recognition receptors, especially TLR-2)
  - Syndrome
    - HNPCC >> FAP
    - Polyps--adenomatous gastric polyps (HNPCC, FAP), Peutz-Jegher syndrome (PJS), hamartomas, Menetrier syndrome

231

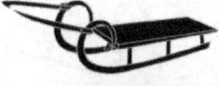

➤ Genetics

- Give examples of common genetic abnormalities in GAC.

The common ($\sim \geq 40\%$ gene frequency) genetic abnormalities in gastric adenocarcinoma are

- o Gene deletion/suppression
    - TP 53
    - FHIT (fragile histidine triad gene)
    - APC (adenomatous polyposis coli) gene LOH (loss of heterogeneity)
    - DCC (deleted in colorectal cancer)

- o ↓ gene expression (due to epigenetic promoter hypermethylation)
    - p16 (marker for poor differentiation)
    - TFF_1 (human trefoil factor 1)
    - $RUNX_3$ (Runt-related transcription factor 3)
    - p27 (associated with a poor prognosis)
    - CDH_1
        - Encodes for E-cadherin (acts as a tumour suppressor gene)
        - Seen in HDGC (hereditary diffuse gastric cancer)

- o ↓ gene expression (due to epigenetic promoter hypermethylation)
    - MLH_1 and MLH_2 (human mut L homolog 1, MSI [microsatellite instability] phenotype)

- o ↑ gene expression (over amplification)
    - COX-2 (cyclooxygenase-2)
    - HGF (hepatocyte growth factor)
    - VEGF (vascular endothelial growth factor)
    - c-Met
    - AIB-1 (amplified in breast cancer)

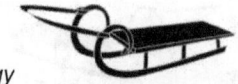

- o DNA aneuploidy
  - – Beta-catenin
  - – EGF/EGFR (epidermal growth factor/epidermal growth factor receptor)

- o Mutations
  - – PIC3A (encodes for a catalytic subunit of PI3K (phosphatidylinositol 3-kinase)
  - – PTPRT (protein-tyrosine phosphatase receptor-type)

- o Microsatellite instability

See Feldman M., et al. Sleisenger and Fordtran's Gastrointestinal and Liver Disease. 9th Edition. *Saunders/Elsevier*, Philadelphia, 2016, Table 54.2, page 908, for a detailed list of genetic abnormalities in gastric adenocarcinoma (GAC).

- • Give the genetic abnormalities which may lead to **diffuse-type** gastric cancer (linitus plastic).

  - o Gene
    - – Deletion/suppression
    - – ↓ expression due to hypermethylation
    - – Amplification/overexpression
    - – Mutations

  - o DNA aneuploidy

  - o Microsatellite instability

- ➢ Endoscopy

- • Give the Japanese and Paris classification of gastric cancer.

Type	Japanese Classification	Paris Classification
0	Superficial, flat tumours with or without minimal elevation or depression	Superficial polypoid, flat/depressed, or excavated tumours
0 – I	Protruded	Polypoid

0–Ip
Protruded, pedunculated

0–Is
Protruded, sessile

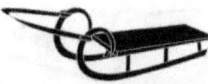

Type	Japanese Classification	Paris Classification
0 – IIa	Superficial and elevated	Non-polypoid and non-excavated, slightly elevated

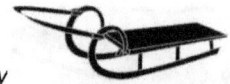

0–IIa
Superficial, elevated

0 – IIb	Flat	Non-polypoid and non-excavated, completely flat

0–IIb
Flat

0 – IIc	Superficial and depressed	Non-polypoid and non-excavated, slightly depressed without ulcer

0–IIc
Superficial shallow, depressed

0 – III	Excavated	Nonpolypoid with a frank ulcer

0–III
Excavated

1	Polypoid tumours that are sharply demarcated from the surrounding mucosa and are usually attached on a wide base	Polypoid carcinomas that are usually attached on a wide base
2	Ulcerated carcinomas that have sharply demarcated and raised margins	Ulcerated carcinomas that have sharply demarcated and raised margins
3	Ulcerated carcinomas that have no definite limits and infiltrate into the surrounding wall	Ulcerated, infiltrating carcinomas that have no definite limits

Type	Japanese Classification	Paris Classification
4	Diffusely infiltrating carcinomas in which ulceration is not usually a marked feature	Nonulcerated, diffusely infiltrating carcinomas
5	Carcinomas that cannot be classified into any of the above types	Unclassifiable advanced carcinomas

- o According to Japanese classification of gastric carcinoma, for the combined superficial types, the type occupying the largest area should be described first, followed by the next type (e.g., IIc+III).
- o Types 0 I and 0 IIa are distinguished from each other by lesion thickness
- o Type 0 I lesions have thickness more than twice that of the normal mucosa and type 0 IIa lesions have a thickness up to twice that of the normal mucosa. Modified from data presented in the Japanese classification of gastric carcinoma and the Paris endoscopic classification of superficial neoplastic lesions.

Printed with permission: Yamamoto H. *Nat Clin Pract Gastroenterol Hepatol* 2007;4(9): pg. 513; and Feldman M., et al. Sleisenger and Fordtran's Gastrointestinal and Liver Disease. 10th Edition. *Saunders/Elsevier*, Philadelphia, 2016, Figure 54.6, page 914.

- ➢ Pathology
    - o Types
        - – Diffuse-type ("linitis plastic") gastric cancer tends to be more closely related to genetic factors than is the case for intestinal-type GAC, which is linked more closely to dietary and environmental factors (e.g., H. pylori infection).

- • Give pathological differences between intestinal and diffuse gastric adenocarcinomas (Lauren classification).

Feature	Intestinal	Diffuse
o Incidence	↓ -ing	Steady
o Low risk areas	-	+
o Worse prognosis	-	+
o Risk factors diet/environment	+	-
o Gland-like tubular structures	+	-
o Singly invasive tumour cells	-	+
o Linitis plastic	-	+

235

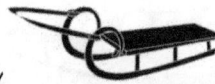

o Another classification
  – Proximal cardia, GE junction
  – Distal fundus, body, antrum
  – Incidence
    ▪ Proximal ↑ ing
    ▪ Distal ↓ ing

• Give sites for metastatic GAC.

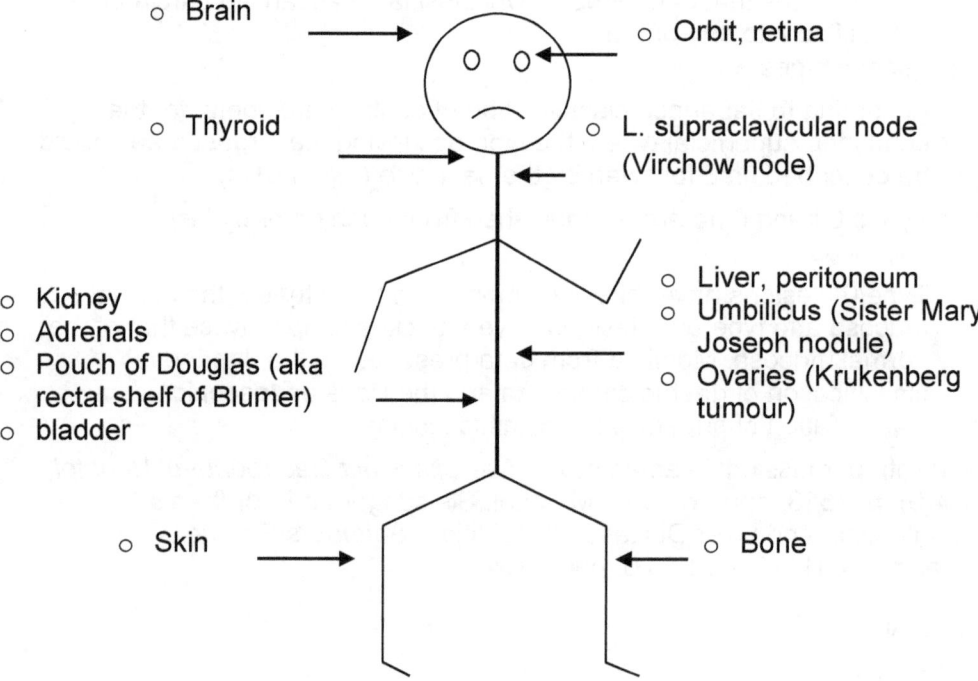

o Brain

o Orbit, retina

o Thyroid

o L. supraclavicular node (Virchow node)

o Kidney
o Adrenals
o Pouch of Douglas (aka rectal shelf of Blumer)
o bladder

o Liver, peritoneum
o Umbilicus (Sister Mary Joseph nodule)
o Ovaries (Krukenberg tumour)

o Skin

o Bone

• Give the generally accepted criteria for EMR (endoscopic mucosal resection) in EGC (early gastric cancer).

  o "the [gastric} cancer is located in the mucosa and the lymph nodes are not included, as indicated by EUS"

  o There is no ulcer scar and the maximum size of the tumour is
    – Type IIa less than 2 cm when the lesion is slightly elevated
    – Type IIb or IIc, less than 1 cm when the tumour is flat (b) or slightly depressed (c)

  o There is no evidence of
    – Multiple gastric cancers, or
    – Simultaneous abdominal cancers

  o "The cancer is of the intestinal type" (i.e., not the diffuse "linitis plastica" type)

Feldman M., et al. Sleisenger and Fordtran's Gastrointestinal and Liver Disease. 9th Edition. *Saunders/Elsevier*, Philadelphia, 2010, page 903.

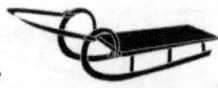

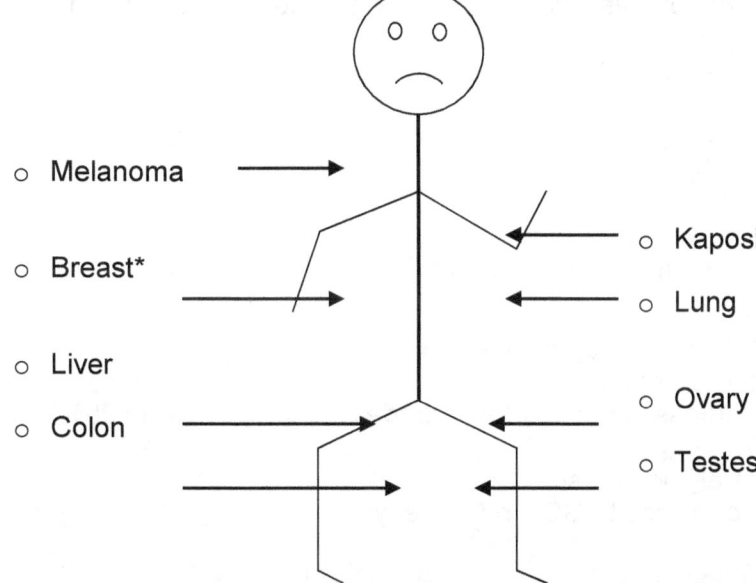

SO YOU WANT TO BE A GI ONCOLOGIST!

- Give primary tumours which commonly metastasis to the stomach.

    o Melanoma

    o Breast*

    o Liver

    o Colon

    o Kaposi

    o Lung

    o Ovary

    o Testes

*Breast cancer is the commonest primary tumour with metastased to the stomach.

- Give pathological **premalignant conditions** for GAC.

    o H. pylori infection may be considered a premalignant condition, and treatment of this infection either early in life (before "point of no return") or in persons who have had EMR (endoscopic mucosal resection) for early gastric cancer may reduce the risk of development or redevelopment of GAC.

    o Chronic atrophic gastritis
      - Risk of progression of chronic atrophic gastritis to GAC
        - 1% per year
        - Depends on the extend of CAG
        - MAG >> corporal atrophic gastritis risk

      - Production of pepsinogens (PG) from oxyntic cells
        - ↓ PGI
        - PG II, normal
        - ↓ PG I/PG II

237

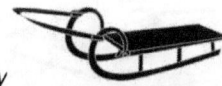

- Intestinal metaplasia (IM)
  - Type I
    - Complete metaplasia
      - Absorptive cells with BBM (brush border membrane)
      - Paneth cells
      - Goblet cells (sialomucins)
  - Type II
    - Incomplete
      - Goblet cells
  - Type III
    - Intermediate
  - Risk of early GCA in type II/III IM. 42% in 5 years
- Dysplasia
  - LGD (low grade dysplasia)
    - Regresses, 60%
    - Progresses to HGD (high grade dysplasia), 10% to 20%
  - HGD
    - Rarely progresses
    - Progresses to GCa in 5% per year

- Adenoma

- Give the risk of gastric polyps progressing to gastric cancer (GCa).

Type	Progression to GCa
Adenoma	3% per 4 yr
FAP (dysplasia in 40%)	
- > 1 cm	1% per yr
- In FAP	Dysplasia in 40%
Ménétrier disease	15%
Hyperplastic, hypersecretory gastropathy(HHG)	Rare

- Give types of gastric adenoma.
  - Intestinal type
  - Pyloric gland
  - Foveolar gland type

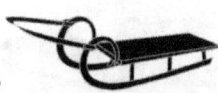

Mastering the Boards: Gastroenterology　　　　　　　　A.B.R. Thomson

- o H. pylori has been declared by the WHO to be carcinogenic, with an attributable risk for gastric cancer of ~60%.

- o In addition to the dietary and life style factors, as well as the molecular factors which represent a genetic basis for non-H.pylori GCa (cytokines [IL-1β, polymorphisms of TNF-α and IL-10), and TLR (toll-like receptors, especially TLR-2), there are molecular factors related to H. pylori which may increase the risk of GCa.

- Give **molecular factors** which increase the risk of carcinogenesis from H. pylori.

  - o Motility
    - – Proteins (Fla A, Fla B) providing for spiral movement of H. pylori

  - o Buffering of gastric acid (↓ H^+ secretion)
    - – Urease gene cluster (Ure A, Ure B)

  - o Adhesion protein
    - – Hop protein (outer membrane proteins)
    - – Adhesion
      - Bab A (encoded by gene Bab A_2)
      - Bab A (binds to blood group antigen Lewis B)

  - o Cag pathogenicity island
    - – ↑ risk (2 - 28x) of GAC with Cag A^+ H. pylori

  - o Molecular needles
    - – TFSS (type 4 secretion system) enhances movement of Cag A^+ bacterial protein into gastric epithelial cells

  - o Vacuolation
    - – Vac A protein, a pore-forming vacuolating toxin, especially in the presence of Cag A^+ H. pylori strains, reduce the activation of T cells, and increase the risk of GAC.

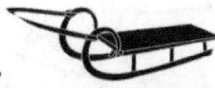

Mastering the Boards: Gastroenterology   A.B.R. Thomson

- Give the approximate annual risk of developing GAC from premalignant lesions.

Condition	Annual Risk	Recommended EGD/Biopsy Follow-up
o Atrophic gastritis (AG)	– 0.1%	▪ None
o Intestinal metaplasia (IM)	– 0.25%	▪ 2-3 years
o Mild to moderate dysplasia (MMD)	– 0.6%	▪ 1 year
o Severe dysplasia (SD)	– 6.0%	▪ Definitive therapy (EMR)

Abbreviation: EGD, esophagogastroduodenoscopy

Adapted from: De Vries AC, et al. *Gastroenterology* 2008;134:945-52.

Early Gastric Cancer (EGC)

➤ Definition
- o Gastric cancer which is T1 and N (EGC is gastric cancer which invades no more deeply into the submucosal, regardless of the involvement of lymph nodes).

➤ Pathology
- o Synchronous and metachronous EGC

	Synchronous EGC (second EGC within 1 year)	Metachronous EGC
– EMR	9%	8%
– Partial gastrectomy	-	2% to 8%

- o EGC with lymph node involvement
  - – Mucosal EGC   2% to 3%
  - – Submucosal EGC 20% to 30%

- Give the effect of the number of perigastric lymph nodes on the long-term survival from early gastric cancer.

# of nodes	Long-Term Survival
0	92-95%
1 to 3	82-88%
4 to 6	73%
> 6	27%

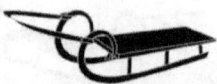

➤ Treatment

    o Staging

- Give the role of MDCT (multi-detector row CT) in staging GAC.

  o MDCT "….appears to have comparable accuracy to EUS in terms of T and N staging of GAC" (Sleisenger and Fordtran's Gastrointestinal and Liver Disease. 9th Edition. *Saunders/Elsevier*, Philadelphia, 2010, page 901; and 10th Edition, 2016, page 916).

  o Test-and-treat for associated H. pylori infection
    - Because H. pylori load falls with development of EGC, biopsies may be false negative
    - Treat for H. pylori infection based on positive serology
    - Treating H. pylori infection in EGC managed by EMR ↓ tumour recurrence at 3-years (OR, 0.35)

  o EMR (endoscopic mucosal resection)

  o EMR/ESR

- Give the standard guidelines for endoscopic therapy (EMR endoscopic mucosal resection, and ESR [endoscopic submucosal resection]) for EGC (early gastric cancer [intestinal type]).

  o High probability of en bloc resection

  o Tumour history
    - Intestinal type adenocarcinoma
    - Tumour confined to the mucosa
    - Absence of venous or lymphatic invasion

  o Tumour size and morphology
    - < 20 mm in diameter, without ulceration
    - < 10 mm in diameter if Paris classification IIb or IIc

  o Expanded criteria for EMR/ESR
    - Mucosal tumour of any size without ulceration
    - Mucosal tumour < 30 mm with ulceration
    - Adjuvant therapy for EGC with positive nodes
    - Observation for T1N0
    - Submucosal tumours < 30 mm confined to the upper 0.5 mm of the submucosal without lymphovascular invasion
    - Successful EMR ~85% (lower success rates with eGC > 2 cm, ulcerated, 1cm, or undifferentiated)
    - 5 year survival rates ~86%

241

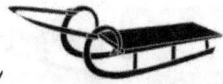

- For incomplete resections
  - Repeat EMR
  - Laser irradiation
  - Heater probe cantery
    - Surgical resection
- If positive lateral margins and negative vertical margins
  - no submucosal or lymphovascular invasion
- Piecemeal resection ↑ risk of recurrence (28%)
  - ESD (endoscopic submucosal dissection)

o ESD complete resection > EMR (83% vs 24%)
  - If positive vertical or lateral resection margins after ESD →
    gastrectomy

- Give the standard guidelines for endoscopic therapy (EMR or ESR) for EGC.

  o PDT (photodynamic therapy)
    - Photofrin II plus argon laser
    - Tissue-destroying

  o Problem: Cannot examine specific to determine if margins are clear

  o Persons with gastric cancer have a 5 year survival rate of only about 25%.

❖ Surgical

- Give the indications for gastrectomy and perigastric regional lymph node
  resection for EGC.

  o Gastrectomy with resection of perigastric regional nodes
    - EGC with positive lateral or vertical margins
    - Laparoscopic lymph node dissection not yet ready for "prime time"
    - 5 year survival rate for EGC treated with gastrectomy ~98%

  o If criteria for EMR are not met → gastrectomy and removal of
    perigastric lymph nodes to ↓ risk of lymph node metastases

  o Type of surgery is determined by site of EGC
    - Upper 1/3   total gastrectomy
    - Lower 2/3   subtotal gastrectomy

  o General indications for gastrectomy with removal of perigastric lymph
    nodes
    - Low probability of en bloc resection with EMR or ESD (i.e., the
      endoscopic resection would be piecemeal)
    - Diffuse rather than intestinal type adenocarcinoma
    - Submucosal tumour size greater than 30 mm, or tumours with ulceration

242

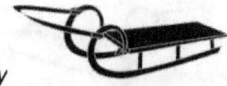

- Evidence of lymphovascular (lymphatic or venous) invasion in the primary tumour, or known/suspected regional lymph node metastases
- Laparoscopic versus open distal gastrectomy give similar outcomes
  - Operative morbidity   22%
  - Operative mortality   0%
  - 5 year survival   96%
  - Disease-specific survival   98%

❖ Chemotherapy/chemoradiation

  o "Chemotherapy for locally advanced gastric cancer without distant metastasis can result in striking of the tumour to the point at which successful curative resection is possible."

  o "Combined chemoradiation after surgical resection appears to be effective at improving progression-free and overall surgical in gastric cancer."

  o After surgical resection for cure of GCa, if these is potential metastasis, intraperitoneal but not systemic chemotherapy may be useful.

  o Post-operative hyperthermic intraperitoneal chemotherapy improves overall survival, as compared with just surgery.

Feldman M., et al. Sleisenger and Fordtran's Gastrointestinal and Liver Disease. 9th Edition. *Saunders/Elsevier*, Philadelphia, 2010, page 904.

Gastric Lymphoma

  o Commonest MALT (mucosa associated lymphoid tissue)

  o Diffuse B cell, or

  o Marginal zone B-cell, or MALT

- Give the distinction between both lymphocytic gastritis and MALT lymphoma both of which are associated with H.pylori infection of the stomach.

  o Lymphocytic gastritis
    - > 25 lymphocytes/100 epithelial cells
    - CD8-positive T lymphocytes
    - Reactive lymphoid follicles
    - Lymphoepithelial lesion of glands
    - Associated with celiac disease

  o MALT
    - Diffuse population of B-cells in lamina propria

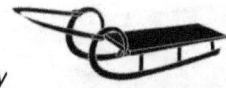

ABBREVIATIONS

5-HT$_3$	5-hydroxytryptamine
AA	Amino acids
ABC	Airway breathing circulation
Ach	Acetylcholine
AG	Atrophic gastritis
AMAG	Autoimmune metaplastic atrophic gastritis
ANG	Acute necrotizing gastritis
ANS	Autonomic nervous system
AP	Action potential
ASA	Acetylsalicylic acid
ASA	American Society of Anesthesiologist
BOM	Bacterial overgrowth syndrome
BOS	Bacterial overgrowth syndrome
BPD	Biliopancreatic diversion
Cag PAI	Cag pathogenicity island
CE	Capsule endoscopy
CNS	Central nervous system
COPD	Chronic obstructive pulmonary disease
COX-2	Cyclooxygenase-2
COXIBs	COX-2 inhibitors
CMV	Cytomegalovirus
CNS	Central nervous system
CT	Concomitant therapy
CTE	CT enterography
CV	Cardiovascular
CVA	Cerebrovascular accident
DBE	Double balloon enteroscopy
DCAG	Diffuse corporal atrophic gastritis
DMN	Dorsal motor nucleus
DU	Duodenal ulcer

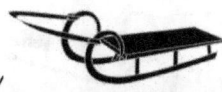

ECa	Esophageal cancer
ECL	Enterochromaffin-like
EGC	Early gastric cancer
EGD	Esophagogastroduodenoscopy
EGFR	Epidermal growth factor receptor
EHT	Endoscopic hemostatic therapy
EMAG	Environmental multifocal atrophic gastritis
EMR	Endoscopic mucosal resection
ENS	Enteric nervous system
EPS	Epigastric pain syndrome
ET	Endoscopic hemostatic therapy
ET	Eradication therapy
EUS	Endoscopic ultrasound
EVB	Esophageal variceal bleed
FAP	Familial adenomatous polyposis
FNA	Fine needle aspiration
GABA	Gamma-aminobutyric acid
GAVE	Gastric antral vascular ectasia
GCa	Gastric cancer
GCP	Gastritis cystica profunda
GERD	Gastroesophageal reflux disease
GET	Gastric emptying test
GI	Gastrointestinal
GIST	Gastrointestinal stromal tumour
GRP	Gastrin related peptide
GU	Gastric ulcer
GVB	Gastric variceal bleed
GVE	Gastric vascular ectasia
GVHD	Graft-versus-host-disease
H2RA	H2 receptor antagonist
HDGC	Hereditary diffuse gastric cancer

246

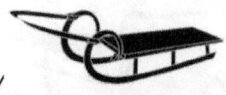

Mastering the Boards: Gastroenterology　　　　　　　　A.B.R. Thomson

HGF	Hepatocyte growth factor
HHG	Hyperplastic, hypersecretory gastropathy
HHT	Hereditary hemorrhagic telegangiectasia
HNPCC	Hereditary nonpolyposis colon cancer
HP-NAP	H. pylori neutrophil-activating protein
HPG	H. pylori gastritis
HSV	Herpes simplex virus
IBS	Irritable bowel syndrome
ICC	Interstitial cells of Cajal
IFN-γ	Interferon-gamma
IM	Intestinal metaplasia
IML	Intermediolateral columns
IMMC	Interdigestive migrating motor complex
IPPN	Isolated pyloric pressure waves "pylorospams"
ITP	Idiopathic thrombocytopenic purpura
LAGB	Laparoscopic adjustable gastric banding
LEs	Liver enzymes
LES	Lower esophageal sphincter
LFTs	Liver function tests
LGD	Low grade dysplasia
LPS	Lipopolysaccharide
MAG	Multifocal atrophic gastritis
MALT	Mucosa-associated lymphoid tissue
MDCT	Multi-detector row CT
MDSCs	Myeloid-derived suppressor cells
MEN	Multiple endocrine neoplasia
MHC	Major histocompatibility
MMD	Mild to moderate dysplasia
mToR	Mammalian target of rapamycin
MU	Marginal ulcer
n	Nerve

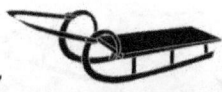

Mastering the Boards: Gastroenterology   A.B.R. Thomson

NA	Nucleus ambiguous
NERD	Non-erosive reflux disease
NFAT	Nuclear translocation of a transcription factor
NNT	Number needed to treat
NO	Nitric oxide
NOD$_1$	Nucleotide-binding oligomerization domain-1
NPV	Negative predictive value
NPY	Neuropeptide Y
NSAIDs	Non-steroidal anti-inflammatory drugs
NUD	Non-ulcer dyspepsia
NVUGIB	Non-variceal upper GI bleeding
OGIB	Obscure GI bleeding
OTC	Over-the-counter
PACAP	Pituitary adenylate cyclase-activating polypeptide
PAMPS	Pathogen-associated molecular receptors
PDT	Photodynamic therapy
PE	Push enteroscopy
PG	Phlegmonas gastritis
PHG	Portal hypertensive gastropathy
PI3K	Phosphatidylinositol 3-kinase
PLR	Positive likelihood ratio
PNS	Parasympathetic nervous system
PONV	Post-operative nausea & vomiting
PP	Plateau potential
PPD	Post-prandial distress
PPIs	Proton pump inhibitors
PPV	Positive predictive value
PR	Pulse rate
PRBC	Packed red blood cells
PTPRT	Protein-tyrosine phosphatase receptor-type
PUD	Peptic ulcer disease

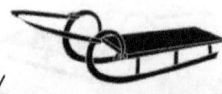

PYY	Peptide YY
RFA	Radiofrequency ablation
RMP	Resting membrane potential
RR	Relative risk
RUNX$_3$	Runt-related transcription factor 3
SBE	Single balloon enteroscopy
RYGB	Roux-en-Y gastric bypass
SBP	Systolic blood pressure
SCF	Stem cell factor
SD	Severe dysplasia
SE	Sleeve gastrectomy
SHR	Endoscopic stigamata of recent hemorrhage.
SIBO	Small intestinal bacterial overgrowth
SIDS	Sudden infant death syndrome
SK	Substance K
SNS	Sympathetic nervous system
SOD	Sphincter of Oddi
SP	Substance P
SSRI	Selective serotonin reuptake inhibitors
SST	Somatostatin
T & T	Test and treat (used in the context of H. pylori infection)
TB	Tuberculosis
TFF$_1$	Trefoil protein
TFM	Tumour-free margins
TGF-α	Transforming growth factor-alpha
TIPS	Transjugular intrahepatic portosystemic shunt
TK	Tyrosine kinase
TLRs	Toll-like receptors
TNF-α	Tumour necrosis factor-alpha
Treg	Regulatory T cells
TS	Tractus solitaries

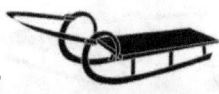

UBT	Urea breath test
UCDA	Ursodeoxycholic acid
UGIB	Upper GI bleeding
VBG	Vertical banded gastroplasty
VEGF	Vascular endothelial growth factor
VIP	Vasoactive intestinal peptides
ZES	Zollinger Ellison syndrome

 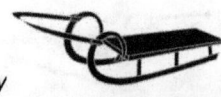

SMALL BOWEL

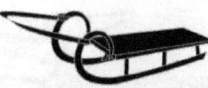

TABLE OF CONTENTS

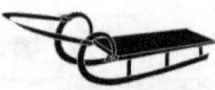

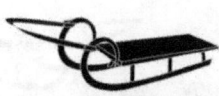

Mastering the Boards: Gastroenterology   A.B.R. Thomson

SMALL INTESTINAL BACTERIAL OVERGROWTH (SIBO) SYNDROME

➢ Microbiology

● Give the usual bacterial presence (10^x/ml) of different sites along the gastrointestinal tract.

   ○ Stomach – 10^3/mL

   ○ Jejunum – 10^4/mL

   ○ Ileum – 10^{6-8}/mL (gram-positive)

   ○ Colon – 10^{10-12}/mL (gram-negative, anaerobic, facultative aerobic)

*note that > 10^5/mL in the proximal small intestine is considered to be abnormal, and is compatible with the diagnosis of SBBO.

➢ Pathgyophysiology

● Give components of the small intestinal mucosal barrier against enteric infection.

Components	Function
○ Lumen	
- Mucus/mucins	▪ Block penetration of ingested antigens
- Proteases: pepsins, pancreatic tryptic enzymes	▪ Breakdown of ingested antigens
- Gastric acid (pH)	▪ Breakdown of ingested antigens
- Bile acids	▪ Breakdown of ingested antigens
- Indigenous microbiotica	▪ Competitive inhibition ▪ *Direct:* competition for essential nutrients and bacterial receptor sites; creation of restrictive physiological environments; secretion of antibiotic-like substances ▪ *Indirect:* chemical modification of bile salts and dietary fats, induction of protective Ig responses, stimulation of peristalsis

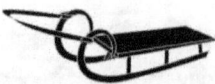

Components	Function

o Epithelium
  - Epithelium:
    glycocalyx (on villi)
	▪ Innate immune response
	▪ Antigen presentation
	▪ Block penetration of ingested antigens (tight junctions)

- Defensins	▪ Antimicrobial peptides
- Trefoil factors	▪ Protection from a variety of deleterious agents (bacterial toxins, chemicals and drugs); provide restitution after mucosal injury
- Secretory-IgA (s-IgA)	
- Paneth cells	▪ Enteric microbial peptides
o Immune system	
- GALT-associated IgA, IgG, IgM (serum)	▪ Clear antigens penetrating gastrointestinal barrier/systemic immunity ▪ Assist in opsonization and phagocytosis of antigens
- Lymphoid follicles in lamina propria (aka Peyer patches)	▪ Clear antigens penetrating gastrointestinal barrier
- Intraepithelial lymphocytes (IEL)	▪ Innate and acquired immune responses
- Mesenteric lymph nodes	▪ Phagocytosis and antigen presentation
- M cells	▪ Overlie lymphoid follicles ▪ Bind, process and deliver pathogens to lymphocytes, macrophages and mucosal lymphoid system ▪ Peyer's patches
– Dendritic cells	
o Muscle - Intestinal peristalsis	▪ Block penetration of ingested antigens

Printed with permission: Acheson DWK. *Best Pract Res Clin Gastroenterol* 2004;18(2):pp 389

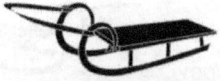

Secretory IgA is the predominant immunoglobulin found in intestinal secretions.

- Give functions of Secretory IgA.

    o Binds bacteria and dietary antigens (thus limiting absorption/immune response)

    o ↑ phagocytosis

- Give the mechanism by which signals from particulate and microbial antigens related to the pathogenicity of luminal microbiota are converged to the intestinal immune system.

    o M cells and mucosal dendritic cells
        – Sampling: TLR (Toll-like receptors, a type of pattern recognition receptor)
        – Signaling; NFkB signals proinflammatory responses

Please see Feldman M., et al. Sleisenger and Fordtran's Gastrointestinal and Liver Disease. 9th Edition. Saunders/Elsevier, Philadelphia, 2010, Table 102.1, page 1992, "Examples of metabolic activities of intestinal microbiota".

➢ Causes/associations

- Give conditions that cause or are associated with small intestinal bacterial overgrowth (SIBO).

    o Atrophic gastritis, pernicious anemia
        – Reduced gastric acid
        – Atrophic gastritis, pernicious anemia
        – Medications (H2 receptor antagonists, proton-pump inhibitors)
        – Gastric surgery

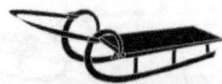

- o Reduced pancreatic and biliary secretion
  - Pancreatic insufficiency
  - Cholestasis

- o Structural abnormalities (neoresevoirs, fistulae)
  - Small bowel diverticulae (not colonic diverticulae)
  - Adhesions
  - Surgical anastomosis and diversions
  - Fistulae (colo-enteric, gastrocolonic)
  - Strictures, webs
  - Absent or incompetent ileocecal valve
  - Defective tight junctions (e.g., celiac disease)

- o Dysmotility syndromes
  - Diabetes
  - Drugs
  - Acute enteric infection
  - Scleroderma
  - Intestinal pseudo-obstruction syndromes
  - IBS-D association, IBS-C association

- o Decreased host defense (decreased immune function)
  - Undernutrition
  - Immune deficiencies particularly absence of secretory immunoglobulin A (IgA)

Abbreviation: SIBO, small intestinal bacterial overgrowth syndrome

➤ Diagnostic tests

• Give tests to diagnose small intestinal bacterial overgrowth (SIBO).

❖ Laboratory

- o Suggestive blood tests: ↓ B12, ↓ Fe, ↑ folic acid (FA), ↑ FA / B12 ratio, ↓ fat soluble vitamins
- o Jejunal
  - Aspiration (>10^5/mL)
  - Luminal bile acids (deconjugated and dehydroxylated)
- o Breath tests
  - CO_2
  - H_2
  - C^{13} glycocholic acid
  - Schilling test (two-step)
  - D-xylose absorption/excretion test

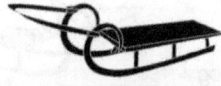

- Stool
  - Weight, fat, bile acids, electrolytes, osmolality

❖ Structural
  - Diagnostic imaging of upper and lower GI tract

Abbreviations: B12, vitamin B12; Fe iron; SIBO, small intestinal bacterial overgrowth syndrome

➢ Treatment

● Give the treatment of the patient with SIBO.
  - Correct any predisposing condition, if possible
  - Nutrition (correction of SIBO complications)
    - Lactose-free, low-residue diet
    - Increase calories/protein if malnourished
    - Micronutrient supplementation – Vitamin B12, fat soluble vitamins (A, D, E and K), calcium, magnesium
  - Drugs
    - Antibiotics versus (gram-neg anaerobes) e.g., metronidazole, tertracycline (not in children), cipro' (not in pregnancy), prebiotics, probiotics
    - Prokinetics
    - Interval or maintenance therapy, where appropriate

Abbreviation: SIBO, small intestinal bacterial overgrowth syndrome

"Never wish life was easier.
Wish you were better."
Jim Rohn

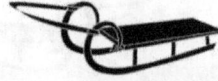

ENTEROHEPATIC CIRCULATION (EHC) OF BILE ACIDS

➢ Bile acid (BA) metabolism

• Give functions of bile acids.

    o Liver   – ↑ hepatic secretion of cholesterol and phospholipids (cholesterol homeostasis)

                  – ↑ bile water flow (choleretic effect)

    o Intestine   – ↑ solubilisation of cholesterol, triglycerides, phospholipids, fat-soluble vitamins

                  – Interact with pancreatic colipase to modify activity of lipase

    o Mucosal defense   – Jejunum   – Bacteriostatic

                  – Ileum   – ↑ expression of antimicrobial genes

    o Stones   – Gallbladder   – ↓ formation of calcium stones

                  – Kidney   – ↓ formation of oxalate stones

    o Metabolic function   – Regulate their own EHC

                  – Signal nuclear and G-protein-coupled receptors → helps to maintain homeostasis of fat, glucose and energy

➢ BA metabolism

    o Size of BA pool   – 2 g to 4 g (50 to 60 mmol per kg body weight)

    o Cycles of BA pool   – Per meal 2 to 3

                  – Per day 6 to 10

    o Absorption of BA per day   – 10 to 30 g (pool size x number of cycles)

    o Colonic loss of BA per day   – 200 to 600 mg

    o Hepatic synthesis of BAA per day to match daily fecal losses   – >> 95%

    o Efficiency of EHC   – (loss/pool size x number of cycles → 500 mg/4g x 10 cycles per day → 0.5 g/40 g x 100%)

                  – Loss ~2%

                  – Recovery (efficiency) ~ 98%

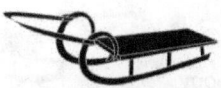

➤ Physiology

  o The rate-limiting stop for the classical pathway of bile acid synthesis and secretion is the enzyme CYP7A1.

  o As the throughput of the bile acids (BA) increases in the cytosol of the ileocyte or hepatocyte, CYP7A, falls and bile acid synthesis and secretion fall.

• Hepatocyte synthesis

• Give the FGF-dependent, SHP-dependent and mitochondrial cholesterol-dependent negative feedback regulation of bile acid synthesis and secretion.

  o Classical ileocyte and hepatocyte CYP7A1 pathway
    – Overall
      ▪ ↑ BA passing through ileocyte → ↓ BA synthesis in hepocyte
    – FGF12: ↑ BA in cytosol of ileocyte → activate FXR → ↑ **FGF$_{12}$** → ↓ hepatic CYP7A1→ ↓ hepatic synthesis of BA
    – **SHP →**
      → ↑ HNF4α ⎱
      → ↓ LRH-1 ⎰ → hepatic CYP 7A1 → ↓ hepatic synthesis of BA

      → Activation of c-Jun (**JNK**) pathway
  o Alternate pathway
    – ↑ cholesterol in mitochondria

Abbreviations: HNF4α, hepatocyte nuclear factor 4α; JNF, c-Jun NH$_2$-terminal kinase; LRH, liver receptor homology; FGF19, fibroblast growth factor-19; FXR, farnesoid X receptor; SHP, small heterodimer partner a nuclear receptor

• Canalicular membrane secretion

  o When bile acids (BA) are conjugated in the liver to the amino acids glycine and taurine, the conjugated BA become more hydrophilic and less hydrophobic, so then passive absorption in the proximal intestine is less.

  o Less passive absorption of conjugated BA in the proximal intestine maintains an adequate concentration of BA in the intestinal lumen to provide for continued solubilisation, digestion and absorption of lipids.

  o As the BA pass along the length of the small intestine, there becomes less and less exogenous or endogenous lipids to be absorbed, and the BA needs to be reabsorbed.

260

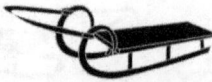

- The reabsorption of bile acids, their return to the liver, resecretion by the hepatocyte, and return to the lumen of the small intestine represents the EHC (enterohepatic absorption of bile acids).

- Microbiotica
  - The endogenous microbiotica in the lumen of the terminal ileum deconjugates the primary and secondary bile acids.
  - Enteric bacteria dehydroxylate Ba (primary ($1°$) $\rightarrow$ secondary ($2°$) BA), and deconjugate $1°/2°$ BA; enteric bacteria also epimerize the 7α-hydroxy group of CDCA (chenic acid), forming UDCA (ursodeoxycholic acid, 3α, 7β – dihydroxy BA).
  - About 95% of BA in the lumen of the intestine are reabsorbed and recycled to the liver, representing the high efficiency of the EHC.
  - The ~5% of the luminal bile acids that are not reabsorbed and recycled spill into the colon bacterial 7α-dehydroxylate in the colon produce $2°$ from $1°$ bile acids:

CA	$\rightarrow$	DCA (50% absorbed by colon)
CDCA	$\rightarrow$	LCA
	$\rightarrow$	UDCA

Abbreviations: BA, bile acid; CA, cholic acid; CDCA, chenodeoxycholic acid (aka chenic acid); DCA, deoxycholic acid; LCA, lithocholic acid; UDCA, ursodeoxycholic acid

➢ Bile secretion

There is bile acid (BA)-dependent and BA-independent bile flow, as well as Na^+-dependent bile acid clearance.

- Give the physiology of bile acid-dependent and independent canalicular secretion of water (bile flow/secretion).
  - Bile acid (BA)-dependent flow
    - Transport of BA across hepatocyte canalicular membrane by
      - BSEP (bile salt export protein)
      - MRP_2 (multidrug resistance-associated protein-2)
      - See "cholehepatic shunt, below

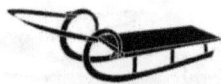

- o BA-independent flow
  - – MRP_2 (multidrug resistance-associated protein 2) transport of GSH (reduced glutathione)
  - – GGTP (gamma glutamyl transpeptidase, which catabolizes GSH in lumen)
  - – AE_2 (chloride [Cl^-] bicarbonate [HCO_3^-] anion exchanger isoform2, which secretes HCO_3^- from cholangiocyte into the lumen of duct

---

SO YOU WANT TO BE A GASTROENTEROLOGIST!

- o Bile acids in the ileocytes bind to and activate FXR (a member of the family of sterol nuclear receptors)

- • Give the functions of FXR (farnesoid X receptor).
  - o BBM
    - – Sodium-dependent bile salt transporter
  - o FXR alters the activity of
    - – Enzymes in the ileocyte cytosol: 7α – hydroxylase
    - – Transporters in hepatocyte
      - ▪ NTCP (sodium-dependent), sinusoidal membrane
      - ▪ BSEP (bile salt export protein), canalicular membrane

- • Give inborn errors of bile acid or phospholipid transport, and for each name the defective transporter.

  - o PFIC type 1
    - – Progressive familial intrahepatic cholestasis
  - o PFIC type 2
    - – BSEP (ABCB11) deficiency
  - o PFIC type 3
    - – MDR3 (ABCB4) deficiency
  - o BRIC (benign recurrent intrahepatic cholestasis) syndrome

---

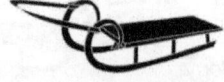

SO YOU WANT TO BE A ROCK STAR GASTROENTEROLOGIST!

- Give the physiological basis for the choleretic effect of UDCA.

  - Unconjugated dihydroxy bile acids such as UDCA are partially reabsorbed from the duct lumen across the luminal membrane of the cholangiocytes.

  - ASBT on the cholangiocyte luminal membrane also quickly shunts conjugated BA back to the hepatocyte for resynthesis.

  - The UDCA quickly returns to the hepatocytes through the periductular capillary plexus.

  - The uptake of the protonated (H^+) unconjugated UDCA generates HCO_3.

  - The UDCA is quickly resecreted into the bile by the hepatocyte canalicular membrane.

  - The HCO_3^- produced from the uptake of the protonated UDCA through the cholehepatic shunt causes a bicarbonate-rich
    - Reuptake of BA by active [ASBT] and by passive process of the luminal membrane of the cholangiocytes choleresis

  - Because this bicarbonate-rich choleresis depends on the uptake of the protonated unconjugated BA, this rapid reabsorption and resecretion of the BA because of uptake by the Cholangiocyte is, of course, causing BA-dependent bile flow.

- In the context of the EHC (enterohepatic circulation) of BA (bile acids), give the difference in the function of hepatocytes in zone I versus zone 3.

	BA Absorption	BA Secretion
- Zone I, periportal	During fasting	Recycle BA
- Zone III, pericentral (aka perivenous)	During feeding	Newly synthesized BA

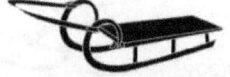

➢ Transport proteins for bile acids in the EHC

Cell Type	BBM/SM	BLM/CM	Cytosol
o Ileocyte	– ASBT (apical sodium bile acid transporter)	▪ OST αβ (organic solute transporter)	– FXR (farnesoid X receptor) – FXF19 (fibroblast growth factor 19)
o Hepatocyte	– NTCP (Na⁺-taurocholate cotransporting polypeptide)	▪ BSEP (bile salt export pump)	
o Cholangiocyte	– ASBT	▪ OST α/β	
o Renal proximal tubular cell	– ASBT	▪ OST α/β	

Abbreviations: BBM, brush border membrane of ileocyte; BLM, basolateral membrane of ileocyte; CM, canalicular membrane; SM, sinusoidal membrane

---

SO YOU WANT TO BE A GASTROENTEROLOGIST!

The liver synthesizes and secretes the primary bile acids (cholic and chenic acid).

- Give the reason why an estimate of the types of bile acids synthesized by the liver cannot be made from assessment of stool bile acids.

  o The conjugated primary bile acids are deconjugated and 7α-dehydroxylate by luminal bacteria to deoxycholic acid (from cholic acid) and lithocholic acid (from chenic acid).

  o And that's the answer! Fecal bile acid is mostly deoxycholic and lithocholic acid, reflecting the action of the colonic microbiotica, and not the secretory pattern of the liver.

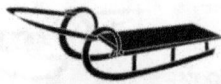

Bile Salt - Induced Diarrhea

- Give the reason why a resection of < 100 cm of ileum result in choleretic diarrhea, whereas a > 100 cm resection results in steatorrhea.

  - The neutral and the acidic pathways for the production of bile acids from cholesterol are capable of increasing their usual secretion rates by ~ 25%.

  - When there is a small reduction in the EHC (enterohepatic circulation [of bile acids [BA]), such as what might occur from an ileal resection of < 100 cm, the hepatic conversion of BA increases, and sufficient BA may be secreted across the CM and into the bile ducts and lumen of the duodenum to maintain a normal CMC (critical micellar concentration [of bile acids]).

  - Bile acid micelles and vesicles form, and lipids are absorbed.

  - Because of the loss of some of the ileum. Some BA escape reabsorption and spill in increased amounts into the colon.

  - In the colon the increased [BA] stimulated cGMP and secretion of Cl⁻, leading to a watery bile-acid induced (choleretic) diarrhea.

- Give the change in pathophysiology which occurs with a loss of > 100 cm of ileum, leading to steatorrhea.

  - When there is a major loss of ileum (> 100 cm), the mount of malabsorbed BA is so great that liver cannot compensate for the large loss of BA by increasing the hepatic conversion of cholesterol to bile acids.

  - Thus, the CMC is not achieved, and fat malabsorption (steatorrhea) occurs.

"Harsh words are heavy and often fall with a big thud,

but a kind word will bounce on and on…"

Anonymous

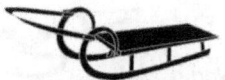

GLUTEN SENSITIVE ENTEROPATHY (GSE, AKA CELIAC DISEASE [CD])

➢ Causes/associations

- Give possible factors which may be useful in the prevention of Celiac disease (CD).

  ○ Breastfeeding
    - CD prevalence is significantly reduced (~50%) when infants are breastfed at the time of gluten introduction.
    - The risk of developing CD decreases by 63% in children breastfed for > 2 months.
    - The mechanism of protection is not yet elucidated.
    - Long-term prospective studies are required to assess this protection from breastfeeding is permanent.

  ○ Timing of gluten introduction
    - Age at first gluten exposure appears to affect CD onset.
    - Continuing breastfeeding with slow gluten introduction could be beneficial.
    - Avoiding early (<4 months) and late (>7 months) introduction of gluten is recommended.

  ○ Viral infections
    - High frequency of rotavirus infection may be correlated with increased risk of CD in predisposed individuals.
    - A peptide recognized by immunoglobulin of CD patient's shares homology with a rotavirus protein (VP-7).
    - A seasonal pattern of CD is observed, with an increased risk of CD in summer- born children.

  ○ Microbiotica and probiotics
    - CD patients have modified intestinal microflora
      • Probiotics may have a minor effect to balance microbiota composition and modulate the immune response

Printed with permission: Macmillan Publishers Ltd: Pinier M. et al. *Am J Gastroenterol* 2010; 105:2551–2561, Box 1, page 2554.

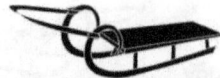

> Pathophysiology

- Give the immunopathogenesis of celiac disease.

  o The toxicity of gluten is due to the gliadins contained in gluten.

  o The main toxic gliadins is prolamin.

    The toxic portion of prolamin is QQQPF (glutamine-glutamine-glutamine-proline-phenylalanine).

  o Gluten is absorbed and passed to lamina propria.

  o Dendritic cells which express HLA-DQ2 or –DQ8 bind gluten.

  o The gluten bound to the dendritic cells is presented to T cells which have the TCR (α/β T cell receptor).

  o The TCR containing T cells (including α/γ TCR in IELs) activate B and other T lymphocytes.

  o The activated B and T lymphocytes produce proinflammatory cytokines.

  o The proinflammtory cytokines (IL-4, -5, -6, -10; IFN (interferon)-γ, TGF (transforming growth factor)-β cause:

    - Enterocyte damage

    - ↑ HLA-DQ2 gene expression

  o The increased and activated B cells produced type 2 tTG (tissue transglutaminase).

  o tTG deaminates neutralizes neutral glutamine residues in gluten to negatively charged glutamic acid residues in DGPs (deamidated gliadin peptides).

  o The DGP increase the injurious T cell responses.

  o ↑ IL-15 ("bridges the innate and adaptive immune responses in celiac disease") causes

    - IEL ↑ IFNα

    - LP CD4+ T cells ↑ response

  o The HLA close II molecules DQ2 and DQ8 are required for but are not sufficient by themselves for the development of CD: 50% of Americans are positive for one of these molecules, but only 1% develop CD. However negative HLA DQ2 or DQ8 rule out CD as a cause of the enteropathy (high negative predictive value).

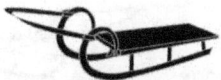

> Clinical

- Give intestinal and extraintestinal conditions associated with celiac disease.

❖ Intestinal tract

- o Mouth
  - – Glossitis
  - – Aphthous ulcers
  - – Poor dentition
  - – Dry mouth
  - – Candidiasis

- o Esophagus
  - – Squamous cell carcinoma
  - – Adenocarcinoma
  - – Eosinophilic esophagitis, esophageal eosinophilic

- o Stomach
  - – Lymphocytic gastritis
  - – Atrophic gastritis

- o Small bowel
  - – Unclassified sprue (sprue-like intestinal disease)
  - – Collagenous sprue
  - – Ulcerative ileojejunitis
  - – Diffuse small intestinal lymphoma
  - – Early aberrant T-cell lymphoma (EATL)
  - – Refractory sprue, types 1 and 2
  - – SIBO (small intestinal bacterial overgrowth)
  - – Adenocarcinoma

- o Colon
  - – Microscopic colitis
  - – IBS
  - – IBD

- o Liver
  - – Autoimmune hepatitis (AIH)
  - – IgG4 autoimmune cholangitis (AIC)
  - – PBC
  - – PSC
  - – Ideopathic transaminitis
  - – Fatty liver

- o Pancreas
  - – 2° insufficiency, diabetes (type I)
  - – IgG4-autoimmune pancreatitis

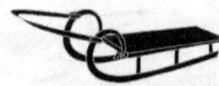

- o Gallbladder, biliary tree
  - – Cholelithiasis
  - – PSC

- o Nutritional abnormalities
  - – Short stature
  - – Osteopenic bone disease
  - – Iron and vitamin deficiencies
  - – Unexplained weight loss

- ❖ Extra-intestinal

  - o Neuropsychiatric and CNS
    - – Chronic fatigue syndrome
    - – Irritability, depression
    - – Peripheral neuropathy
    - – Epilepsy (with intracranial calcifications)
    - – Gluten ataxia syndrome (gait and limb ataxia), paresthesia
    - – Night blindness
    - – Autism (controversial)

  - o Teeth
    - – Dental enamel defects

  - o Skin
    - – Follicular hyperkeratosis, dermatitis
    - – Petechiae, ecchymoses
    - – Dermatitis herpetiformis (granular IgA deposits)
    - – Edema
    - – Glossitis
    - – Cheilosis
    - – Aphthous ulcers
    - – Acrodermatitis enterohepatica
    - – Spoon nailing
    - – Clubbing

  - o Heart
    - – Cardiomyopathy

  - o Lung
    - – Fibrosing alveolitis
    - – Bird fancier lung

  - o Hematopoietic
    - – Iron deficiency anemia
    - – Thrombobocytosis
    - – Howell-Jolly bodies
    - – Hyposplenism
    - – IgA deficiency

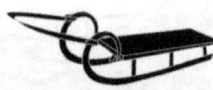

- – Hypersegmented PMNs
- – Megaloblastic anemia (B12, folic acid)
- – Lymphoma
- – Macrocytic anemia
- – Deficiency
  - ▪ B12
  - ▪ Folate

- o Musculoskeletal
  - – Atrophy, tetany, weakness, myalgias gluteal wasting
  - – Autoimmune connective tissue disorders: Sjorgren syndrome, RA, lupus
  - – Osteoporosis

- o Endocrine
  - – Secondary hyperparathyroidism
  - – Insulin-dependent DM, (T1DM)
  - – Autoimmune thyroid disease
  - – Autoimmune adrenal disease

- o Obstetrical/gynecological (reproductive)
  - – Amenorrhea
  - – Infertility
  - – Miscarriage
  - – Postpartum hemorrhage
  - – ↑ risk of celiac disease in child

- o Renal
  - – IgA nephropathy

- o Genetic disorders
  - – Down syndrome
  - – Turner syndrome
  - – Williams syndrome (elf-faced)

- o Pediatrics
  - – Delayed puberty
  - – Slow growth

Abbreviations: AIC, autoimmune cholangitis; AIH, autoimmune hepatitis; CD, celiac disease; DM, diabetes mellitus; IBS, irritable bowel syndrome; PBC, primary biliary cirrhosis; PSC, primary sclerosing cholangitis; RA, rheumatoid arthritis.

Adapted from: Green PHR, Rostami K, Marsh MN. *Best Pract Res Clin Gastroenterol* 2005;19(3): pg 39.; and Crowe SE. *2007 AGA Institute Postgraduate Course*: pg. 25.

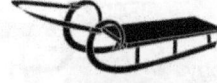

Dermatitis Herpetiformis (DH)

- o A celiac-like enteropathy responsive to gluten withdrawal is seen in 90% o persons with dermatitis herpetiformis (DH).

- o These persons have IgA precipitation in the dermoapidermal junction characteristic granular/speckled deposits

- o A pruritic papulovascular rash is seen on extensor surfaces as well as on the buttocks, trunk, neck and scalp.

- Give differences between linear IgA disease, and the usual granular/speckled IgA deposits around the skin lesion in DH.

  - o Linear IgA disease occurs in ~10% of persons with DH-like papulovascular skin lesions

  - o This condition differs as follows from the normal DH with granular/speckle IgA deposits:
    - ↑ IgA anti-basement membrane antibody in blood
    - Absent tTG or EMA (endomyseal antibody)
    - HLA susceptibility genes other than HLA DQ2 or DQ8
    - No gluten-sensitive enteropathy

Celiac Clinical Tips

- o Growth failure may occur in children with undiagnosed celiac disease, and catch-up growth may be incomplete after introducing a gluten-free diet. Anti-pituitary antibodies (APA) suggestive of autoimmune hypopituitorism (based on lymphocytic hypophysitis) occur in 42% of newly diagnosed celiac youths (30% high and 70% low titer of APA), and may also be associated with low level of IGF-1.

- o In Europe, the standard mortality rate of persons with symptomatic celiac disease is increased and varies from 1.26 in Finland to 3.6 in Sicily.

➢ Diagnosis

- Give why there is no "best test" to diagnose celiac disease.

  - o Not just GI symptoms
    - Some patients have just extra intestinal features
    - Some patients have just positive serology (false-positive or true-positive)

  - o Not just EGD
    - There are numerous causes of "scalloping of the mucosa"

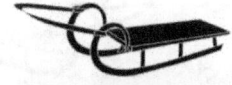

- o Not just serum anti-glutaminase (tTG)
  - False-negatives
    - Person has not recently been on a gluten free diet, NPO, on immunosuppressants or had a bone marrow transplantation
  - False-positive may be seen in IBD, chronic liver or autoimmune disease, or severe HF (heart failure)
- o Not just small bowel mucosa biopsy
  - An inadequate number of biopsies may have been taken (need 4 to 6 duodenal or jejunal mucosa biopsies)
  - The mucosal biopsy may be compatible with celiac disease, but there are no features which are pathognomic, and other conditions must be excluded
  - There are many conditions which have ↑ IEL (intraepithelial lymphocytes) +/- VA (villous atrophy or small bowel mucosal biopsy
- o Not just response to gluten withdrawal
  - There are reports of what is being called "non-celiac gluten sensitivity"

- ➤ Laboratory
- • Give clinical indications for serological testing for CD.
  - o Positive family history
  - o Autoimmune endocrine disorders
    - Insulin-dependent diabetes mellitus
    - Autoimmune thyroid disease
    - Autoimmune adrenal disease
  - o Autoimmune connective tissue disorders
    - Sjogren syndrome
    - Rheumatoid arthritis
    - Systemic lupus erythematosus
  - o Hepatobiliary conditions
    - Primary sclerosing cholangitis
    - Primary biliary cirrhosis
    - Autoimmune cholangitis
    - Elevated transaminases
  - o Other gastrointestinal disorders
    - Lymphocytic gastritis
    - Microscopic colitis
  - o Miscellaneous conditions
    - IgA deficiency
    - IgA nephropathy
    - Down syndrome, Turner syndrome

Printed with permission: Crowe SE. *2007 AGA Institute Postgraduate Course*: pg. 25.

272

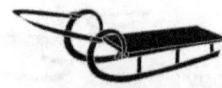

IgA tTG (tissue transglutamase) serology is >95% sensitive for CD, especially when there is a high titre

- Give clinical conditions which are associated with false positive or false negative, **serologic testing** for CD (anti-tTG).

    o False-negative
    - True false negative
    - IgA deficiency
    - Children < 2 years
    - Recent gluten free diet

o GI conditions with
- ↑ risk of IgA deficiency
- Pernicious anemia
- Giardiasis
- Secondary deficiency of disaccharidases

    - TPN (NPO, with no gluten taken by mouth)
    - Current or recent use of steroids, immunosuppressives, anti-TNFs
    - Previous hematopoietic stem cell transplantation

    o False-positive
    - Autoimmune diseases (may be associated with CD which is in a latent phase)
    - Liver diseases
    - Inflammatory bowel disease (IBD)
    - Silent (occult), or potential (latent) celiac disease
    - Heart failure (New York class 3 or 4)

    o Note- some persons with autoimmune disorders, liver disease, or inflammatory bond disease may have a false-positive anti-positive or may have a true positive and have associated C12

Adapted from: Green PHR, et al. *Best Pract Res Clin Gastroenterol* 2005; 19(3): pg 391.

Clinical Tips

    o In the patient with IgA deficiency who is being assessed for celiac disease, request an IqGDPE serological test

    o Treating isolated IgA deficiency with IgA is **not** recommended, because it is not required

- Give a second and even more important reason why IV immunoglobulin should not be used to treat isolated IgA deficiency.

    o Persons with IgA deficiency may have IgG or IgE antibodies to the IgA in the IV immune globulin (anti-IgA antibodies), to which they could have a severe anaphylactic reaction.

    o If patient fails to respond to a confirmed diagnosis of CD, they probably do not have CD, or they have an associated condition which masks satisfactory symptom improvement.

    o If the patient responds to a confirmed gluten-free diet, then recurs while still on a GFD, look for complications of CD (primary or secondary non-responsive celic disease [NRCD]).

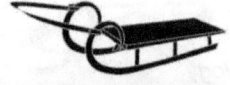

- ➢ Endoscopy

  - ○ Scalloping or absence of duodenal folds on EGD alerts the endoscopist to the possibility of celiac disease, and triggers the recognition of the need to take at least 6 mucosal pinch biopsies from D2 and/or D3 (second and third part of duodenum).

  - ○ The endoscopic features of CD (scalloping of the muscosal folds, less prominent folds, fissules, and a nodular/ mosaic pattern) are only 59% sensitive but 92% specific for CD.

- • Give causes of duodenal scalloping other than celiac disease.

  - ○ Other "sprues"   – Tropical sprue
  - ○ Infections   – Giardiasis
                         – HIV infection
  - ○ Immune   – Eosinophilic enteritis
  - ○ Systemic disease – Amyloidosis

- ➢ Histopathology

- • Give the early subtle histopathological changes of celiac disease.

  - ○ Villus enterocytes – Reduced BBM
                          – Cuboidal/squamoid shape
                          – Cytoplasm more basophilic
                          – Basal polarity of nucleic lost
                          – Lysosomes large
                          – Endoplasmic reticulum decreased
                          – Vacuoles in cytoplasm and mitochondria
  - ○ Crypt cells   – ↑ mitosis
  - ○ Tight junctions   – Abnormal
  - ○ Immunocytes   – ↑ IEL
                          – ↑ CD8+ T cells
                          – ↑ lymphocytes (> 40/hpf)
                            ▪ IgA, IgM, IgG producing
                            ▪ ↑ CD4+ T cells in lamina propria
                          – ↑ PMNs and eosinophils
  - ○ Severe celiac disease on duodenal biopsy
    - – May look like colon, but if you see Brunner's glands – Must be duodenum

Abbreviations: BBM, brush border membrane; IEL, intraepithelial lymphocytes; PMN, polymorphonuclear cells

274

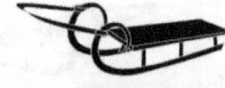

- Give conditions causing malabsorption that are usually **excluded** by a normal small bowel biopsy.

  o Sprue (actually, not always – patchy, treated, immunosuppression, potential – anti tTG positive: small bowel biopsy maybe truly normal histologically normal, or histologically normal in the biopsies taken, but disease is patchy so lesions were "missed" due to sampling error)

  o Hypogammaglobulinemia

  o α-β-Lipoproteinemia

  o Whipple disease (except in <u>very</u> rare circumstances with only CNS infection)

- Give differential diagnoses of a "sprue-like" small bowel biopsy in a patient suspected of having CD (villous shortening, ↑ IEL).

  o Celiac disease and its variants

  o Infection
    - Cryptococcus
    - Giardia lamblia
    - Giardiasis
    - Histoplasmosis
    - HIV (immunodeficiency syndromes)
    - MAC (Mycobacterium-avium complex infection)
    - Post viral gastroenteritis
    - Small intestinal bacterial overgrowth (stasis syndrome)
    - Strongyloides
    - Topical sprue (infectious agent suspected)
    - Whipple disease

  o Infiltration
    - Amyloidosis
    - Benign tumour
    - Malignant immunoproliferative small intestinal disease (IPSID, i.e., alpha chain disease), lymphoma
    - Mastocytosis
    - Waldenstrom macroglobulinemia
    - Xanthelasma

  o Immune conditions
    - Crohn disease
    - Eosinophilic gastroenteritis
    - Graft-versus-host disease
    - Hypogammaglobulinemia

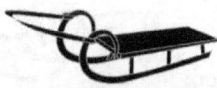

- o Food
  - − Food protein hypersensitivity (rye, barley, egg, fish, rice, poultry, cow's milk, soy, other proteins)
  - − Oats-induced villous atrophy
  - − Folate, cobalamin, zinc deficiency
  - − Protein-calorie malnutrition

- o Drugs, radiation
  - − NSAIDs, colchicine, neomycin, chemotherapy, MMF
  - − The calcium channel blocker
  - − Radiation

- o Miscellaneous
  - − Zollinger-Ellison syndrome
  - − mesenteric lymph node cavitation syndrome
  - − α-β-Lipoproteinemia
  - − lymphangiectasia
  - − microvillus inclusion disease (children)

Abbreviations: CD, celiac disease; IPSID, immunoproliferative small intestinal disease

Adapted from: Freeman HJ. *Can J Gastroenterol* 2008;22(3): pg 277.

- • Give causes other than refractory CD for **villous shortening** in the presence of normal numbers of IELs (villous shortening, N-IELs).

  - o Autoimmune enteropathy

  - o Common variable immunodeficiency syndrome

  - o Crohn disease

  - o Eosinophilic gastroenteritis

  - o HIV/AIDS

  - o Immunoproliferative small intestinal disease

  - o Radiation enteritis

  - o TPN (total parental nutrition)

  - o Tuberculosis (including atypical)

  - o Whipple disease

Printed with permission: Daum S, et al. *Best Pract Res Clin Gastroenterol* 2005; 19(3): 415.

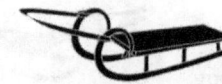

> Villous shortening, ↑ IELS
>
> Common conditions
>
> - o Celiac disease
> - o Tropical sprue
> - o Collagenous sprue
> - o Cow/soya milk intolerance
> - o Post-infection diarrhea

- Give conditions other than celiac disease where there may be an increased numbers of small intestinal intraepithelial lymphocytes (IELs), on the small bowel mucosal biopsy, without villous shortening.

  ↑ IELs, No Villous Shortening

  - o Celiac disease
  - o Tropical sprue
  - o Autoimmune diseases/conditions
  - o Microscopic colitis
  - o Crohn colitis
  - o Non-steroidal anti-inflammatory drugs (NSAIDs)
  - o Small intestinal bacterial overgrowth (SIBO)

Abbreviations: CD, celiac disease; IELs, intestinal intraepithelial lymphocytes

Printed with permission: Collins P, Wahab PJ, Murray JA. *Best Pract Res Clin Gastroenterol* 2005;19(3): pg 344.; and Daum S, Cellier C, Mulder CJJM. *Best Pract Res Clin Gastroenterol* 2005;19(3):pg. 415.

"The ends justify the means.
This is the modern dilemma."
Machia velli

277

 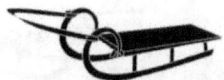

- Give factors which support the diagnosis of CD in patients with an increased density of intraepithelial lymphocytes (IELs) but no villous shortening, on the small bowel mucosal biopsy.

  - o Family history of celiac disease
    – Increased risk of CD to approximately least 15% of first-degree relatives are affected (1/100 → 15/100)

  - o Concomitant autoimmune conditions
    – Increased risk of CD to ~ 5%

  - o HLA DQ2 or DQ8 positive
    – Sensitivity 84%, specificity 91%

  - o Increased density of villous tip IELs
    – Sensitivity 84%, specificity 95%

  - o Increased density of $\gamma\delta$ + IELs
    – High sensitivity, low specificity, high negative predictive value

  - o Gluten dependence/ response
    – Should be ascertained by gluten challenge after gluten-free diet

Printed with permission: Collins P, Wahab PJ, Murray JA. *Best Pract Res Clin Gastroenterol* 2005; 19(3): pg 347.

- Give the histological features which may be used to distinguish the conditions which may be associated with a "sprue-like" lesion from celiac disease.

Cause of Malabsorption	Histological Features
o Abeta-lipoproteinemia	- Large lipid droplets
o Amyloidosis	- Congo red-stained deposits with apple-green birefringence in polarized light
o Collagenous sprue	- Collagenous band below atrophic epithelium
o Crohn disease	- Epitheloid granulomas, and characteristic focal inflammation
o Eosinophilic gastroenteritis	- Eosinophilic infiltration
o Infection (enteric)	- Organism seen on histological examination (e.g., giardia lamblia, strongyloides, TB, HIV)
o Lymphangiectasia	- Ectatic lymph vessels, fat in lymphatics
o Lymphoma	- Clonal expansion of lymphocytes
o Mastocytosis	- Diffuse infiltration with mast cells
o Mycobacterium-avium complex infection (MAC)	- Acid-fast bacilli, foam cells, PAS positive diastase sensitive staining in macrophages
o Whipple disease	- Acid-fast bacilli, foam cells, PAS positive, diastase resistant staining in macrophages

Adapted from: Freeman HJ. *Can J Gastroenterol* 2008; 22(3): pg. 277.

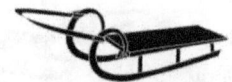

- Give the differential diagnosis of PAS positive staining on small bowel biopsy.
    - Lymphatic ectasia
    - MAC (Mycobacterium-avium complex) infection
    - Whipple disease (diastase resistant)
    - α_1 antitrypsin deficiency

- Give causes of small bowel biopsy showing "vacant spaces" which stain positive with a lipid stain.
    - Abetalipoproteinemia
    - Cholesterol embolization
    - Lymphangiectasia

- ➤ Treatment
    - The patient with proven celiac disease (CD) must be on a gluten-free diet for life
    - Associated nutrient deficiencies are treated
    - Associated intestinal and non-intestinal conditions are treated
    - After instituting a gluten-free diet, 90% of CD patients lose their symptoms and signs, and anti- tTG normalizes, even with low level or episodic intake of gluten

- Give the acceptable foods, and the foods to avoid for CD patients.

    - Acceptable foods
        - Corn, rice, buckwheat products, potatoes
        - Wine, and distilled alcoholic beverages
        - Fruit and vegetables
        - Meat
        - Nuts
        - Dairy products (unless lactose-intolerant)

    - Foods to avoid
        - Wheat, rye, barley*
        - Triticale (wheat-rye hybrid)
        - Millet and sorghum
        - Oat products (if there is cross-contamination)
        - Hydrolyzed vegetable protein
        - Beer, lager, stout, malt

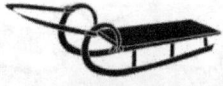

- Give common sources of food which may be hidden gluten.

  - Foods and beverages
    - Bouillon/soups
    - Candy
    - Communion wafers
    - Drink mixes/herbal tea
    - Gravy/sauces
    - Imitation meat/seafood
    - Salad dressings/marinades
    - Nutritional supplements
    - Self-basting turkeys
    - Soy sauce
    - Fat replacers
    - Contamination
    - Malt alcohol/vinegar
  - Medications
    - Medications (pills and capsules)
  - Contamination
    - Play-Doh®
    - Lipstick/lip balms
    - Airborne flour
    - Glues and pastes
    - Chewing gum

Abbreviation: CD, celiac disease

Adapted from: *Sleisenger & Fordtran's gastrointestinal and liver disease: Pathophysiology/Diagnosis/Management* 2006: pg 2295; and 2010, pg. 1813; 10th Edition, 2016, Box 107-3, page 1865.

  - Prevalence of conditions associated with CD, which may result in an apparent complete response to gluten-free diet; IBS (18%); lactose intolerance (9%); microscopic colitis (7%); or bacterial overgrowth syndrome (6%)

Abbreviations: CD, celiac disease ; DPG, deamidated gliadin peptide; NRCD, non-responsive CD; tTG, transglutamase

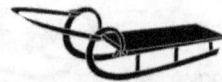

A patient with previously well-controlled biopsy-proven CD while on a gluten-free diet (GFD), develops recurrent diarrhea.

- Give causes or conditions specific to CD that could explain this clinical scenario.
    - Diet
        - Non-adherence to GFD
        - Unintentional gluten intake
        - Zinc deficiency, folate/B12 deficiency
        - Primary lactose intolerance (lactase deficiency)
        - Lactose/fructose malabsorption
        - Severe malnutrition
    - Small intestinal manifestation of sprue
        - Refractory celiac disease (RCD)*
        - Collagenous colitis
        - Small bowel adenocarcinomans
        - Early abberrant T cell lymphoma (EATL)
        - Lymphoma of small bowel
        - Ulcerative jejunoileitis
    - Other GI complications of CD
        - Primary pancreatic deficiency
        - Loss of stimulus for pancreatic enzyme secretion; unmasked pancreatic insufficiency
        - Cholestatic liver disease
        - Small bacterial overgrowth (SIBO)
        - Diarrhea-predominant irritable bowel syndrome (IBS-D)
        - Microscopic colitis
    - Non-intestinal complications
        - Diabetes
        - Thyroid disease (hypo- [SIBO] or hyperthyroidism[rapid transit])
        - Adrenal insufficiency
    - Wrong initial diagnosis (including unclassified sprue**)
    - A second disease

*refractory celiac disease requires evidence of an initial response to a gluten-free diet. **with unclassified sprue (or sprue-like intestinal disease), no initial response to a gluten-free diet was documented.*

Abbreviation: CD, celiac disease; EATL, early abberrant T cell lymphoma; GFD, gluten-free diet; IBS-D, predominant irritable bowel syndrome

Adapted from: Freeman HJ. *Can J Gastroenterol* 2008; 22(3): pg. 277.

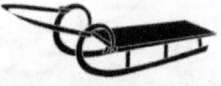

Non-Responsive Celiac Disease (NRCD)

➤ Definition

- o NRCD (non-responsive celiac disease) is defined as "..... the persistence of symptoms, signs, or laboratory abnormalities typical of celiac disease despite adherence to a gluten-free diet for at least six months" (Feldman M., et al. Sleisenger and Fordtran's Gastrointestinal and Liver Disease. 9th Edition. Saunders/Elsevier, Philadelphia, 2010, page 1815)

➤ Demography

- o 10% of celiac disease patients develop 1° or 2° NRCD, usually due to non-adherance to the receommended gluten-free diet (36%)
- o 10% of those with NRCD, and 1% of those with CD, develop refractory celiac disease (RCD)

➤ Types

- o Primary
- o Secondary

Refractory Celiac Disease (RCD)

➤ Definition

- o RCD is defined as ".... Symptomatic, severe small intestinal villus atrophy that mimics celiac disease but does not respond to at least six months of a strict gluten-free diet and is not accounted for by other causes of villus atrophy or overt intestinal lymphoma" (Feldman M., et al. Sleisenger and Fordtran's Gastrointestinal and Liver Disease. 9th Edition. Saunders/Elsevier, Philadelphia, 2010, page 1816).

➤ Types

- o Type I RCD
  - – Normal intra-epithelial T cell lymphocytes (IELs: no clonal T cell expansion)
  - – 5 year survival rate, 90%
- o Type II RCD
  - – Clonal T cell expansion
  - – Monoclonal rearrangement of the TCR gene
  - – Presence of abnormal intra-epithelial IELs which lack the usual T cell markers (CD4, CD8, IL-2R)

282

 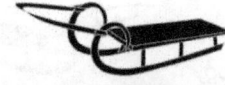

- Associated with
  - Ulcerative ileo jejunitis
  - Necrotizing mesenteric lymphodenopathy
  - T-cell enteropathy
- ↑↑ IL-15 may be responsible for this lymphomatous transformation
- 5 year survival rate < 50% (1 yr mortality rate ~ 70%), despite nutritional support, steroids (including budesonide), immunosuppressants, anti-TNF or stem cell transplantation

➢ Immunopathogenesis

- Give the immunopathogenesis of RCD (refractory celiac disease).
  - ↑ IL-15 in mucosa of small intestine → ↓ SMAD3 dependent TGF-β signaling in T lymphocytes
  - Initial normal expression of T cell surface markers (CD3+, CD8+, CD4-) and normal TC (T-cell receptors, polyclonal plasma cell immunophenotype) (still normal cytologically)
  - ↓ TGF-β signaling
    - Continued intestinal inflammation in celiac small intestine
  - T cells become aberrant, becoming phenotypically abnormal (on flow cytometry determination), with immune dysregulation including monoclonal expansion, CD3 in the cytoplasm, CD108 on the surface of the T cells, loss of TCR, CD3, CD8, CD4 (on flow cytometry determination)
  - Once > 29% of T cells are abnormal, the RCD I is said to have progressed to RCD II
  - EATL (enteropathy-associated T-cell lymphoma) is on a continuum with RCD II, both of which are associated with HLA-DQ2 homozygosity
  - EATL is said to have occurred when
    - The T cells are cytologically abnormal
    - Tumour masses develop
  - In RCD II, steroids, azathioprine, infliximab are ineffective against the aberrant monoclonal T cells, and 2-CDA (cladribine) or ASCT (autologous stem cell transplantation) may be necessary

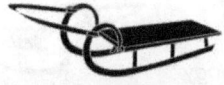

> Clinical Challenge

A patient from the Middle East develops symptoms of malabsorption. Serology for tTG is negative. IPSID (immunoproliferative small intestinal disease) needs to be ruled out.

- Give the blood testing and small bowel biopsy changes which support the diagnosis of IPSID.
  - o Blood – abnormal alpha heavy chain immunoglobulin
  - o Biopsy – marked infiltration of the lamina propria with lymphocytes and plasma cells

IPSID does not respond to gluten withdrawal, and is associated with the risk of the development of Mediterranean lymphoma. Because the early stages of IPSID can be treated, it is important to make the diagnosis.

- Give the specific treatment for IPSID.
  - o IPSID may be treated early with a prolonged cause of tetracycline, which act against the associated infection with Campylobacter jejuni, which may have a role to play in IPSID.
  - o If a lymphoma develops, treat with chemotherapy, or total abdominal irradiation.

> Treatment
  - o Diet – high calorie, high protein, low fat, with supplements of MCTs
  - o Correct associated nutrient and electrolyte deficiency, e.g., folic acid, vitamin B12, fat soluble vitamins
  - o Tetracycline 250 mg qid for 6 mon (repeated courses may be necessary)
  - o For the causes and treatment of tropical malabsorption, please see Sleisenger and Fordtran's Gastrointestinal and Liver Disease, 10th edition, 2010, Table 108.2, page 1883.

Ulcerative Jejunoileitis
  - o A rare complication of celiac disease characterized by intestinal ulceration and stricture

  - o ↑ risk of malignant transfunction to diffuse or multifocal EATL (enteropathy-associated T cell lymphoma)
    - – A strict gluten-free diet for 5 to 10 years markedly reduces the risk of EALT as well as small bowel adenocarcinomas
    - – Type 2
      - • IEL's are phenotypically abnormal
      - • IEL's lack the usual CD8 expression

Abbreviations: GFD, gluten free diet; IELs, intra-epithelial T cell lymphocytes; NRCD, non-responsive CD; RCD, refractory celiac disease

284

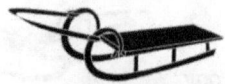

TROPICAL SPRUE

➤ Definition

  o "Tropical sprue is a primary ..... malabsorption syndrome that occurs in visitors to or residents of the tropics" (Feldman M., et al. Sleisenger and Fordtran's Gastrointestinal and Liver Disease. 10th Edition. Saunders/Elsevier, Philadelphia, 2016, page 1874).

➤ Histopathology

  o The EM (electron microscopy) demonstration in small bowel biopsies of viral particles resembling human enteric coronaviruses is likely not related to the pathogenesis.

  o EM also shows degeneration of cells in the crypts.

➤ Clinical

  o Hyperpigmentation of the palms, knuckles and buccal mucosa is a curious clinical association, thought to be due to an attered metabolism of melanin secondary to vitamin B12 deficiency.

  o Vitamin B12 deficiency is common because of the villous atrophy occurs in the distal small intestine.

  o Coma and colonic pseudo-obstruction are two addition interesting clinical features.

➤ Treatment

  o Antibiotic treatment (tetracycline 250 mg qid for 6 months, plus supplements of vitamin B12 and folic acid).

Please see Sleisenger and Fordtran's Gastrointestinal and Liver Disease. 10th Edition. Saunders/Elsevier, Philadelphia, 2010, Table 108.1, page 1877, "Clinical Features of Tropical Malabsorption and Their Causes".

SO YOU WANT TO BE A GASTROENTEROLOGIST!

• Give the specific therapy for tropical sprue and the benefits of folic acid.

  o Specific therapy is tetracycline 250 mg po qid or doxycycline 100 mg po OD, for 6 mon

  o Folic acid does more than treat the deficiency of this vitamin, with correction of associated anemia and glossitis, and fascilitating the correction vitamin B12 deficiency

  o Folic acid helps correct the villorophy and malabsorption

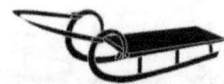

Mastering the Boards: Gastroenterology   A.B.R. Thomson

WHIPPLE DISEASE

➤ Definition

  o A systemic infection caused by Tropheryma whipplei, has "foamy macrophage" in the submucosal of the small or large (rare) intestine, and these stain PAS-positive, diastase sensitive macrophage staining.

➤ Causes/associations

  o Caused by chronic infection of Tropheryma whipplei, a rod-shaped bacterium

  o T. whipplei 16S rRNA is mostly extracellular, and below the basement membrane

➤ Immunopathogenesis

  o ↓ Th1 and ↑ Th2 immune response

  o ↑ IL-16 and nucleosomes (suggesting ↑ apoptosis) from macrophage and monocytes

➤ Clinical

  o 10% of Whipplei patients have secondary infection from Giardia lamblia.

  o ~ 25% have CNS infection, rarely without intestinal, joint or heart involvement, and CSF cytology and stereotactic biopsy of lesions shown MRI or CT scan may be necessary.

  o Lymphadenopathy
    – Peripheral – lymphadenitis
    – Abdominal – granulomatous reaction and fat deposits

MCP Tip

• Give "buzzwords" for tropheryma whipplei infection (Whipple disease) in addition to PAS-positive, diastase-resistant foamy macrophages.
  o Cerebellar ataxia plus diarrhea

  o Pericarditis, pleurisy in middle-aged male

  o Nystagmus plus oculomastocatory nysrythmia

  o Arhtralgias

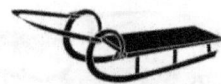

➢ Laboratory
   o Performance characteristics of PCP analysis of saliva and stool: when both are positive, sensitivity is 65% and specificity is 95% for intestinal involvement with Tropheryma whipplei.

➢ Diagnostic imaging
   o Diagnostic imaging shows malabsorption pictures as well as lymphadenopathy (peripheral, mesenteric and retroperitoneal)

➢ Histopathology
   o The PAS (periodic acid-Schill)-positive, diastase resistant inclusions in the phagolysosomes of the "foamy" macrophage are filled with glycoprotein, possibly representing bacterial remnants of their cell walls.

   o Lipid droplets and lymphangiectasia are common in the small bowel, and the PAS-positive diastase-resistant material in the macrophage is glycoprotein.

287

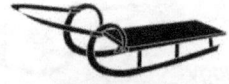

- Give causes of PAS-positive sensitive macrophage staining.
  - Whipple disease (diastase resistant)
  - Mycobacterium aviam complex (MAC enteritis)
  - Alpha-1 anti-trypsin deficiency
  - Lymphatic ectasia

- ➢ Treatment

  - Induction   – Ceftriaxon
    - 2 gm IV od (10 to 14 days)
    – Penicillin G
    - 6 to 24 million units IV daily, plus
    – Streptomycin
    - 1 gm IM od

  - Long-term (for at least 1 yr)   – Trimethoprim/sulfamethoxazole
    - 160/800 mg po bid
    – For other antibiotic choices, please see Feldman et al., Gastrointestinal and Liver Disease, Ninth Edition, 2010, Table 106-1, page 1841

SO YOU WANT TO BE A GASTROENTEROLOGIST!

Tropheryma (T) whipplei is sensitive to tetracycline antibiotics, but is not recommended for use.

- Give the reason why tetracycline is not recommended for use to treat T. whippeli

  - T. whipplei may invade the CNS, and tetracycline does not cross the blood brain barrier, and should not be used
  - Curiously, T. whipplei may occur just in the CNS

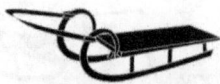

CROHN DISEASE

(Please also see Colon chapter, ulcerative colitis)

➤ Demography

    ○ Incidence   – $10/10^5$ per year in USA/Canada and Northern Europe

    ○ Prevalence   –   > $200/10^5$
                  –   Female-to-male ratio of 1.3:1

➤ Terminology

• Give the meaning of the following terms for adults with Crohn disease.

Term		Definition
○ Active disease		- CDAI >150
○ Remission		- Change in CDAI $\geq$ -100, CDA1$\leq$150
○ Relapse		- CDAI > 150 & ↑ CDAI by 70
○ Early relapse		- Relapse < 3 months after achieving remission on previous therapy
○ Pattern of relapse		- Infrequent $\leq$ 1 relapse/year - Frequent $\geq$ 2/year
○ GCS refractory disease*		- Active disease despite full dose GCS for 4 weeks
○ GCS dependent disease*		- Unable to reduce GCS below the equivalent of prednisone of 10 mg/day (budesonide 3 mg/d) with 3 months of starting GCS, without recurrent active disease - Relapse within 3 months of stopping GCS (early relapse)
○ Morphological recurrence[†]	0	No lesions
	1	<5 aphthous ulcers
	2	>5 aphthous ulcers with normal mucosa between the lesions, or skip areas of larger lesions, or lesions confined to the ileocolonic anastomotic lining (< 1 cm)
	3	Diffuse aphthous ileitis with diffusely inflamed mucosa
	4	Diffuse ileal inflammation with larger ulcers, nodules or narrowing

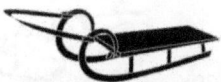

- o Extent
  - - Localized: < 30 cm in extent
  - - Extensive: >100 cm in total extent

- o Colitis unclassified
  - - (do not use the term "indeterminate colitis" which is used for operative specimens) A change in diagnosis from Crohn colitis to UC during the first year; occurs in 10-15% of cases.

- o Risk factors for recurrence
  - - Smoking, prior appendectomy, family history of IBD, perhaps the use of OCA, NSAIDs, antibiotics, pregnancy, ± stress

assumes exclusion of disease-specific complications.
[†] *hyperemia and edema alone are not signs of recurrence*

Abbreviations: CDAI, Crohn disease activity index; GCS: glucoscorticosteroids; NSAIDs, non-steroidal anti-inflammatory drug; OCA, oral contraceptive agent; UC, ulcerative colitis

➢ Immunopathogensis
  - o Rational for suggesting that genetic changes are important
    - – "It is estimated that known genetic associations account for only about 20% of the genetic variance underlying, susceptibility to inflammatory bowel disease" (Abraham & Cho, NEJM 2009;361: 2066-78)
    - – Familial clustering of cases of IBD
    - – Twin studies
      - ▪ Concordance rate among monozygotic twins, 67% (for UC, only ~15%)
    - – NOD2 (Nucleotide Oligomerization Domain 2) (host- microbiome interactions)
    - – Components of the IL-23 type 17 helper T cell (Th 17) pathway
    - – ATG 16 G1, the autophagy gene, as well as the immunity- related GTPase M protein (IRGM) intracellular components such as organelles, apoptotic bodies, and microbes
  - o Mutations
    - – Intestinal macrophages secrete cytokines and chemokines in response to intestinal bacteria. This process of post-translational modification may be impaired in some persons with CD, as well as there being a reduced recruitment of neutrophils to the tissue for destruction and removal of the organisms in the autophage lysosomes.
    - – This may possibly be associated with NOD_2 receptor mutations which reduce the acute inflammatory response to enteric organisms, and thereby exacerbating and amplifying the chronic response.

290

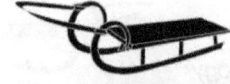

- The NOD2 mutations are associated with reduced transcription of IL-10, leading to an enhancement of the granulomatous reaction, which in course is a feature of CD.
- This defect in the transport of vesicles in the macrophage may be linked to mutations in IREM and ATE 16L1, autophagy related genes which may be abnormal in CD.
- NOD_2 mutations are also associated with higher loads of bacteria colonization of the crypts, and thereby higher bacterial loads.

- Give the defective innate immunity, abnormal autophagia, and excessive response in adaptive immunity which occur in Crohn disease, and contribute to the pathogenesis of this chronic inflammatory condition.
   - ↑ type or amount of luminal antigens which stimulate an inflammation and sustain an abnormally increased immune response
   - Microbiome (microorganisms which inhabit the GI tract)
      - Persons with CD and UC have a reduced number and diversity, as compared with controls, of the mucosa-associated phyla Firmicutes and Bacteroidetes
   - ↑ intestinal permeability ("leakiness") to antigens
   - Lumen
      - Acid
      - Blie
      - Pancreatic enzymes
      - Mucus
   - Motility
   - BBM
      - Tight junctions
      - α-defensins
      - Toll like receptors
      - Cell matrix adhesion
      - Epithelial cell development or proliferation
      - Restitution of epithelial cells after injury
      - Stress of the endoplasmic reticulum
   - MALT/GALT
      - B cells secretory immunoglobulins
      - Dendritic cells
      - T cells (Peyer's patches, mesenteric lymph nodes, lymphoid follicles) when activated produce integrin a4B7 and CCR9 (a chemokine receptor)
      - Pattern recognition receptors (innate immune cells) Intestinal vasculature-adhesion molecules (selections, integrins) and chemokines (secreted cell attractants)
      - Leukocyte migration

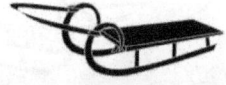

o Mucosal repair and barrier function
  - Polymorphisms in proximity to the gene encoding EP_4 ($PTGE_4$) in CD
o In NOD2 homozygotes there are
  - ↓ defensin production by crypt Paneth cells
  - ↓ sensing of intracellular bacteria or antigens
o Abnormal antigens are taken up by APC (antigen presenting cells), such as dendritic cells, macrophages
o Autophagy of antigen in proteasomes is abnormal
o MHC lass II cells presents antigen with abnormal epitope to CD3 receptor of T cells
o Interaction become active once exposed to binding of costimulatory signals:
  - TNF to TNF-R
  - CD40 to CD40 ligand
  - B7 to CD28
o The p40 subunit on IL-20 and IL-23, together IL-6 and TGF-β lead to differentiation of T cells into Th-17
o ↑ NFkB in mononuclear cells lead to ↑ IL-1, -6 and TNF, as well as adhesion molecules and chemokines.
o TNF causes
  - ↑ synthesis of proteins noted above
  - With IFN-α, causes ↑ MHC class II expression on epithelial cells
  - ↑ neutrophil activation
o The Th1 and Th17 immune response is increased further through leucocyte trafficking
  - Mononuclear expression of adhesion molecules
  - Rolling of leucocytes (WBC) along endothelium through expression of selectins and integrins
  - Integrins bind to intestinal receptors

Integrins	Ligands	Site of Binding
• α4β7	– Mucosal adhessin	Endothelium of venules in LP (Mad CAM-1)
• αEβ7	– Cellular E-cadherin	IELs (intraepithelial lymphocytes)

o Monocytes and granular cells in LP (, lamina propria) release proinflammatory substances which initiate and maintain inflammation:
  - Prostaglandins
  - Leukotrienes
  - Nitric oxide (NO)
  - Reactive oxygen species (ROS)
  - Proteases
    ▪ Collagenase
    ▪ Matrix metaloproteasis

292

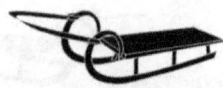

- Give the role of NOD2 in the pathogenesis of Crohn disease.
  - NOD2 (nucleotide-binding oligomerization domain 2) gene (aka CAR15 [caspase-recruitment domain 15)
    - "carriage of disease-associated allelic variants on both chromosomes confers an odds ratio for Crohn disease of 17.1...., and heterozygous persons have an odds ratio of 2.5 ...... for the disease" (Sleisenger and Fordtran's Gastrointestinal and Liver Disease. 9th Edition. Saunders/Elsevier, Philadelphia, 2016, page 1992)
    - Associated with
      - Younger onset
      - Ileal disease
      - Structuring
    - About 25% of CD patients have abnormal NOD2/CARD5 but penetrance is < 1%
  - NODs acts as an intracellular sensor, binding to muramyl dipeptide of bacterial dipeptide
  - NOD2 is expressed in Paneth cells, which are in the crypts and produce defensins
  - Defects in NODs impair the normal antibacterial responses to luminal antigens
    - Autophagy
    - Innate immune response
  - Altered expression of autophagy-related genes
  - ATG 16L1 (autophagy-related 16-like 1 gene)
  - IRGM (immunity related GTPase family member M)
  - IL-23 and IL-23R

- ➢ Clinical manifestations (approximate)
  - Diarrhea   90%
  - Pain   90%
  - Bleeding   50%
  - Weight Loss   85%
  - Fever   60%
  - Malaise   40%
  - Perianal disease 35%
    - Perianal disease occurring before intestinal inflammation, 24%
    - Proximal intestinal Crohn disease and distal disease
      - Early 1/3, no
      - Late 3/3, yes

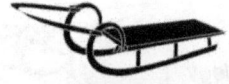

- Others
  - Intra-abdominal abscess in ~25% of Crohn patient during the lifetime of their disease
  - Angular cheilitis, 8%
  - PSC (primary sclerosing cholangitis) does occur in Crohn disease (4%), especially Crohn colitis
  - Complications of weight loss, malnutrition, osteoporosis

CLINICAL CHALLENGE

- In the context of the patient with Crohn disease, give the meaning of the Melkersson-Rosenthal syndrome.
  - The Melkersson-Rosenthal syndrome is the presence of recurrent swelling of the tongue in the patient with Crohn disease.

SO YOU WANT TO BE AN IBD-OLOGIST!

- Give the mechanism of the lung conditions associated with Crohn disease.
  - Crohn disease is associated with reactive airway disease ("asthma") and with COPD (chronic obstruction pulmonary disease, because of the "... commonality of bronchus-associated lymphoid tissue and gut-associated lymphoid tissue" (Feldman M., et al. Sleisenger and Fordtran's Gastrointestinal and Liver Disease. 9th Edition. Saunders/Elsevier, Philadelphia, 2010, page 1955).

➢ Diagnosis

- Give tools to assess disease activity of CD.
  - Suspicion of ↑ risk
    - Young males
    - Previous surgery
    - Fistulizing/stenotic CD
    - Smoking
    - Ileum > 20 cm involvement
    - Proximal intestinal disease
    - ≥ 2 previous attacks requiring treatment with corticostroids

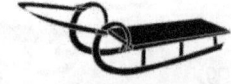

- o Symptoms
  - CDAI (Crohn disease activity index)
  - No correlation between CDAI and CDEIS (endoscopy score)
  - Lehman score – complications
  - Quality of life score
- o Laboratory
  - CRP
  - Fecal calprotectin
  - L/M (lactulose/mannitol) urinary excretion test
- o Endoscopy
  - No previos surgery
    - Simplex index
  - Post-resection
    - Rutgeerts index
  - Confocal microscopy
  - Biopsy grading
  - Mucosal healing
- o Diagnostic imaging
  - Cross-sectional imaging (CTE) is being replaced by MR enterography (MRE)
  - CT enterography (CTE)
  - WBC flux into gut (colon-good in CD-colitis, UC; not useful in SB-CD)
  - Ultrasound findings suggesting active IBD
    - Wall thickening
    - Inflammatory fat
    - Lymphadenopathy
  - Complications (strictures)
- o Colour doppler US (aka colour doppler)
  - Inflammation induces neoangiogenesis
  - Active vs inactive CD 200% ↑ vascularity
  - ↑ blood flow → ↑ inflammation
  - Fractional blood volume
    - Peak intensity
    - AUC (area under curve)
    - Area under wash in (AUWI) and washout (AUWO)

Source: Lakatos PL, et al. Am J Gastroenterol 2012; 107: 579-588.

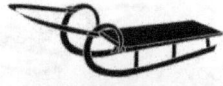

Mastering the Boards: Gastroenterology   A.B.R. Thomson

- Give the performance characteristics of CT enterography (CTE) for CD.
  - Performance characteristics of CTE for the diagnosis of CD
    - Sensitivity, 82%
    - Specificity, 89%

- Give the three criteria on CTE which correlate best with the endoscopic evidence of active CD.
  - CTE and the best criteria for diagnosis of active CD:
    - Mural enhancement
    - ↑ attenuation (↑ density of perenteric fat)
    - "comb" sign (segmental dilation of the vasa recta of a loop of intestine)

➤ Endoscopy

- Give macroscopic features on colonoscopy which suggest the diagnosis of CD.
  - Confluent deep linear ulcers, aphthoid ulcers
  - Deep fissures
  - Fistulas
  - Cobblestoning
  - Skip lesions (segmental disease)
  - Strictures
  - Rectum typically spared

➤ Histopathology
  - Thickening of the intestinal wall
  - Fat wrapping of mesentery
  - Aphthous ulcers
    - Focal areas of immune activation → lymphoid aggregates which destroy the underlying M cells which express HLA-DR
    - Coalesce to from ulcers
      - Stellate
      - Serpiginous
      - Copplestoning
  - Granuloma
    - Collections of
      - Histiocytes
      - Lymphocytes
      - Eosinophils
      - Giant cells

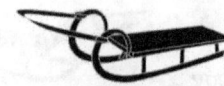

- No central necrosis
- "the presence of lymphoid aggregates in the submucosal and external to the muscularis propria is a reliable sign of Crohn disease even when granulomas are not seen" (Sleisenger and Fordtran's Gastrointestinal and Liver Disease. 10th Edition. Saunders/Elsevier, Philadelphia, 2016, page 1998).

o Hypertrophy of mesenteric adipose tissue ("creeping fat")
  - Associated with
    ▪ Active inflammation
    ▪ TNF produced by adipocytes
    ▪ Lymphoid aggregates and transmural inflammation

o Pyloric metaplasia

➢ Laboratory

• Give blood, stool, or urine tests in Crohn disease which suggest the possibility of a higher risk of future symptomatic relapse.

o Blood
  - CRP
    ▪ ↑ CRP (> 20 mg/L), ↑ ESR (> 15), (8X ↑ risk of relapse if both markers positive: negative predictive value 97%)
    ▪ ↑↑↑ CRP – suspect abscess
    ▪ CRP may be used to guide therapy and follow-up

o ↑ α_2 globulin, α glycoprotein, ↑ TNF

o Stool markers (calprotectin, lactoferrin, TNF – related to extent and degree of ulcerated intestinal surface, with high predictive value for colonic inflammation, and for upcoming clinical relapse

o ↑ urine lactulose/mannitol excretion ratio (intestinal permeability test)

SO YOU WANT TO BE AN IBD-OLOGIST!

• Give the serological markers which predict a specific phenotype of Crohn disease.

Serological Marker	Crohn Phenotype
o ASCA (anti-Saccharomyces cerevisiae antibody)	o Small intestine
o Anti-cBiR1	o Stricturing and interally penetrating disease
o Anti OmpC (anti – E. coli outer membrane porin C	o Perforation (fistula)
o pANCA (perinuclear anti-neutrophil cytoplasmic antibodies)	o "UC-like" Crohn disease

---

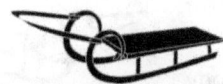

> Differential

- Give the features used to make a distinction between ulcerative colitis (UC) and Crohn disease (CD).

Feature	UC	CD
Clinical Features		
o Malaise, fever	+	+++
o Abdominal pain	+	+++
o Diarrhea	+	+++
o Rectal bleeding	+++	+
o Weight loss	+	++
o Signs of malnutrition	+	++
o Perianal disease	+	++
o Abdominal mass	O	++
o Risk of colorectal cancer	+++	++
Intestinal Complications		
o Stricture	Rare (exclude CRC)	Common
o Fistulas	Very Rare	Common
o Sepsis	Uncommon	Common
o Toxic Megacolon	May occur	Uncommon
o Perforation	Uncommon	Uncommon
o Hemorrhage	Common	Uncommon
o Rate of malignancy	Increased	Increased
Radiological Features		
o Mucosal Ulceration	Superficial	Superficial
o Fissures	Never	Characteristic
o Strictures or fistulas	Rare	Common
o Ileal involvement	Never ("backwash ileitis")	Narrowed/common
o Distribution	Continuous, Symmetric	Discontinuous, Asymmetric

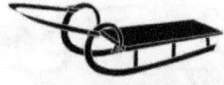

Feature	UC	CD
• Endoscopic Features		
○ Aphthous and linear ulcers	Rare	Common
○ Cobblestone appearance	Never	Common
○ Pseudopolyps	Common	May Occur
○ Distribution	Continuous	Discontinuous
○ Rectal Involvement	Characteristic	Occasionally occurs
• Histopathology		
○ Crypt	-Distorted -Abscesses	-Normal or focally distorted abcesses
○ Inflammation type	-Acute and chronic -Continuous between and within biopsies	-Normal or chronic -Patchy between and within biopsies
○ Depth	-Superficial	-Transmural
○ Granuloma	-No	-Yes

Please see Sleisenger and Fordtran's Gastrointestinal and Liver Disease. 9th Edition. Saunders/Elsevier, Philadelphia, 2016, Table 115-2, page 2008, "Differentiating Crohn Colitis from Ulcerative Colitis".

- Give differential diagnoses of small bowel and colonic Crohn disease.

<u>Small Bowel – CD</u>

○ Backwash ileitis in ulcerative colitis

○ Latrogenic (drugs)
  – Ischemic (oral contraceptives, ergotamine, amphetamines, phenylephrine, cocaine)
  – NSAID-related ulcer or stricture

○ Gynecological disorders
  – Ectopic pregnancy
  – Endometriosis
  – Ovarian cyst or tumour
  – Ovarian torsion
  – Pelvic inflammatory disease
  – Tubo-ovarian abscess

<u>Colon – CD</u>

– Acute self-limited colitis
– Indeterminate colitis
– Ulcerative colitis
– Behçet disease
– Microscopic colitis
– Collagenous colitis
– Lymphocytic colitis
– Diversion colitis
– Pouchitis
– Diverticular disease associated segmental colitis
– Graft-vs-host disease
– Solitary rectal ulcer syndrome

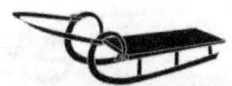

Small Bowel – CD

- o Ileitis associated with spondyloarthropathy
- o Infection
  - Actinomycosis israelii
  - Anisakis simplex
  - Cryptococcosis
  - Cytomegalovirus
  - Histoplasma capsulatum
  - Mycobacterium avium complex
  - Mycobacterium tuberculosis
  - Neutropenic enterocolitis
  - Salmonella
  - Yersinia enterocolitica
  - Yersinia pseudotuberculosis
- o Infiltrative disorders
- o Amyloidosis
- o Eosinophilic gastroenteritis
- o Other inflammatory disorders
  - Appendiceal abscess
  - Appendicitis
  - Cecal diverticulitis
- o Neoplasms
  - Carcinoid tumour
  - Cecal or ileal adenocarcinoma
  - Lymphoma
  - Lymphosarcoma
  - Metastatic cancer
- o Lymphoid nodular hyperplasia
- o Torsion of the appendiceal epiploica
- o Vascular disorders
  - Behçet syndrome
- o Ischemia (radiation, drugs); acute enteritis, chronic enteritis, stricture; chronic mesenteric ischemia); focal segmental ischemia
- o Henoch-Schönlein purpura

Colon – CD

- o Infection
  - Viral
    - Cytomegalovirus (CMV)
    - Herpes (HSV)
  - Bacterial
    - Aeromonas hydrophila
    - Campylobacter jejuni
    - Chlamydia trachomatis
    - Clostridium difficile
    - Escherichia coli (0157:H7)
    - Listeria monocytogenes
    - Neisseria gonorrhoeae
    - Salmonella species
    - Shigella species
    - Staphylococcus aureus
    - Syphilis
    - Vibrio perahaemolyticus
    - Yersinia enterocolitica
  - Protozoan
    - Amebiasis (ENT amoeba histolytica)
    - Balantidiasis
    - Schistosomiasis
  - Fungal
    - Histoplasmosis
    - Candidiasis
- o Iatrogenic (drugs)
  - Amphetamines
  - Cocaine
  - Enemas
  - Ergotamine
  - Gold
  - Laxatives
  - Nonsteroidal anti-inflammatory drugs (NASIDs)
  - Methyldopa
  - OCA
  - Penicillamine
  - Phenylephrine
- o Ischemia (radiation, drugs)

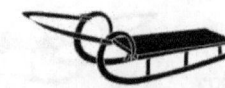

Small Bowel – CD	Colon – CD
o Vasculitis (Churg-Strauss syndrome, giant cell Arteritis, lymphomatoid granulomatosis, polyarteritis nodosa, rheumatoid vasculitis, systemic lupus erythematosus, Takayasu arteritis, Thromboangiitis obliterans, Wegener granulomatosis)	o Infiltration
	- Amyloidosis
	- Chronic granulomatous disease
	- Eosinophilic colitis
	- Neutropenic colitis
	- Sarcoidosis
	o Neoplasms
	o Lymphoid nodular hyperplasia
	- Carcinoid tumour
	- Cecal or ileal adenocarcinoma
	- Lymphoma
	- Lymphosarcoma
	- Metastatic cancer

Abbreviation: CMV, cytomegalovirus; HSV, herpes simplex virus; NSAID, nonsteroidal inflammatory drug

Printed with permission: *Sleisenger & Fordtran's gastrointestinal and liver disease: Pathophysiology/ Diagnosis/Management, 8th Edition,* 2006: pg. 2475.; and 10th edition, 2016, page 2514.

➤ Treatment

   o The therapeutic approach to patients with Crohn disease is changing rapidly, with the "step-up" approach being replaced by "step in early" with biological used early in patients with high risk disease.

- Give the natural history of corticosteroid therapy for CD.

	30 Day	1 Year
o Failure of steroid withdrawal (relapse at dose reduction or within 30 days after end of treatment)	25%	-
o Prolonged Response	32%	49%
o GCS Dependence	28%	22%
o Surgery	38%	29%
o Induction of clinical remission (4-16 wk)	75%	

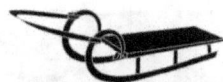

- Give immunosuppressive agents commonly used in gastroenterology or hepatology (for example for Crohn disease, ulcerative colitis, autoimmune hepatitis), and for each give their mode of action, common toxic effects, and recommended monitoring.

Agent	Mode of Action	Monitoring	Toxic Effects
o Cyclosporine (CyA), tacrolimus	– Calcineurin inhibitor: which suppresses IL-2-dependent T cell proliferation	- Blood level (CyA, cholesterol, magnesium, creatinine) - BP - BS	- Renal - Neurologic - Hyperlipidemic - Hypertension - Hirsutism
o Sirolimus (Rapamycin)	– Inhibition of mTOR, which disrupts IL-2 induced intracellular signaling in lymphocytes	- Blood level	- Neutropenia - Thrombocytopeni - Hyperlipidemia
o Prednisone	– Alter gene transcription of steroid response elements (SRE); cytokine inhibitor (IL-1, IL-2, IL-6, TNF, and IFN gamma)	- BP - BS - Annual eye exam - DEXA scan	(see previous question)
o Azathioprine	- Inhibition of T and B cell proliferation by interfering with purine synthesis (↓DNA/RNA)	- White blood cell count - Liver enzymes	- Bone marrow suppression - Hepatotoxicity
o Mycophe-nolate mofetil (Cellsept)	- Inhibition of T and B cell proliferation by interfering with purine synthesis	- White blood cell count	- Diarrhea - Bone marrow suppression
o Methotrexate	- Folate antimetabolite (↓DNA)	- Liver biopsy after 1,500 mg (only 2 years maintenance therapy)	- Hepatic fibrosis - Bone marrow suppression

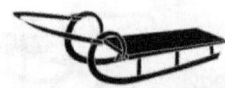

Agent	Mode of Action	Monitoring	Toxic Effects
o OKT3	- Blocking of T cell CD receptor, depletion o effector T cells and T regs, preventing stimulation by antigen	CD3⁺ count	- Cytokine release syndrome - Pulmonary edema - Increased risk of infections
o IL-2 receptor blocker	- Competitive inhibition of IL-2 receptor on activated lymphocytes	None	- Hypersensitivity reactions with basiliximab

Abbreviations: BP, blood pressure; BS, blood sugar; DEXA, DEXA scan for bone mineral density; IFN, interferon; IL, interleukin; LEs, liver enzymes; MTOR, mammalian target of rapamyacin; TNF, tumour necrosis factor

Adapted from: Martin P, and Rosen HR. *Sleisenger & Fordtran's gastrointestinal and liver disease: Pathophysiology/Diagnosis/Management* 2006: pg. 2049.

➤ Prognosis
- o At any given point in time following the first year of the disease
  - – Activity
    - ▪ High 10%
    - ▪ Low 25%
  - – Remission
    - ▪ 65%

- o Predictors of future severe Crohn disease
  - – Young < 40 yr
  - – Steroid use early
  - – Resection early
  - – Clinical:
    - ▪ perianal disease at the time of diagnosis
    - ▪ early need to use steroids
    - ▪ age under 40 years
  - – Mutation in NOD$_2$/CARD 15 (ileal stricture, future need for surgical resection)
    - ▪ HLA-DRB1* 0103 allele
    - ▪ Increasing number of abnormal serological markers (such as pANCA, ASCA, AMCA, ALCA, anti-omp-c, anti-CB$_{1R1}$, anti-I$_2$

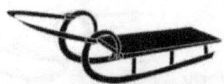

Azathioprine (AZA) and 6-MP

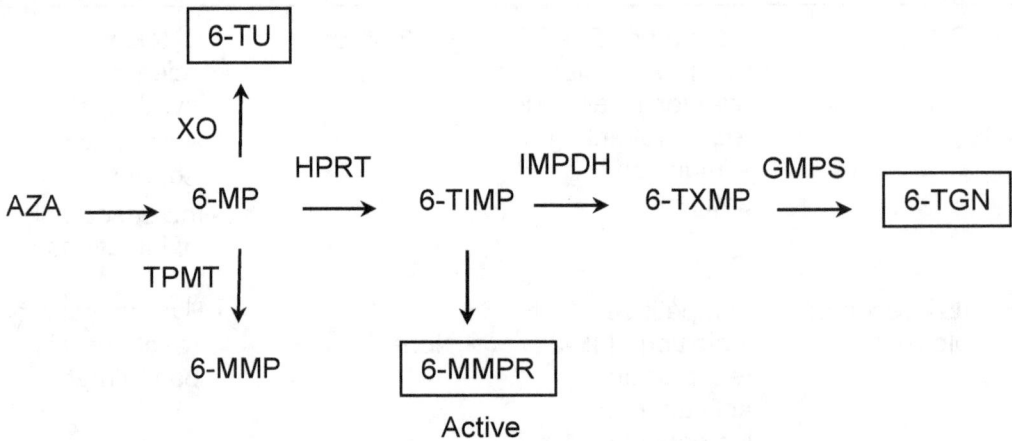

Abbreviations: 6-MMP, 6-methylmercaptopurine; 6-MMPR, 6-methylmercaptopurine ribonucleotide 6-MP, 6-mercaptopurine; 6-TIMP, 6-thioinosine 5'-monophosphate; 6-TU, 6-thiouric acid; AZA, azathioprine; HPRT, hypoxanthine phosphoribosyl transferase; TPMT, thiopurine methyltransferase; XO, xanthine oxidase

Azathioprine (AZA) Tips

- o In persons with reduced TPMT activity (1 in 300), the risk of myelotoxicity when using the standard rather than a reduced dose of AZA/6-MP is increased 4-fold.

- o In support of measuring AZA metabolites (such as 6-TG), weight-based dosing of AZA/6-MP still underestimates the dose 50% of the time (Morales A, Salguti S, Miao CL, et al. *Inflamm Bowel Dis* 2007;13:380-5).

- o Even persons with normal TPMT activity may develop myelotoxicity.

- o Even persons starting on low doses of AZA with a view of gradual dose escalation may develop myelotoxicity.

➤ Adverse effects

- In discussing with a patient the risk of starting azathioprine, give potential risks and their likelihood of occurrence.

  o 3% of allergic reaction including pancreatitis and hepatitis, usually within the first month intolerance to medication (i.e., headache, nausea, malaise) that requires drug withdrawal in 10%
  o 20-25 % risk of leucopenia
  o Drug interaction: allopurimol, 5-ASA
  o Increase levels of 6-TG; possible increased immunosuppression ad risk of malignancy when given with anti-TNF therapy
  o Increase in relative risk of small bowel lymphoma (controversial)
  o Lack of response

- Give different ways of monitoring during azathioprine therapy to reduce the risks of adverse effects.

  o Gene assay that measures the thiopurine methyl transferase (TPMT) genotype(mutation)
  o TPMT enzyme assay
  o 6-TGN (metabolic products) (6-thio guanine nucleotides, active metabolite)
  o Access CBC, liver enzymes

- Give the clinical interpretations of the following blood concentrations of azathiopurine metabolites.

6-TGN	6-MMP	Clinical Interpretations
o ↓	– ↓	▪ Non-adherent, or ▪ Under-dosed (sub-therapeutic)
o N	– ↑	▪ ↑ risk for ↑ liver enzymes
o ↑	– ↓	▪ Responder, refractory ▪ ↑ risk of leucopenia
o ↑	– ↑	▪ Over-dosed

Abbreviations: 6-TGN, 6-Thioguanine nucleotides; 6-MMP, 6-methyl mercaptopurine; MP, Mercaptopurine

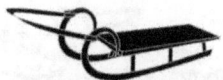

- Give the approximate percentage of patients reported from meta-analysis of trials of AZA/6-MP to achieve and to maintain remission in CD.

	AZA/6-MP	Placebo	TG	OR	NNT
o Achieve remission*	54	33	21	2.36	5
o Maintain remission	67	52	15	2.16 4.13*	7

* 17 weeks necessary; **, optimal dose, 2.5 mg/kg

- o Threshold level of 6-TG of 230 to 260 pmol / 8×10^8 RBC to achieve remission with TG of 26% (62% vs 36% placebo); aim for a ratio of 6-MMP: 6-TG of < 10

Abbreviations: OR, odds ratio; NNT, number needed to treat; TG, therapeutic gain

- o 50% of IBD patients are exposed to AZA (azathioprine) in the first 3 year after diagnosis.

Methotrexate (MTX)

➢ Adverse effects
  - o Hepatic fibrosis
    - With mean cumulative dose of MTX > 2.5 g, only minimal hepatic toxicity
    - Risk of hepatic fibrosis with MTX: ↑ by alcohol, obesity, diabetes
  - o Reproduction
    - Women
      - Abortifacient, teratogenic
    - Men
      - Toxic to sperm
  - o Lung
    - Rare cases of interstitial pneumonitis

- Give gastrointestinal complications of immunosuppression with azathioprine or methotrexate (not including glucocorticosteroids).
  - o Infection
    - CMV, HBV, HSV, EBV (PTLD)
    - Candida albicans, tropicalis
    - Yersinia enterocolitica
    - C. difficile
    - Microsposidia
    - Strongyloides stercoralis
    - H. pylori
    - TB (including reactivation)

306

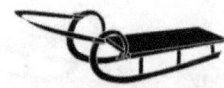

- o Mucosal injury
  - – Diarrhea
  - – Ulceration
    - ▪ AZA or MMF-induced slowing of intestinal cell turnover
    - ▪ May also result of concomitant intake of other medications, e.g., NSAIDs, steroids,
- o Colon: diverticular disease → diverticulitis
- o Perforations (upper or lower GI tract)
- o Liver
  - – Hepatitis
  - – Methotrexate-associated fibrosis/cirrhosis
- o Biliary tract
  - – Thickened gallbladder wall
  - – Sludge
  - – Stones
  - – Dilated ducts
  - – Hydrops

> **Big Dangers of MTX**
> - o Teratotoxicity
> - o Pneumonitis/fibrosis
> - o Hepatic fibrosis
> - o Leukopenia

- o Pancreatitis
  - – Acute (AZA, CyA; CS may also be from complications of CMV, hypercalcemia, cholelithiasis)
- o GI malignancy
  - – Lymphomas (including MALT lymphoma, hepatosplenic lymphoma)
  - – Kaposi sarcoma
  - – Colorectal cancer (CRC)
  - – Post-transplant lymphoproliferative disorder (PTLD; EBV- associated)
  - – Cervical dysplasia

Abbreviations: AZA, azathioprine; CS, corticosteroids; CyA, cyclosporin A; EBV, Ebstein Barr virus; PTLD, post-transplant lymphoproliferative disorder

Adapted from: Helderman J, and Goral S. *J Am Soc Nephrol* 2002; 13: 277-87.

Anti-Tumour Necrosis Factor-α (anti-TNF or ATNF)

- ➢ Indications
  - o Generally indicated for
    - – Inflammatory disease failing to respond to steroids and immunosuppressants
    - – Unclear whether patients at high risk of severe disease are candidates for early anti-TNF treating

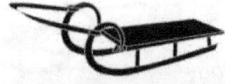

A.B.R. Thomson

- Start high or step-up therapy in IBD – the hope is that if the patient is treated early with effective therapy (anti-TNF)
  - There will be
    - ↓ rate of progression of IBD.
    - ↓ use of corticosteroids
  - Three shortcomings of SONIC study
    - Open-label
    - No comparative group of early anti-TNF vs early immunomodulator
    - Episodic rather than regularly scheduled anti-TNF
    - No stratification for who was likely to develop disabling, complicated or severe disease
    - Used IBD symptoms, not mucosal changes
- Possible future outcome considerations
  - Treat to target (mucosal healing), rather than just symptoms
  - We may underestimate the needs to treat when we don' treat the asymptomatic patients with continued "smoldering inflammation"
- Important to follow literature on value of accessing inflammatory activity of disease and to make the target to endoscopic mucosal healing, or mucosal plus histological healing
- Response and secondary failure after anti TNF-α therapy
  - Approximately 1/3 of primary responders lose response over course of 6-12 months
    - Change in behavior of disease
    - Development of antibodies to therapy
  - If anti-TNF therapy is added to AZA or MTX because of failure to respond to these immunosuppressants, then it would appear to be reasonable to stop immunosuppressant once the anti-TNF therapy has been started, especially since withdrawal of aziothioprine and continuation of the infliximab (IFX) alone has no effect on the continued response to IFX, as compared to patients on both IFX and AZA. This issue remains controversial.
  - For patients with secondary loss of response to IFX, switching to ADA gives "recapture" remission rates of 21% at 4 weeks and 40% at one year ; switching from IFX to certolizumab pegol at 6 weeks gives a "recapture" response of 60% and remission of 40%.

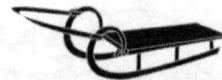

> Terms

- Give a definition for primary and secondary infliximab failures (IFX) in patients with inflammatory bowel disease (IBD); outline their proposed mechanisms.
    - Primary
        - No response to induction therapy, possibly due to
            - High pre-treatment TNF-α levels
            - Inadequate dose of IFX (low trough IFX concentration), or
            - TNF-α independent inflammatory pathways
    - Secondary
        - Loss of symptomatic response after initial successful induction therapy
        - Mechanisms
            - Antibody to IFX (especially with on-demand IFX infusions)
            - Increased clearance (rapid metabolism) of IFX
            - Inadequate dose of IFX (low trough IFX concentration) non-TNFα dependent inflammatory pathways
            - Development of IBD-related complications e.g., stricture, abscess
            - Non-IBD related symptoms e.g IBS, SIBO, bile acid wastage, c. difficile infection

Adapted from: Toruner M, et al. Presented at DDW 2006; and van Asche et al. *Gastroenterology* 2007; 132:A-103.

Anti-TNF results overall

- Remission   35%
- Maintenance (1 yr) 25-30%
    - Stratify patients by objective measures of inflammation
        - CRP, mucosa lesions on endoscopy
    - "don't stop drugs that work"
        - 25% of patients who respond to TNFB that are then stopped will recur

> **Cautions: Trial Design**
> - Many of the ATNF trials had an initial 2 wk lead-in period, and only those persons who improved on therapy were continued or the randomized portions of the study to determine rates of remission and maintenance of remission

- Anti-TNF therapy vs placebo:
    - Failure to achieve remission 43% vs 70% RR 0.72; NNT (to achieve 1 remission), 4
    - 5 mg/kg per day – equivalent benefit as 10 mg/kg per day
    - After induction dosing of infliximab (0, 2, 6 weeks), continue dosing every 8 weeks.
    - Results of Act 1 and Act 2 studies (Infliximab)

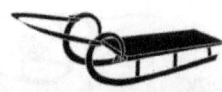

	Duration of Treatment, weeks	Clinical Response		Mucosal Healing
		Anti-TNF	PL	
o Response	8	64% and 66%	29%	55%
- Remission	30	39% and 32%	15%	57%
o Response	54	45% and 44%	20%	22%
- Remission	54	34%	17%	

Abbreviation: PL. placebo

A patient has an increased risk of infection if they are being treated with immunosuppressants or anti-TNF therapy.

- Give conditions associated with an increased risk of infection in the patient who is not receiving immunosuppressants or biologicals (anti-TNF therapy).

  o Granulocytes (chronic granulomastous disease)
    - ↑ risk of invasion skin infections

  o Cell-mediated defects (e.g., HIV infection, ↓ CD4 T cells)
    - Viral or fungal infections

  o Immunoglobulins
    - Encapsulated bacteria

  o CFTR (cystic fibrosis)
    - Infection of sinuses and lung

  o Complement deficiency
    - Neisseria meningitides gonorrhea

Adapted from: Board Basics 3, 2012, page 9.

  o Antibodies to anti-TNF agents
    - ANA (antinuclear antibodies) develop in 50% of anti-TNF blockers of these, 30% develop anti-dsDNA (a double-stranded)

- Give the approximate frequency (per 10^5) of the serious side effects of anti-TNF agents in Crohn disease.

Event	Estimated Frequency per 10^5
o Non-Hodgkin lymphoma (baseline)	20
- On immunosuppression	40
- Also on anti TNF in perspective	60
o Tuberculosis infection	50
o Death from sepsis	40

Adapted from: Siegal, Corey A. *2009 ACG Annual Postgraduate Course* 2009:267-9.

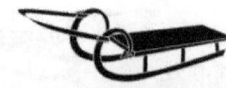

- ➤ In perspective

  - ○ Surgery is commonly needed in persons with Crohn disease' 18% in the first year after diagnosis, and 80% after 20 years. The operative mortality is $80/10^5$, compared with a $40/10^5$ mortality rate for dying of sepsis from anti-TNF therapy.

  - ○ NHL (non-Hodgkin lymphoma)

Group	Incidence (per 10^5 patient-year)
– General population	1.9
– Crohn disease on	
• Immunomodulators	1.7
• Anti-TNF blocker	6.1
– Standardized incidence rates	3.23

  - ○ Meta-analysis has shown that the rate of non-Hodgkins lymphoma (NHL) is $61/10^5$ patient years in persons on anti-TNF therapy plus immunomodulators, a rate similar to that from the use of immunomodulators (Siegel CA, et al. *Clin Gastroenterol Hepatol* 2009)

  - ○ Baseline risk of lymphoma in IBD is approximately $20/10^5$ (standardized incidence rate, SIR).

  - ○ Patients with IBD on a thiopurine analog such as azathioprine have an adjusted hazard ratio of lymphoproliferative disorders of 5.28, as compared to those who have never been on this class of drugs, and this number returns to normal if the thiopurine is stopped.

  - ○ The risk is about the same for persons on azathioprine or a biologic who develop extranodal hepatosplenic T-cell lymphoma (HSTCL).

  - ○ The number of persons needed to heal with azathioprine / G mercaptopurine per year to cause one case of lymphoma is 4,357, compared to 2,380 for an anti – TNF drug.

  - ○ Do not use risk data from patients with rheumatoid arthritis (RA).

Please see: Chami G, Feagan BG. Chapter 63. In: Therapeutic Choices. Grey J, Ed. 6th Edition, Canadian Pharmacists Association: Ottawa, ON, 2011, Table 1: Drugs Used for the Treatment of Inflammatory Bowel Disease, page 847-853.

- • Give common anti-TNF medication-associated skin rashes.

  - ○ Psoriatic lesions ± pus

  - ○ Eczematous lesions

  - ○ Lupus-like lesions

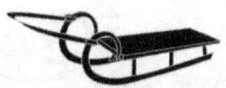

- Give relative contraindications to anti-TNF therapy.
  - Pre-existing severe immunosuppression
  - Allergy to anti-TNF
  - Intestinal stenosis
  - Fistulizing disease with abscess
  - Fistulae to bladder
  - Untreated active infection (TB, HBV, HCV)
  - Multiple sclerosis (MS), optic neuritis
  - Congestive cardiac failure (New York grade III, IV)
  - Lymphoma
  - Acute liver failure
  - Cancer in the past

Abbreviations: HBV, hepatitis B viral infection; HCV, hepatitis C viral infection; MS, multiple sclerosis; TB, tuberculosis

➤ Combination therapy
  - Immunomodulators decrease risk of HAHAs (human antihuman antibodies) but may ↑ risk of NHL or infection

- Give the advantages and disadvantages of adding concomitant immunomodulators to anti-TNF therapy in Crohn disease (CD).

Advantages	Disadvantages
o ↓ Antibodies (at least to infliximab)	− ↓ duration of response (with episodic therapy)
o Benefit in steroid-dependent CD (SONIC)	− No difference in short- or long-term responses to induction + maintenance therapy in refractory CD (ACCENT, CHARM, PRECISE)
o ↓ acute/delayed infusion reactions	
o ↓ immunogenicity	− No benefit with steroid-induction (COMMIT)
	− ↑ long-term toxicity ▪ ↑ risk of infections, including serious infections
	− High cost

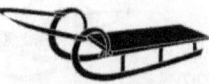

> The debate is settled!
>
> "Give immune suppressants with TNF-α therapy."
>
> Dr. B. Fegan, 2013

- o What to think of when TNFB is not working?
  - Poor compliance
  - Inadequate dose or too long interval between dosing possibly because of ↑ loss of ATNF through inflamed bowel
  - Developed antibodies to ATNF drug
  - Disease not driven by TNF (different disease driver)
  - Wrong diagnosis of cause of symptoms
- o The severity of IBD is determined by the general course of the disease and not by the severity of the flare
- o Remember that there is often a disconnect between symptoms and what is happening to the inflammation in the mucosa.

- Give risk factors associated with time-to-relapse in patients with Crohn disease who are in clinical remission on maintenance therapy with both infliximab and anti-metabolites, and then who stop infliximab.
  - o Patient
    - No previous surgical resection
    - Male sex
  - o Laboratory
    - Hemoglobin level ≤ 145 g/L
    - Leukocyte count > 6 x 10^9 per L
    - CDEIS > 0
    - hsCRP level ≥ 5 mg/L
    - Fecal calprotection level ≥ 300 μg/g`
  - o Drugs
    - Infliximab trough level ≥ 2 mg/L
    - Corticosteroids use 6-12 months before infliximab discontinuation
  - o Clinical relapse rate (%) as a function of the number of risk factors
    - < 4 risk factors: < 20%
    - 4 risk factors: ~ 40%
    - 5-6 risk factors: ~ 80%
  - o > 6 risk factors: 100%

Printed with permission: de Chambrun GP, et al. IBD in 2011: Advances in IBD management--towards a tailored approach. Nat Rev Gastroenterol Hepatol. 2012;9(2):70-2. Box-1.

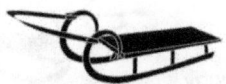

- Give the risk of treatment-associated opportunistic infections in IBD.

	Odds Ratio
o Any medication (5-ASA, AZA/6MP, Steroids, MTX, Infliximab)	3.50
o 5-ASA	0.98
o Corticosteroids	3.4
o AZA/6MP	3.1
o MTX	4.0
o Infliximab	4.4
o One medication	2.7
o Two medications	9.4

- Give live vaccines which should **not** be given while the IBD patient is on anti-TNF therapy.

❖ Non-oral
  - o Bacilli Calmette-Guerin (BCG)
  - o Herpes Zoster Virus (HZV)
  - o Inhaled nasal influenza
  - o Japanese encephalitis
  - o Measles, mumps, rubella (MMR)
  - o Rotavirus
  - o Vaccinia (smallpox)
  - o Varicella
  - o Yellow fever

❖ Oral
  - o Polio
  - o Typhoid

- Give the recommended dosing for adalimumab or certolizumab pegol, in patients with Crohn disease.

❖ Adalimumab
  - o 160 mg subcutaneously (SC) on day 1 of week 0, followed by 80 mg SC on day 1 of week 2.
  - o Patients who respond to this two week induction regimen should continue on a maintenance regimen of 40 mg SC every other week.
  - o Patients who have suboptimal response to 40 mg SC every other week may increase frequency of dosing to 40 mg SC weekly, or increase their dose to 80 mg every other week.
    - − Subsequent response in 4-week nonresponders has not been established.
  - o Episodic dosing has not been evaluated, and may increase immunogenicity

314

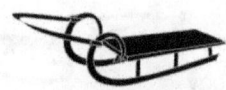

- ❖ Certolizumab pegol
  - o Recommended dosing is 400 mg SC at weeks 0, 2, and 4 and then end 4.
    - − No evidence of benefit for additional treatment at week 6 for nonresponders
  - o Patients who respond to the induction regimen should continue on maintenance dosing with 400 mg SC every 4 weeks.
    - − Additional dosing schedules have not been evaluated in IBD but anticipate similar recommendations to other anti-TNFs regarding higher dose/reduced interval treatment. In patients with rheumatoid arthritis, changing the maintenance dosing schedule to 200 mg SC every 2 weeks increases drug exposure by approximately 50%

"Debunking" Some CD Therapies
  - o No evidence for
    - − Fish oil supplements
    - − SCFA (short-chain fatty acid) enemas (only useful in diversion colitis)
    - − Transdermal nicotine patches to maintain remission (for UC patients who smoke and have mildly active UC, using nicotine patches may be beneficial while the patient stops smoking
    - − Heparin
  - o Elemental, hydrolyzed and polymeric formulas are equally effective in the treatment of IBD (Zachos M, et al *Cochrane Database Syst Rev* 2007:CD000542.) (Or, 0, 33)

  - o Miscellaneous
    - - Best results for maintenance therapy in Crohn disease-stop smoking

  - o Still "on radar screen": more data needed
    - − Methotrexate in doses > 12.5 mg per week
    - − Budesonide MMX
    - − Trichuris suis (helminthes, from pigs)
    - − Oral phosphatidylcholine
    - − Anti-integrin antibodies
    - − Thiazolidinediones (rosiglitazone)
    - − Antibodies against IL-12, IL-23
    - − MAd CAM (mucosal addressin cell adhesion molecule-1)

Abbreviation: NHL, non-Hodgkins lymphoma

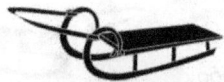

Symptom Recurrence in CD

A patient with CD (Crohn disease) develops diarrhea.

- Give causes of the diarrhea which relate to CD or its complications.
    - Active CD
    - Mesalamine-(5-ASA) associated diarrhea
    - SIBO (small intestinal bacterial overgrowth from associated dysmotility, fistula, stricture)
    - Enteric infection
    - Bile salt malabsorption (choleretic diarrhea)
    - Steatorrhea
    - Temporary lactase deficiency (lactose intolerance)

Because it is increasingly recognized that "attacks " or flares of IBD may be associated with enteric infection, anticipate the MCQ examining where you appreciate this association and are prepared to act upon this association, rather than the reflex action of placing every IBD patient with recurrent symptoms on corticosteroids, immunosuppressants , or biological.

- Give micro-organisms which may cause what appears to be a recurrence of IBD.

    - Toxin Bacteria
        - Campylobacter
        - Clostridium difficile
        - Escherichia Coli O157: H7
        - Salmonella
        - Shigella
        - Yesinia

    - Ova and parasites
        - Including Entamoeba histolytica, especially in
            - First Nations persons, or
            - Patients visiting from endemic areas including Southern USA

    - Viruses
        - CMV (cytomegalovirus)
        - HSV (herpes simplex virus)

316

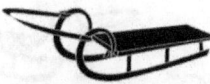

- Give risk factors for the development of **osteopenia/osteoporosis** in inflammatory bowel disease (IBD).
  - Demographics
    - Low bone mineral intensity peak in patients with pediatric onset of IBD
    - Increasing age
    - Female gender
    - Immobilization
    - Smoking
    - Family history of osteoporosis
  - Nutrition
    - Malnutrition
    - Malabsorption of vitamin D, calcium and Vitamin K
    - Low body mass index
  - Drugs
    - Use of corticosteroids
  - Inflammation
    - Chronic inflammatory state
    - Type of IBD (CD vs UC, small intestinal involvement)
  - Metabolic
    - Previous fragility fracture
    - Hypogonadism

Abbreviations: IBD, inflammatory bowel disease; CD, Crohn disease; UC, ulcerative colitis

Adapted from: Ghishan FR & Kiela PR. *AJP-Gastrointest Liver Physiol* • 2011;300: G191-G201 Table 1, page G192.

"Whoever said that old age was "The Golden Years" was already demented."

Grandad

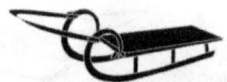

Clinical Scenario

A 25 year old female has had ileal Crohn disease for 3 years and has been taking no medications for the past 2 years. She smokes 1 pack of cigarettes per day. She presents to your office with 1 month of abdominal pain and diarrhea. You get a small bowel follow through and it reveals a short segment of ileal disease. You prescribe entocort 9 mg/day. You see her again in 1 month and she feels completely well and you begin tapering her entocort. *

- Give options for further therapy at this time.
    - Taper entocort to 6 mg/day, then to 3 mg then stop before 12 months
    - Taper entocort completely off and leave her on no medications
    - Taper entocort off and use Pentasa® 4 gm/day
    - Start azathioprine or 6-mercaptopurine as maintenance agents
    - Start methotrexate as a maintenance agent (advise contraception)
    - Start anti-TNF, with or without immune suppression (controversial)
    - Stop smoking (equivalent to immunosuppression)
    - Discuss contraception, pregnancy planning
    - Antibiotics, probiotics
    - Surgery
    - Symptom control
    - Education, including Crohn and Colitis Foundation (CCFC)

- Give the treatments for **calcium oxalate kidney stones**.
    - Fluids
        - Adequate intake of water by mouth
    - Reduce oxalate absorption
        - Reduce intake of oxalate (cranberry juice, chocolate, etc.)
        - Oral calcium supplements to bind oxalates in the gut lumen
        - Colectomy, if indicated for other reasons
    - Increase renal excretion
        - Correct metabolic acidosis
    - Bind luminal bile acids with binding agents (e.g., cholestyramine)

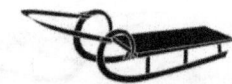

- Give examples of drugs used to treat IBD which have potentially serious **interactions with other drugs**.

    o 5-ASAs-increase INR, 6-TG and methotrexate (MTX); decreases digitalis levels

    o Allopurinol-increases 6-TG

    o ACE inhibitors-increase 6-MP-associated risk of anemia, leucopenia

    o Methotrexate (MTX) levels are reduced by tetracycline, and increased by penicillin 5-ASAs and NSAIDs; folic acid deficiency worsens MTX toxicity

    o Metronidazole increases the effect of statins, sildenafil, calcium channel blockers, and ↑ INR

    o Anti-TNF therapy causes 6.4 fold increase in mortality rate in persons with pre-existing pulmonary disease

    o Steroids cause osteoporosis by changing the optimal ratio of Rank-L relative to OPG/ OCIF; this effect of steroids is greatest in the first 6 months of their use

Abbreviations: MTX, methotrexate; OCIF, osteoclastogenesis inhibitory factor; OPG, osteoprotegerin

IBD and Pregnancy

   o Fertility
     - Colectomy and ileoanal anastamosis increases infertility 3-fold
     - The incidence of abnormal PAP smears is increased in women with IBD

   o Clinical course
     - ↑ active disease- not confirmed more recently
     - In a community based study from northern California, the activity of IBD at conception usually carries through the pregnancy as well as postpartum period
     - Poor outcome of pregnancy – Not confirmed more recently

   o Delivery
     - Although the only contraindications to vaginal delivery in Crohn disease is active perianal disease, the likelihood of having a Caesarean section is increased 1.5 times above that of non-IBD women.
     - Having an extensive episiotomy at delivery may contribute to the 18% risk of a woman developing perianal disease after childbirth.

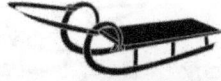

Mastering the Boards: Gastroenterology   A.B.R. Thomson

- o Outcomes
  - The transmission of IBD from parent to child is low
    - One parent with IBD; transmission risk is 7%
    - Both parents have IBD, 37% risk of transmission
  - Flexible sigmoidoscopy during pregnancy does not increase the risk of premature labour.
- o Breastfeeding
  - Breastfeeding may or may not be a risk factor for the development of Crohn disease in the infant.
  - Only 29-44% of IBD patients breastfeed their infant (compared to an American standard of 60%).
  - 43% of those mothers who breastfeed their babies flared, possibly because 74% of those who flared had stopped maintenenace medications.
- o Medications – FDA category
  - There have been no reports of hepatosplenic T-cell lymphoma in IBD patients on monotherapy with anti-TNF therapy
  - Avoid use of methotrexate, thalidomide
- o Family counselling
  - Discuss with family note of IBD in the child

"Success is peace of mind which is a direct result of self-satisfaction in knowing you did your best to become the best you are capable of becoming."

John R Wooden

 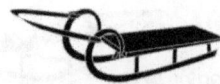

- Give a classification of the **safety of medications** used in patients with IBD who are **pregnant +/- breastfeeding**.

Drug	FDA Category	Recommendations for Breastfeeding
Adalimumab	B	LHD
Amoxicillin/clavulanic acid	B	Probably compatible
AZA/6-MP	D	LHD
Balsalazide	B	Yes
Ciprofloxacin	C	LHD
Corticosteroids	C	Yes
Cyclosporin	C	**No**
Diphenoxylate	C	**No**
Infliximab	B	LHD
Loperamide	B	Yes
Mesalamine	B	Yes
Methotrexate	**No**	**No**
Metronidazole	B	**No**
Olsalazine	C	LHD
Rifaximin	C	LHD
Sulfasalazine	B	Yes
Tacrolimus	C	LHD
Thalidomide	**No**	**No**

> - During **pregnancy and lactation, No**
>   - Thalidomide
>   - Methotrexate
> - During **breastfeeding, No**
>   - Thalidomide
>   - Metronidazole,
>   - Cyclosporine
>   - Dephenoxylate

Abbreviation: LHD, limited human data

Printed with permission: Kane SV. *2008 ACG Annual Postgraduate course book*: pg. 27.

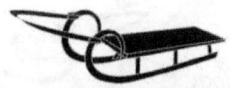

Mastering the Boards: Gastroenterology   A.B.R. Thomson

- Give the causes, diagnostic procedures, and the management of the patient with Crohn disease (CD) who presents with subacute, small bowel obstruction (SBO).

  - Causes
    - Active CD
    - Stricture
    - Fruit pits
    - Gallstone ileus
    - Enterolith

  - Diagnostic procedures
    - Plain abdominal films
    - Conventional CT
    - CT enterography
    - MRI enterography
    - Small bowel (gastrograffin) x-ray
    - Abdominal ultrasound
    - Doppler ultrasound
    - FDG-PGT (18F- flurodeoxyglucose positron emission tomography [PET])
    - Capsule endoscopy (penalty, because of suspected stricture)

  - Management
    - Treatment of inflammatory CD (avoid anti-TNF)
    - Through-the-scope balloon dilation
    - Adjuvant steroid injection into inflammatory narrowing
    - Expandable metal stents
    - Stricturoplasty
    - Open or laparoscopic surgical resection

Abbreviations: PET, positron emission tomography

For additional details on SIBO in conditions other than Crohn disease, please see later section "Small bowel obstruction."

- Give major causes of small or large intestinal **ileus** in any patient, and not necessarily one with Crohn disease.

  - Infection
    - Intra-abdominal or systemic sepsis

  - Inflammation
    - Appendicitis, diverticulitis, perforated duodenum
    - Lower lobe pneumonia

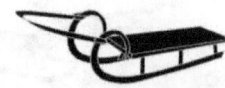

- o Ischemia
  - Mesenteric arterial embolus or thrombosis, mesenteric venous thrombosis, chronic mesenteric ischemia
- o Metabolic
  - ↓ K^+, Na^+, Ca^{2+}, Mg^{2+}
  - ↑ Ca^{2+}, Mg^{2+}
- o Trauma
  - Laparotomy, laparoscopy
    - Lower rib fractures
  - Lumbar compression
    - Fracture
- o Drugs
  - Narcotics, phenothiazines, diltiazem, anticholinergic agents, clozapine
- o Miscellaneous
  - Bands and adhesions
  - Herniation
  - Gallstone ileus

Adapted from: *Sleisenger & Fordtran's gastrointestinal and liver disease: Pathophysiology/Diagnosis/Management* 2006: pg. 2671.

- • Give the classification of gastrointestinal **fistulae**, based on anatomy, output volume, and etiology.

Scheme	Classification
o Anatomical location	– Internal, external – Low, high – Simple, complex
o Output volume	– Pancreatic 　▪ Low (<200 mL/day) 　▪ High (≥200 mL/day) – Intestinal 　▪ Low (<500 mL/day) 　▪ High (≥500 mL/day)
o Etiological	– Underlying disease

Printed with permission: Messmann H, et al. *Best Pract Res Clin Gastroenterol* 2004, pg. 811.

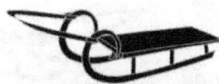

- In the patient with Crohn disease and **perianal fistulae** (PF), give a classification, 6 diagnostic tests, as well as medical and/or surgical treatments.

➢ Diagnostic tests

- o Digital rectal examination (DRE)
- o EUA (examination under general anaesthesia)
- o Pelvic ultrasound
- o Pelvic CT
- o Pelvic MRI
- o Sigmoidoscopy/colonoscopy
- o EUS
- o Barium studies (fistulogram, sinogram)
- o Cystoscopy

- Give the patient-related and fistula-related characteristics associated with spontaneous closure of gastrointesinal fistulae.

  - o Patient characteristics
    - – Young (< 40 years)
    - – Well nourished
    - – Cause of fistulae
    - – Anastamosis characteristics – anastamotic breakdown
    - – Low output (mL/day) <500

  - o Fistula characteristics
    - – Lateral fistula
    - – Fistula tract >2 cm
    - – Non-epithelialised fistula tract
    - – No incomplete disruption
    - – No abscess near leakage
    - – No distal obstruction
    - – Enteral defect <1 cm
    - – Fistula site: Oropharyngeal, esophageal, duodenal stump, pancreatobiliary, jejunal
    - – Late post-operative leakage
    - – Adjacent bowel healthy
    - – No severe systemic diseases

Printed with permission: Messmann H., et al. *Best Pract Res Clin Gastroenterol* 2004, pg. 811.;Hoffman KM, et al. *Best Pract Res Clin Gastroenterol* 2005; 19(5): 677.

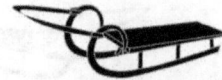

> Treatments
  o Medical
    – Drugs used to treat Crohn disease
    – CO_2 laser ablation
    – Hyperbaric O_2
    – Injection of silver microspheres with antibiotic

  o Surgery
    – Seton placement
    – Glue
    – Fistulotomy
    – Endorectal advancement flap
    – Fecal diversion
    – Proctocolectomy

Abbreviations: DRE, digital rectal examination; EUA, examination under general anaesthesia; EUS, endoscopic ultrasound; PF, perianal fistulae

Nutrition in CD

> Demography
  o The prevalence of malnutrition is increased in IBD: 6.1% in Crohn disease, 7.2% in ulcerative colitis, vs 1.8% in non-IBD controls (275-5)
  o The adjusted odds ratio for malnutrition in IBD is 5.57 (95% CI 5.29-5.86), with a greater risk of malnutrition in those with fistulizing CD (or 1.65; 95% CI: 1.50-1.82), and in IBD patients who had undergone bowel surgery (or 1.37; 95% CI: 1.27-1.48).
  o Malnutrition was also associated with a longer length of hospital stay, increased hospital mortality (or 3.49: 95% CI: 2.89-4.23) and double to hospital costs.

• Give the approximate frequency of nutritional deficiencies in IBD (Crohn disease and ulcerative colitis).

  o High (~ 70%)
    – Weight loss

  o Medium (~ 40%)
    – Anemia
    – Folic acid
    – Hypoalbuminemia
    – Iron
    – Vitamin B12
    – Vitamin D
    – Zinc

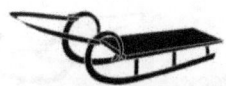

- o Low (~ 25%)
  - – Calcium
  - – Magnesium
  - – Selenium
  - – Vitamins A, E, K

Adapted from: Seidner, Douglas L. *2009 ACG Annual Postgraduate Course*: 271-6.

- Give the mechanisms of developments of nutritional disorders in CD.
  - o ↓ intake
    - – Anorexia, nausea, vomiting
    - – Misinformed diet choices
    - – Food intake-associated abdominal pain
  - o ↓ Digestion/absorption
    - – Reduced absorptive surface (e.g., shortened small intestine due to prior resection, diseased segments)
    - – Bacterial overgrowth (e.g., associated with strictures and bypassed loops, stasis)
    - – Bile salt deficiency after ileal resection (e.g., impaired micelle formation and steatorrhea)
    - – Lactase deficiency (e.g., associated with small bowel disease)
    - – Drug-induced malabsorption
      - ▪ Cholestyramine (e.g., bile acids; fat; fat-soluble vitamins, including vitamin D and K)
      - ▪ Sulfasalazine (e.g., folic deficiency associated with reduced absorption and increased requirement related to hemolysis)
      - ▪ Steroids (e.g., calcium absorption, and patient mobilization)
      - ▪ Methotrexate (e.g., nausea/vomiting)
    - – Increased nutrient loss
      - ▪ Protein-losing enteropathy
  - o Diarrhea fistula losses of electrolytes, minerals and trace elements zinc, iron, calcium, magnesium, selenium
  - o Gastrointestinal blood loss (e.g., iron loss)
  - o ↑ requirements
    - – Chronic inflammatory disease
    - – Fever
    - – Abscess
    - – Superimposed infection
    - – Surgery
  - o ↑ losses
    - – Diarrhea
    - – Protein losing enteropathy

Printed with permission: Griffiths AM. *Best Pract Res Clin Gastroenterol* 2004;18(3): pg.519.

326

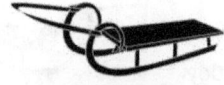

SMALL INTESTINAL MOTILITY

- o Smooth muscle contractions reduce the diameter and/or shorten the length of the small intestine
- o Actin and myosin contractile filaments are attached to dense bands within the myocytes
- o There is a need for the Ca^{2+}_i (intracellular calcium) to increase in order for the myocyte to shorten
- o This Ca^{2+}_i comes from
  - – L-type Ca^{2+} channels
  - – Release of Ca^{2+} from sarcoplasmic reticulum membrane via IP3 receptor-operated Ca^{2+} channels
- o Ca^{2+} binds to calmodulin
- o Calmodulin activates myosin light chain kinase
- o Myosin light chain kinase phosphorylates MLC20 (20 kDa light chain of myosin)
- o MLC20 has three functions to facilitate
  - – Actin binding to myosin
  - – Cross-bridge cycling
  - – Development of mechanical force
- o MLC phosphatase reduces phosphorylate of MLC20
- o Reduced phosphorylation of MLC20 reduces MLC20-associated functions, noted above, and thereby causes muscle relaxation causes slow waves to propagate predominantly abroad" (Feldman M., et al. Sleisenger and Fordtran's Gastrointestinal and Liver Disease. 10th Edition. Saunders/Elsevier, Philadelphia, 2016, page 1680).
- o "...a gradient of slow wave intrinsic frequencies.

- • Give a comparison of patterns of small intestinal vs colonic motility which occur with feeding and with fasting.
  - o Small intestinal motility
    - – Feeding pattern
      - ▪ "continuous low, varying-amplitude, ungrouped phasic contractions, the activity of which depends on the quantity and composition of the ingested food" (Sleisenger and Fordtran's Gastrointestinal and Liver Disease. 10th Edition. Saunders/Elsevier, Philadelphia, 2016, page 1692)
  - o Fasting pattern
    - – Four phases of the MMC (migrating motor complex) which occurs every 1 to 2 hours between meals, and continues to push food and fluid distally

327

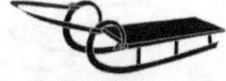

I   no contractions, but smooth muscle oscillations

II   smooth muscle contractions, intermittent

III smooth muscle contractions, continuous, 11/min proximally, and pushing luminal contents distally

IV no contractions

- o Colonic motility
  - – Feeding pattern
    - ▪ Segmental (mixing) activity
  - – Fasting (propulsive) pattern
  - – HAPC (high-amplitude propagated contractions, aka mass movements)
  - – LACA (low-amplitude contractile activity)

SO YOU WANT TO BE A GASTROENTEROLOGIST!

- Give the physiological explanation for **"the law of the intestine"**.
  - o Stimulus in the lumen of the intestine acts on the enterochrommaffin cells to release 5-HT
  - o 5-HT$_{1P}$ and 5-HT$_3$ act on IPANs (intrinsic primary afferent neurons) in the submucosal plexus
  - o IPANs release 5-HT$_4$ which act on the interneurons in the myenteric plexus
  - o These interneurons contain receptors for opiod, SS (somatostatin) and GABA (γ-amino butyric acid)
  - o The portion of the intestine just proximal to the stimulus releases interneuron Ach (acetylcholine) and SP (substance P)
  - o The portion of the intestine just distal to the stimulus releases interneuron VIP (vasoactive intestinal peptide) and NO (nitric oxide)
  - o The net result is the "law the intestine": proximal contraction, distal relaxation

---

- **Intestinal Cells of Cajal** (ICC)
  - o Function of ICC
    - – Pacemakers
    - – Transduction of excitatory and inhibitory neural signals to myocytes
  - o There are three groups of ICCs in the small intestine
    - – ICC-DMP (deep muscle plexus)
    - – ICC-MY (myenteric plexus; pacemaker cells)
    - – ICC-IM (intramuscular plexus)

328

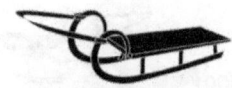

Mastering the Boards: Gastroenterology   A.B.R. Thomson

- o ICC MY
    - – Produce slow waves in myocytes → activity of other ICCs is entrained
    - – Propagation of slow waves through gap junctions of myocytes
- o Nerves from ENS (enteric nervous system)
    - – Target ICC MY, with response to myocytes
- o Enteric motor neurons
    - – Excitatory
        - ▪ M2, M3 acetylcholine receptors
        - ▪ SP (substance P) receptors for NK1
    - – Inhibitory
        - ▪ NO (nitric oxide), and
        - ▪ VIP (vasoactive intestinal peptide) activate receptor on non-receptor mechanisms to
            - – Open K^+ channels
            - – Class Ca^{2+} channels
            - – Cause relaxation

- **Neurons Involved with Small Intestinal Motility**
    - o Intrinsic   – Afferent
        - ▪ Submucosal plexus – mucosal and submucosal plexus, also joined by interganglionic fascicles
        - ▪ Myenteric plexus – primary, secondary, tertiary plexus
        - ▪ Deep plexus – neurons responding to mechanical stimulation and mucosal chemical stimulation
        - – Efferent
            - ▪ Excitatory transmitters
                - – Fast   Acetylcholine
                - – Slow   Substance P
            - ▪ Inhibitory
                - – Fast   VIP
                - – B-NAD (B-nicotinamide adenine dinucleotide)

    - o Extrinsic   – Afferent

Small intestine (physiological regulation) → nodose and jugular ganglia → brainstem

Spinal afferents (pain) → perivascular nerves → prevertebral ganglia → postganglionic sympathetic motor neurons → splanchnic nerves thoracic dorsal postganglia → dorsal roots → thoracic spinal nerves

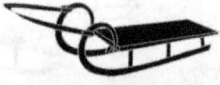

329

- Give the **regulation** of intestinal motility, the secretion of mucus, and blood flow, through the PINES (paracrine, immunologic, neural, and endocrine systems) controls.
  - o Minute-to-minute regulation in response to mechanical or chemical stimuli in the intestinal lumen activate receptors which activate PINES
  - o Mediators may be released from mast cells (e.g., histamine), from submucosal immunocytes (e.g., prostaglandins, leukotrienes) reactive oxygen metabolites and from intestinal mesenchymal cells such as myofibroblasts (cytokines, chemokines, eicosanoids, growth factors)
  - o Acid or volume in the lumen stretch the intestine and activates TRVP1 (vanilloid receptor) or capsaicin-sensitive afferent neurons, which stimulate the submucosal neurons
  - o The immunocompetent cells in the LP (lamina propria) forming the GALT (gut-associated lymphoid tissue) are comprised of
    - – T lymphocytes, 60%
    - – B cells and plasma cell, 25%
    - – Macrophages, 10%
    - – Mast cells and PMNs (polymorphonuclear leukocytes especially eosinophils), 5%
  - o Stimulation of these immunocytes causes release of inflammatory mediators
  - o When here are ↑ PMNs as with inflammation, the PMNs respond to chemoattractants, pass in an integrin-dependent process from blood vessels into the intercellular space between colonocytes, and cause adenosine-mediated secretion

- Give **clinical tests** of small intestinal motility.
  - o Multichannel manometric recordings of IDMC (interdigestive motor cycle)
  - o Intracellular measurements of electrical potential
  - o Intraluminal manometry
  - o Intraluminal impedence (MII, multichannel intraluminal impedance)
  - o Contrast fluoroscopy
  - o Ultrasonography
  - o MRI
  - o Breath tests of small intestinal transit

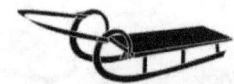

DIARRHEA

- Definition
  - Abnormal loss of water and electrolytes from the intestinal tract due to decreased absorption and increased secretion, translated to the patient as an increase in frequency and volume of stools

Sodium (Na^+) / H_2O Absorption

- Give the effect of systemic pH on Na^+ / H_2O transport.

  - Metabolic acidosis
    - ↑ electroneutral NaCl absorption
  - Metabolic alkalosis
    - ↓ electroneutral NaCl absorption
  - In the short term, the number of SGLT1 transporters is increased by PKA- and PKC-dependent processes.
  - PKC and MAP kinase (integrin-activated protein kinase) signaling pathways are induced by glucose to cause the recruitment of cytosolic GLUT2 to the BBM.
  - GLUT2 recruited to the BBM facilitates the transport of glucose and fructose across the BBM, especially when the luminal concentration of these monosaccharides is high.

SO YOU WANT TO BE A GASTROENTEROLOGIST!

- Give the **"standing-gradient hypothesis"** in the context of understanding how a glass of water is absorbed.

  - The movement of solutes such as Na^+, glucose and amino acids by the enterocyte BBM (brush border membrane) produce small increases in the osmolarity in the intercellular and subepithelial spaces.
  - This causes water to move across the BBM (such as with glucose transport by SGLT1), as well as through TJs (tight junctions).

The movement of Na^+ and H_2O with glucose, as mediated by BBM SGLT1, is the basis of the benefit of ORS (oral rehydration solutions).

- Give the relative amount of Na^+ and H_2O which moves through this water channel.
  - "...about 175 molecules of water can be transported per ion or mole of solute." (Sleisenger and Fordtran's Gastrointestinal and Liver Disease. 10th Edition. Saunders/Elsevier, Philadelphia, 2016, page 1718).

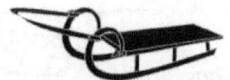

- Give the physiological pathways that ↑ NaCl and water **absorption** and signaling molecules for each pathway.

  - ↓ cAMP
    - Norepinephrine
    - Epinephrine
    - Dopamine
    - Enkephalins
    - Neuropeptide Y
    - Somatostatin

  - Coupled transport
    - Glucose, galactose, fructose
    - Amino acids, dipeptides/tripeptides
    - Short-chain fatty acids

  - Other pathways
    - Aldosterone
    - Glucocorticosteroids
    - Somatostatin
    - GLP-2

Adapted from: Freeman HJ, and Thomson ABR. *First Principles of Gastroenterology* 2005. pg. 190.

> **Chloride (Cl⁻)/H₂O secretion**

Cyclic AMP, cyclic GMP and intracellular calcium (Ca^{2+}_i) are involved in the secretion of chloride by intestinal crypt cells.

- Give the steps which are involved in the transduction of an external signal into a charge in cellular function, such as occurs with secretagogues.

  - An agonist (stimulatory or inhibitory) binds to the membrane receptor for adenylate cyclase or for guanylate cyclase

  - Guanylate cyclase is activated, through inhibitory or stimulatory G proteins (Gi and Gs, respectively; guanine nucleotide regulatory proteins),

  - For example, VIP and prostaglandins activate receptors which bind to Gs, whereas somatostatin activates GI.

  - An increase in intracellular, cGMP activates PKG II (protein kinase II), and ↑ cAMPi activates PKA (protein kinase A)

  - PKG II acts through GKAP (G kinase-anchoring proteins) or through AKAP (A kinase-anchoring proteins) to activate phosphorylation of specific target proteins to activate membrane channels or transporters.

Adapted from: Sleisenger and Fordtran's Gastrointestinal and Liver Disease. 10th Edition. Saunders/Elsevier, Philadelphia, 2016, page 1721-3.

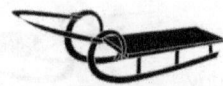

- Give the classes of Cl⁻ channels.
  - CFTR1 (cystic fibrosis transmembrane conductance regulator)
  - ClC2, salvage pathway for Cl⁻ transport in CF, and target for the laxative, lubiprostome
  - CLCA (Ca-activated Cl⁻ channel), involved in rotaviral-associated diarrhea
  - Mutations in SLC26A3 result in congenital Cl⁻ diarrhea

> **Regulation** of Na^+ / H_2O secretion

- Give the mechanisms in health and disease of control of Na+ / H_2O secretion by the small bowel and colon.
  - The presecretory factors may be classified by their mechanism of action.
  - The eicosanoids include arachidonic acid, prostaglandins and leukotrienes.
  - The eicosanoids act through cAMP and Ca^{2+}_i to stimulate electrogenic Cl⁻ secretion and inhibit electroneutral Na absorption
  - Acetylcholine
    - M3 receptors
    - Released from enterochromaffin cells (95%), and from serotoninergic neuron of the myenteric plexus
    - ↑ Ca^{2+}_i (intracellular calcium)
    - Inactivated by SERT (serotonin reuptake transporter) on enterocytes and neurons
  - Neurotensin
    - ↑ Ca^{2+}_i
  - VIP, secretin, PHL (peptide histidine leucine), PHM (peptide histidine methionine)
    - ↑ cAMP
    - ↑ cGMP
  - Microbial pathogens
    - Vibrio chlorae
      - Enterotoxin
        - ↑ cAMP
        - ↑ CFTR activity
        - ↓ NHE3
      - ZOT (zonula occludens toxin)
      - Channel-like protein
    - E-coli, Yersinia enterocolitica
      - Enterotoxins
        - ↑ cAMP
        - ↑ CFTR
        - NHE3
    - Rotavirus
      - NSP4 (enterotoxin)
        - ↓ BBM disaccharides
        - ↓ BBM SGLT1 (mature enterocytes)

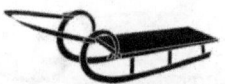

- o Clostridium difficile toxins A and B
  – Rho family disrupts the perijunctional actin-myosin ring
- o C. perfringers enterotoxin
  – Disrupts fibrils of TJ (tight junctions)
- o EPEC, EHEC, ETEC, Salmonella, Shigella
  – ↑ galanin receptors → ↑ Ca^{2+}-dependent Cl^- secretion
- o Bile acids
  – CDCA (chenodeoxycholic acid, a 7α-dihydroxy bile acid)
    - ↑ cAMP
    - ↑ Ca^{2+} and PKC cascade

Please see Sleisenger and Fordtran's Gastrointestinal and Liver Disease. 9th Edition. Saunders/Elsevier, Philadelphia, 2010, Table 101-3, page 1729.

- Give the effects of aldosterone, glucocorticosteroids and catecholamines on Na^+ / H_2O absorption by the small bowel and colon.
  - o Aldosterone – colon
    – ↑ ENac
    – ↑ Na^+/K^+ ATPase
    – ↑ SGKi
    – ↑ K^+ absorption and secretion

  - o Glucocorticosteroids – small and large intestine
    – Low concentration Na^+ absorption
      - ↑electroneutral
      - ↓ electrogenic
    – High concentration Na^+ absorption
      - ↑electroneutral
      - ↓ electrogenic

  - o Catecholamines, (dopamine, epinephrine) encepalins, somatostatin
    – ↑ G α1 cascade
    – ↓ cAMP cascade
    – ↑ electroneutral Na+ absorption
    – ↓ secretion

Please see : Feldman M., et al. Sleisenger and Fordtran's Gastrointestinal and Liver Disease. 10th Edition. Saunders/Elsevier, Philadelphia, 2016, Table 101-1, page 1728, "Agents that Stimulate Intestinal Absorption of Fluid and Electrolytes".

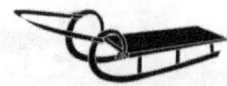

- Give the physiological pathways that ↑ NaCl/water secretion, and for each pathway, give signaling molecules.

  o ↑ cAMP
    - Vasoactive intestinal polypeptide
    - Adenosine
    - Prostaglandins
    - Histamine
    - Bradykinin

  o ↑ cGMP
    - Nitric oxide
    - Guanylin
    - Uroguanylin

  o ↑ Ca_i, and/or activate protein kinase C
    - Acetylcholine
    - Serotonin
    - Substance P
    - Histamine
    - Bradykinin
    - ATP
    - Adenosine
    - Neurotensin

  o Other pathways
    - Interferon-γ
    - TNF-α
    - Interleukin-1 (IL-1)
    - Interleukin-6 (IL-6)
    - Epidemal growth factor (EGF)

Adapted from: Freeman HJ, and Thomson ABR. *First Principles of Gastroenterology* 2005. pg. 190.

Potassium (K^+)

- Give the mechanism by which K^+ channels modulate the hyperpolarization of the cell interior resulting from Na^+, K^+-ATPase on the basal membrane (BM) of the enterocyte or H^+, K^+-ATPase on the apical membrane (AM) of the parietal cell, and promote Cl^- secretion.

  o BM, small and large intestine
    - cAMP-activated KCNE3/KCNQ1 channels
    - Ca^{2+}-calmodulin-activated KCNN4 channels

  o AM, colon
    - KCN MA1 channels

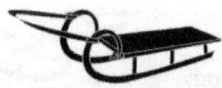

Bicarbonate (HCO_3^-)

- o When a patient has diarrhea, HCO_3^- is the major anion lost in the stool, being secreted by electrogenic and electroneutral processes, linked to the inward movement of Cl^- through NHE distributed along the length of the small and large intestine.
- o SLC (solute carriers) include
  - − SCL4 for HCO_3^-, and
  - − SCL26, the multifunctional anion exchange family (e.g., Cl^-, HCO_3^-, sulfate, oxalate)
- o Examples of SLC26 include
  - − SLC26A3 (aka Cl^-/HCO_3^- exchanger, or DRA [down-regulated adenoma]) in the AM (apical membrane) of colonocytes, and
  - − SLC26A6 (aka PAT1 [putative anion transporter 1], expressed in AM of enterocytes > colonocytes]

SO YOU WANT TO BE A GASTROENTEROLOGIST!

Acetylcholine (Ach), neurotensin, bile acids and SP (substance P), among others, activate secretion through ↑ Ca^{2+}_i, achieved by
- − ↑ passage of Ca^{2+} into cell
- − ↑ release of Ca^{2+} from Ca_i^{2+} stores

- • Give an explanation of the process of Ca^{2+} -induced diarrhea.
  - o SP → ↑ Ca^{2+} entry through Ca^{2+} channels
  - o Ach
    - − Binds to M3 receptors
    - − Activates Gaq (a class of G proteins)
    - − Gaq stimulates PLC (phospholipase C)
  - o Neurotensin, bile acids also ↑ PLC
    - − PLC hydrolyzes PIP2 into IP3 (inositol IP3) and DAG (diacylglycerol)
      - ▪ PIP2 -----PLC----> IP3 + DAG
    - − DAG is also produced from phosphatidic acid (PA) through tyrosine kinase receptors and the activation of PLD (phospholipase D)
      - ▪ PA -----PLD----> DAG
    - − DAG → ↑ PKC (protein kinase C)
    - − IP3 → binds to IP3R (IP3 receptors) to release Ca^{2+} from intracellular Ca^{2+} stores
    - − Ca^{2+}
      - ▪ Activates Ca^{2+} channels
      - ▪ Binds to calmodulin (CAM) to activate Ca^{2+}- calmodulin TK
    - − PKC and Ca^{2+} and CAM TK → ↑ activity of membrane channels and Cl^- transporters

---

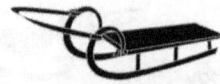

- Give a **classification of drugs** used in gastroenterology which are associated with diarrhea.

    o Esophagus/stomach
    - – Magnesium-containing antacids, PPIs, H2RAs
    - – Misoprostol

    o Small bowel
    - – Prokinetics
    - – Antiabsorptives
    - – 5-ASA, immunosuppressants

    o Colon
    - – Laxatives osmotic
    - – Magnesium citrate
    - – Antibiotics
    - – Cholinergics

    o Liver
    - – Lactulose (PSE) for hepatic encephalopathy
    - – Herbs

    o Heart
    - – Beta blockers

    o Chemotherapy

➤ Clinical

- Give symptoms or signs that would confirm your suspicion of dehydration from diarrhea.

o CNS	–	Lethargy
	–	Thirst
o Eye	–	Dry
	–	Sunken
o Lung	–	Tachypnea
o CVS	–	↑ HR (tachycardia)
	–	↓ BP (including postural hypotension)
	–	↓ JVP (jugular venous pressure)
o Skin	–	Dry
	–	↓ turgor
o Kidney	–	↓ urination

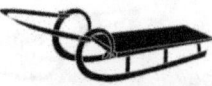

SO YOU WANT TO BE A GASTROENTEROLOGIST!

If the **stool osmotic gap** is > 50 mOsm/kg in a patient with diarrhea, the cause of the diarrhea is likely excessive osmotically active agents in the stools (lactose, fructose, sorbitol, magnesium).
- Give the formula to calculate stool osmolality from stool electrolytes

$$2 \times (Na^+ + K^+) = \text{stool osmolality (mOsm/kg)}$$

- A little trick-if the stool osmolality is increased and the stool pH is acidic (pH < 5), give the likely class of substances that is causing the diarrhea.
    - When carbohydrates are malabsorbed, they increase the stool osmolality and cause diarrhea.
    - The malabsorbed carbohydrates are metabolized by the colonic luminal bacteria, forming short chain fatty acids (SCFA) which render the pH of the stools acidic (pH < 5).

Giardiasis is a common cause of chronic diarrhea. Small bowel mucosal biopsy will show the organism, and there will be a marked infiltration of plasma cells in the lamina propria in response to the infection. Giardiasis is more common in CVID **(chronic variable immunodeficiency).**

- Give the histopathological feature on small bowel mucosal biopsy in the patient with chronic diarrhea from giardiasis that the patient has CVID.
    - Giardiasis normally causes a dense plasma cell infiltration in the submucosal in response to the infection
    - In CVID the plasma cell infiltration will be absent

"There are up-sides, down-sides and all kinds of sides (!)"

Grandad

338

- Give signs and symptoms of systemic illnesses to be considered in the person with diarrhea.

Sign or Symptom	Diagnosis to be Considered
o Systemic – Marked weight loss	▪ Malabsorption ▪ Inflammatory bowel disease ▪ Cancer ▪ Thyrotoxicosis
o Joint – Arthritis	▪ Ulcerative colitis ▪ Crohn disease ▪ Whipple disease ▪ *Yersinia* infection
o CNS – Neuropathy	
o CVS – Postural hypotension	▪ Diabetic diarrhea ▪ Addison disease ▪ Idiopathic orthostatic hypotension ▪ Autonomic dysfunction

o Hematology
   – Eosinophilia
   – Lymphadenopathy
	▪ Eosinophilic gastroenteritis
	▪ Parasitic infection
	▪ Lymphoma
	▪ Whipple disease

o Skin
   – Flushing
   – Hyperpigmentation
	▪ Malignant carcinoid syndrome

o GU – Proteinuria	▪ Diabetic diarrhea ▪ Amyloidosis

o GI
   – Peptic ulcers
 	
   – Endocrine
	▪ Zollinger-Ellison syndrome
	▪ Whipple disease
	▪ Celiac disease
	
	▪ Addison disease
	▪ Pancreatic cholera
	▪ Diabetic mellitus

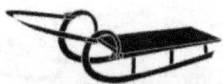

- Give features which help to differentiating chronic organic diarrhea from functional diarrhea.

Feature	Organic Diarrhea	Functional Diarrhea
The patient		
o Weight loss	– Often present	▪ Absent
o Duration of illness	– Variable (weeks to years)	▪ Usually long (>6 mon)
o Emotional stress	– No relation to symptoms	▪ Usually precedes or coincides with symptoms
The stools		
o Quantity of stool	– Variable but usually >200 g in 24 h	▪ Usually small (<200 g in 24 h)
o Blood in stool	– May be present	▪ Absent (unless from hemorrhoids)
o Fatty stools	– May be present	▪ Absent
o Timing of diarrhea	– No special pattern – May occur at night	▪ Usually in the morning or after meals ▪ Not usually at night
Other symptoms		
o Fever, arthritis, skin lesions	– May be present	▪ Absent
o Cramping abdominal pain	– Often present	▪ May be present

This distinction between organic and functional causes of chronic diarrhea may be useful in assessing the patient with IBS (irritable bowel syndrome), versus other types of colonic disorders.

"Remember that you are not called to do extraordinary things, but ordinary things with love."

Mother Theresa

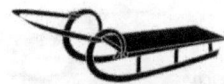

TRAVELLERS' DIARRHEA

- Give foods and/or beverages which are generally safe, often safe and often unsafe with respect to the risk for developing Travellers' Diarrhea (TD).

Generally safe	Often safe	Often unsafe
o Food and beverages served steaming (>59°C) hot	– Tortillas and breads or toast containing butter or sauces	▪ Fruits and vegetables with intact skins: berries, tomatoes
o Bottled carbonated drinks including soft drinks and beer	– Fruit juices which may have been augmented with tap water	▪ Hot sauces on tabletop ▪ Moist foods served at room temperature including vegetables and meats
o Bottled water with intact seal apparent on opening	– Use of tap water to rinse mouth and toothbrush without swallowing it	▪ Any food served buffet-style that is maintained at room temperature
o Syrups, jellies, jams, honey		
o Fruits that are peeled	– Foods serviced on airplanes in developing regions	▪ Tap water even at hotels claiming filtration systems
o Dry items such as bread and rolls		▪ Large quantities of ice
o Any foods carefully prepared in one's own apartment or hotel	– Few ice cubes	▪ Hamburgers not served hot or at fast food service restaurants with rapid turnover of prepared hamburgers

Printed with permission: Dupont H.L. *Aliment Pharmacol Ther* 2008; 27: pg. 744.

- Give the major enteropathogens causing "Travellers' Diarrhea".
  - o Bacteria
    - – Aeromonas and Plesiomonas
    - – Campylobacter jejuni
    - – Enteroaggregative E. coli (EAggEC)
    - – Enteroinvasive E. coli (EIEC)
    - – Enteropathogenic E. coli (EPEC)
    - – Enterotoxigenic Eschenchia coli (ETEC)
    - – Mycobacterium tuberculosis (and Mycobacterium bovis)
    - – Salmonella

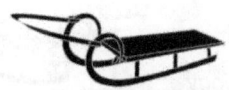

- o Viruses
    - Enteric adenoviruses (types 40, 41)
    - Measles virus
    - Human immunodeficiency virus
    - Rotavirus
- o Protozoa
    - Ciliophora
        - Balantidium coli
    - Coccidia
        - Cryptosporidium parvum
        - Isosprora belli
    - Cyclospora – Cyclospora cayetanensis
    - Mastigophora
        - Giardia lamblia
    - Microspora
        - Enterocytozoon bieneusi
        - Encephalitozoon intestinalis
- o Helminths
    - Strongyloides stercoralis
        - Schistosoma

Printed with permission: Farthing MJG. *Sleisenger & Fordtran's gastrointestinal and liver disease: Pathophysiology/ Diagnosis/Management* 2006: pg 2308.

- Give causes of prolonged diarrheal illness after travel.

    - o Infection
        - Aeromonas
        - Antibiotic-associated diarrhea (AAD), Cl. difficile infection
        - Cryptosporidium
        - Entamoeba histolytica
        - Escherichia coli (enteroinvasive)
        - Giardia
        - Missed second infection
        - Onset of chronic (presumably viral) enteritis/colitis
        - Persistent bacterial infection
        - Persistent protozoal infection

    - o Diet/Drugs
        - Change in diet
        - Excess alcohol intake
        - Drugs

    - o Other Diseases
        - Unmasked lactase deficiency, celiac disease, IBD, (microscopic lymphocytic/collagenous colitis)
        - Tropical sprue
        - Post-infectious diarrhea-predominant IBS (D-IBS)

342

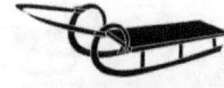

Abbreviations: AAD, antibiotic-associated diarrhea; D-IBS, diarrhea-predominant IBS; GSE, gluten sensitive enteropathy; IBD, inflammatory bowel disease.

Please see Sleisenger and Fordtran's Gastrointestinal and Liver Disease. 10th Edition. Saunders/Elsevier, Philadelphia, 2016, Table 110-1, page 1924 and Table 110-9, page 1925.

Salmonellosis

- Give conditions which predispose to Salmonellosis.
  - Achlorhydria
  - Hemolytic anemia
  - Immunosuppression
  - Malignancy
  - Schistosomiasis
  - Ulcerative colitis

Please see Feldman M., et al. Sleisenger and Fordtran's Gastrointestinal and Liver Disease. 9th Edition. Saunders/Elsevier, Philadelphia, 2010, Table 107.9, page 1862.

- Give carbohydrate-containing foods that may be absorbed incompletely in the healthy human small intestine, and provide the name of the substrate responsible for colonic gas production.

Food	Malabsorbed Carbohydrate
Dairy products (milk, ice cream, cottage cheese, yogurt)	– Lactose
Soft drinks, honey	– Fructose
Legumes (baked beans, soy beans)	– Stachyose, raffinose
Dietetic candies and chewing gum	– Mannitol, sorbitol, xylitol
Complex carbohydrates (wheat, corn, potatoes)	– Resistant and retrograded starch
Grains, fruits, vegetables	– Fibre (hemicellulose, pectin, gums) mucilage

Adapted from: *Sleisenger & Fordtran's Gastrointestinal and Liver Disease: Pathophysiology/ Diagnosis/ Management*, 10th Edition. Saunders/Elsevier, Philadelphia, 2016, Table 17-1, page 245.

- Give clinical syndromes seen with Salmonella.
  - Gastroenteritis
  - Bacteremia
  - Typhoid fever
  - Localized infection
  - Carrier stage

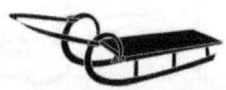

Please see Feldman M., et al. Sleisenger and Fordtran's Gastrointestinal and Liver Disease. 9th Edition. Saunders/Elsevier, Philadelphia, 2010, page 1863-5.

Clinical Pearl

- Give causes of recurrent severe abdominal pain in a person with a history of a family member who is similarly affected with frequent episodes of abdominal pain.

  o Hereditary angioedema
    - Autosomal dominant ↓C1 esterase activity
    - Clinical
      - Triggers
        - Viral infection
        - ACE inhibitor
        - Spontaneous (unknown)
      - Peripheral/visceral edema
      - Swelling of tongue and periorbital regions

  o Familial Mediterranean Fever (FMF)

  o Crohn disease
    - Mouth ulcers (aphthous)
    - Tongue swelling

  o Irritable bowel syndrome (IBS)

- Give the fate of the dietary carbohydrates which are malabsorbed.
  o The short-chain fatty acids (SCFA) include acetate, proprionate and butyrate, which are formed from the bacterial metabolism of undigested carbohydrate in the colon.
  o SCFAs are > 95% ionized and are absorbed by carriers such as NHE3, SLC16A1 (MCT1 [monocarboxylate transporter family])
  o For example Cl^- butyrate exchangers and SCFA – HCO_3^- exchangers are linked to the absorption of Na^+ and H_2O
  o Protonated SCFA (H^+ derived from the acid microclimate, resulting from NHE3 exchange of Na+ into the cell and H^+ moved to the external side of the apical membrane of the colonocyte, across which they diffuse into the adenocyte where they are used for metabolic fuel of the colonocytes, as well as for calories for the host from carbohydrate.

344

 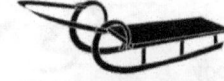

- Give what is the examiner thinking when they add information to the clinical scenario.

Added Information	Think of
o Infectious causes of **terminal ileitis**.	– MAC – Yersinia – Campylobacter – Cryptosporidium
o Enteritis + acid-fast staining	– TB – MAC – Isospora belli – Cryptosporidium
o HIV-associated diarrhea	– Haiti – Charcot Leyden crystals in stool
o Foamy macrophage on small bowel biopsy	– MAC – Tropheryma Whippelii

o Recurrent abdominal pain plus family	– Mediterranean origin
	  ▪ FMF (Familial Mediterranean Fever)
	  ▪ IPSID (immunoproliferative small intestinal disease)

o Campylori jejuni infection plus lymphoma	– IPSID
o Giardiasis	– No plasma cell infiltration in submucosal on mucosa biopsy – CVID (common variable immunodeficiency)

Source: Spiegel BM. Slack Incorporated 2009, page 92-94; also please see: Maclean C. Chapter 55. In: Therapeutic Choices. Grey J, Ed. 6th Edition, Canadian Pharmacists Association: Ottawa, ON, 2011, Table 2, page 731-733; and Fedorak RN, et al. Chapter 57. In: Therapeutic Choices. Grey J, Ed. 6th Edition, Canadian Pharmacists Association: Ottawa, ON, 2011, Table 2, page 759-761.

Cryptosporidiosis

Cryptosporidiosis occurs in both immunocompetent and immunocompromised patients, and causes watery diarrhea. Because the Cryptosporidium infection usually involves the terminal ileum, there may be vitamin B12 deficiency.

- Give the CD4 counts at which cryptosporidiosis is likely to occur, at what level the infection should be treated, and with what.

  - o CD4
    - – < 180, cryptosporidiosis occurs in 10% of HIV-infected persons with diarrhea
    - – < 50, nitazoxanide

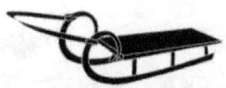

NEOPLASMS

➢ Pathological types

• Give a classification of benign and malignant small intestinal tumours.
  o Epithelium
    - Adenoma
    - Adenocarcinoma
  o Vascular
    - Angiosarcoma
    - Hemangiomas
  o Neural
    - Neurofibroma
    - Neurofibrosarcoma
    - Neurilemmoma
    - Spinal cells (Interstitial cells of Cajal)
    - Schwannomas
  o Neuroendocrine tumours (NET; aka "carcinoid" tumours, now an archaic term)
  o Muscle
    - Leiomyoma (40%)
    - Leiomyosarcoma
  o Fat
    - Lipoma (20%; usually in ileum)
    - Liposarcoma
  o WBC (Lymphoma)
    - Low-grade B cell lymphoma
    - Immunoproliferative small intestinal
    - Enteropathy-associated T-cell lymphoma (EATL)
  o Gastrointestinal stromal tumour (GIST)
    - May be both endo- and exogastric, giving a dumbbell shape
  o Lymphatic-lymphangioma
  o Fibrous tissue
    - Fibroma
    - Fibrosarcoma
  o Desmoid tumours
    - Endo- or exogastric (into or away from lumen, respectively)
    - Exogastric dislace rather than invade adjacent tissue
  o Metastases
    - Ovary
    - Endometrium
    - Colon
    - Periampullary lesions

Please see Sleisenger and Fordtran's Gastrointestinal and Liver Disease. 10th Edition. Saunders/Elsevier, Philadelphia, 2016, Table 125-1, page 2197.

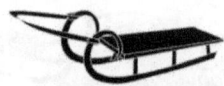

➤ Diagnostic Imaging

• Give the performance characteristics of diagnostic imaging (barium studies and CT scanning) to diagnose small bowel tumours.

	Demonstration of Small Bowel Tumour	Sensitivity	Specificity
o UGIS-SBFT	30% to 44%		
o Barium enteroclysis	90%		
o CT/SPEC	99%		
o MDCT-E	100%	100%	95%

Abbreviations: UGIS-SBFT, upper GI series with a small intestinal follow-through; MDCT-E, multidetector CT enteroclysis

➤ Commonest malignant tumours of the small intestine

  o 95% comprised of
    – Adenocarcinoma, 47%
      ▪ Duodenum
        – Sessile
        – Villous
      ▪ Ileum
        – Polypoid
    – Carcinoid, 28%
    – Sarcoma/GISTs, 13%

➤ Risk Factors

About ½ of malignant small bowel tumours are sessile adenocarcinoma of the duodenum followed by ¼ being ileal polypoid NET ("carcinoids").

• Give risk factors for malignant small intestine tumours.

  o The patient   – Older
                   – Male
                   – African ancestry

  o Diet   – Sugar
                   – Red meat

  o Associated   – Crohn disease (with or without immunosuppression or
    intestinal   TNF-α blocker)
    diseases   – Celiac disease (adenocarcinoma, as well as NHL [non-
                     Hodgin lymphoma])
                   – Polyposis syndrome
                     ▪ FAP (familial adenomatous polyposis)
                     ▪ HNPCC (hereditary non-polyposis colorectal cancer)
                     ▪ PJS (Peutz-Jeghers syndrome)
                     ▪ JP (Juvenile Polyposis)

347

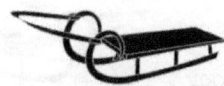

➢ Endoscopy

• Give the EUS (endoscopic ultrasound) correlation of the TNM (tumour, node [regional lymph node] and distant metastases) classification of small intestinal tumours.

TNM Classification

Tis   In situ carcinoma

T1 Invasion into lamina propria or submucosal

T2 Invasion into muscularis propria

T3 Invasion into subserosa

T4 Invasion through visceral peritoneum, or into other organs or structures

➢ Anatomical layers (on EUS)

Layer EUS

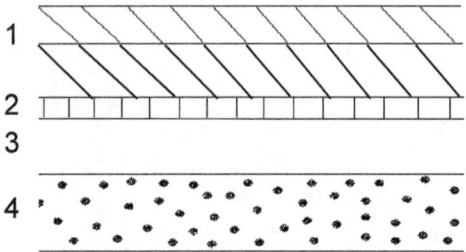

1   Mucosa - White/hypoechoic

2   Muscularis mucosae (MM) – **Dark** on EUS

3   Submucosa – White on EUS

4   Muscularis propria (MP) – **Dark** on EUS

5   Serosa – White on EUS

Gastrointestinal Stromal Tumours (GIST)

➢ Demography

     o GIST is common in (~85% of stromal tumours)

     o Site
         – Stomach   ~70%
         – Small bowel   ~25%
         – Colon/rectum   5%
         – Formed from interstitial stromal tissue

     o Malignant potential
         – All GISTs > 10 mm

348

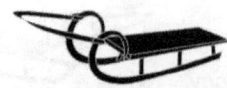

➢ Genetics

  o Genetic mutational activation of genes
    – KIT
    – PDGFRA
    – DC117

➢ Laboratory

  o C-kit (a stem cell factor receptor) Marker for GIST (~99%)
    – CD34 (a hematopoietic cell progenitor cell antigen) (70%)
    – Smooth muscle actin (20% to 30%)
    – S 100 protein (marker of neural differentiation)

➢ Diagnostic Imaging

  o PET 85% to 100% sensitive for 1-2% GIST

➢ Endoscopy

  o EGD

  o EUS characteristics which are ~ characteristic

  o EUS plus FNA

- Give endoscopic features of GISTs which suggest that they are benign vs malignant.

GIST Features	Benign	Malignant
o Endoscopy (EGD)	Smooth bump	Ulcerated (has broken through the mucosa)
o EUS heterogeneous	-	+
o Irregular margins	-	+
o Cystic spaces	-	+
o > 4cm	-	+
o Lymphadenopathy	-	+

➢ Differential

- Give the features that distinguish between a leiomyoma, a glomus tumour, and a GIST tumour.

Feature	Leiomyoma	Glomus	GIST
Positive for smooth muscle actin	+	-	-
Positive for CD117 (c-kit)	-	-	+
Vimention	-	+	-

349

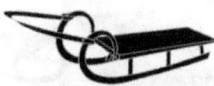

- o Duplication Cysts
    - – Embryological remnants of an accessory stomach
    - – EUS
        - ▪ Spherical
        - ▪ Hypo-/anechoic
    - – Complications
        - ▪ Obstruction
        - ▪ Development of
            - - Carcinoids
            - - Gastric cancer

- ➢ Treatment

    - o Surgical
        - – Laparoscopic resection is possible
        - – Segmental resection for ≥ 2 cm; leaving the tumour pseudocapsule intact
        - – Obtain negative tumour resection margins

    - o TK (tyrosine kinase) inhibitors, e.g., imatimib
        - – Used as adjuvant or neoadjuvant therapy (before surgical resection)
        - – GISTs ≥ 3 cm
        - – ↓ GIST recurrence is post-op year 1
        - – Duodenal GIST
            - ▪ Duodenectomy if possible (no involvement of papilla of Vater)
            - ▪ Pancreaticoduodenectomy otherwise
            - ▪ Neoadjuvant therapy with imatinib (a TKI) may be beneficial for duodenal GIST
        - – Jejunum/ileal GIST
            - ▪ Segmental resection with TFM (tumour-free margins)
            - ▪ Do not resect regional lymph nodes

Neuroendocrine tumours (NET) (aka "carcinoid")

➢ Site

- Give the distribution along the length of the small and large intestine the type of the neuroendocrine cells, and their cellular product.

    - o The neurosecretory granules in the cytoplasm of neuroendocrine cells are stained black with the Grimelius stain.

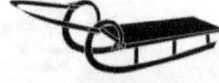

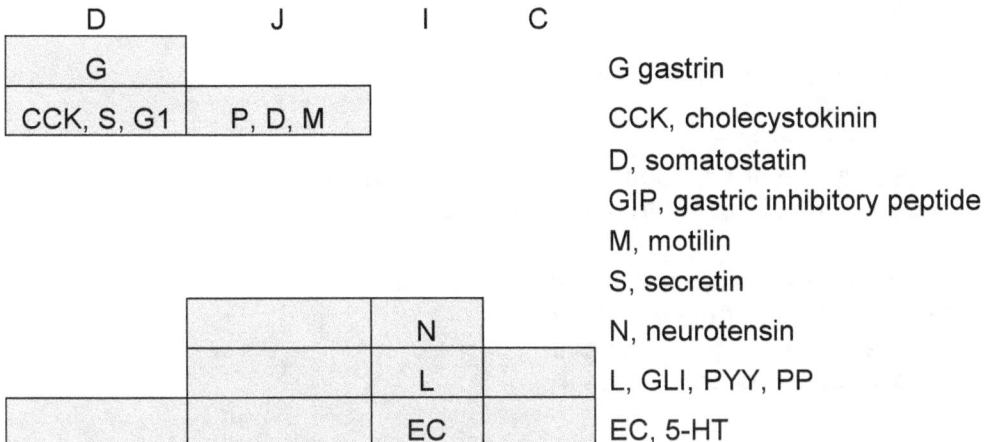

D	J	I	C
G			
CCK, S, G1	P, D, M		

G gastrin

CCK, cholecystokinin

D, somatostatin

GIP, gastric inhibitory peptide

M, motilin

S, secretin

		N		N, neurotensin
		L		L, GLI, PYY, PP
		EC		EC, 5-HT

Adapted from: Sleisenger and Fordtran's Gastrointestinal and Liver Disease. 9th Edition. Saunders/Elsevier, Philadelphia, 2010, Table 96.1, page 1620.

- o Chromogragm A suggests the diagnosis, making the granular material stain brown

➤ Endoscopy

- o Endoscopy appearance – polyps
  - – K67 shows classification of NET

➤ Treatment

- Give the treatment of the three types of neuroendocrine (NET; aka carcinoid) tumours based on the measurement of the fasting serum gastrin concentration.

Type	Gastrin	Association	Malignant	Treatment
1	↑↑	Atrophic gastritis	Low	Endoscopic surveillance
2	↑↑↑	Gastrinoma-ZES	Low	Removal when > 2 cm
3	N	Sporatic	High	Resection, even when small

Schwannoma

- o S-100 positive
- o EUS layer 4

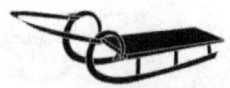

Pancreatic Rest (aka ectopic pancreas, aberrant pancreas, heterotopic pancreas)
➢ Endoscopy
 o EGD
 – Cystically dilated exocrine cells
 – May undergo malignant degeneration
 – Submucosal tumour
 – Usually in antrum, duodenum, proximal small bowel
 – Central umbilication (from a draining duct)
 o EUS
 – Hypoechoic area rom pancreatic acinar cells
 – Anechoic area from draining duct
 – Heterogeneous/fuzzy margins
 – Layer 3 or 4, or both 3 plus 4

➢ Diagnostic imaging

• Give the characteristics of the CT scan which suggests pancreatic rest rather than another type of submucosal tumour, and indicate how certain you can be.

 o CT findings
 – Seen in duodenum, antrum or pylorus
 – Flat and oval shape
 – Fuzzy, poorly-defined border
 – Endoluminal growth
 – Mucosa over the submucosal tumour is markedly enhanced
 – Performance characteristics, depending upon number of above CT scan findings

Number of CT Findings	Sensitivity	Specificity
2	100%	83%
3	100%	100%

GI Lymphoma
 o GALT
 – "extranodal marginal zone B cell lymphoma of gut-associated lymphoid tissue"
 – Nodular lymphoid hyperplasia
 – Variable immunodeficiency
 – Selective IgA deficiency
 – Giardiasis associated
 o Celiac disease
 – B cell lymphoma
 – EATL (enteropathy associated T cell lymphoma)
 – *celiac-like lesion close to edge of biopsy showing lymphoma
 o Small intestine
 – IPSID (immunoproliferative small intestinal disease)

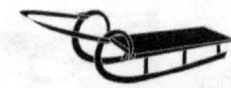

SMALL BOWEL OBSTRUCTION

- ➢ Definition
  - o Intestinal obstruction is the "impairment to the aboral passage of intestinal contents" (Feldman M., et al. Sleisenger and Fordtran's Gastrointestinal and Liver Disease. 9th Edition. Saunders/Elsevier, Philadelphia, 2010, page 2105).

- ➢ Types
  - o Partial, or complete
  - o Simple, or strangulated (including closed-loop obstruction)
  - o Small bowel, or colon

- ➢ Causes
  - o There are numerous causes of SBO; please see Sleisenger and Fordtran's Gastrointestinal and Liver Disease. 10th Edition. Saunders/Elsevier, Philadelphia, 2016, Box 123-1, page 2155, "Causes of Intestinal Obstruction". Also please see Feldman M., et al. Sleisenger and Fordtran's Gastrointestinal and Liver Disease. 9th Edition. Saunders/Elsevier, Philadelphia, 2010, Table 120.1, page 2124, "Factors that Contribute to Ileus" as well as Feldman M., et al. Sleisenger and Fordtran's Gastrointestinal and Liver Disease. 9th Edition. Saunders/Elsevier, Philadelphia, 2010, Table 120.5, page 2128, "Commonly Associated with Acute Colonic Pseudo-obstruction".

- • Give causes of small and large bowel obstruction.

  - o Adhesions, hernias, strictures from IBD, gallstone ileus, mesenteric artery syndrome, small bowel tumours, metastatic cancer, cystic fibrosis, volvulus, Crohn disease
  - o Colon cancer, volvulus, diverticulitis, ileus, narcotics ileus, mesenteric ischemia, IBD with stricture, Ogilvie syndrome, adhesions, intussusception, endometriosis

- ➢ Clinical course
  - o MR ~ 5%
  - o Recurrence 30-50% over 10 yrs
  - o In the patint with a small bowel obstruction, give the significance of severe, continuous pain
    - – Feculent vomitus
      - ▪ Bacterial overgrowth from obstruction
    - – Fistula from small to large bowel

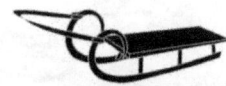

- o Abdominal film and SBO and no air in colon
  - SBO is complete
- o Ischemia
  - Thick bowel wall
  - Pneumatosis intestinalis

- In the context of small bowel obstruction (SBO), give the meaning of the small bowel **feces** sign, **whirl** sign, and the **beak** sign.
  - o Small bowel feces sign — "mottled admixture of particulate matter and gas within the dilated bowel proximal to a low-grade obstruction or in the setting of intestinal ischemia
  - o Whirl sign — "tightly twisted mesentery around a collapsed bowel segment", seen in closed-loop small bowel obstruction
  - o Beak sign — "fusiform tapering in the longitudinal section of bowel at the site of obstruction"

Feldman M., et al. Sleisenger and Fordtran's Gastrointestinal and Liver Disease. 9th Edition. Saunders/Elsevier, Philadelphia, 2010, page 2109

- Give potential severe complications of bowel obstruction.
  - o Perforation
  - o Septicemia
  - o Hypovolemia
  - o Death

➢ Diagnostic Imaging

  - o Plain abdominal films
    - Sensitivity of plain abdominal films for SBO is poor only about 75% (this means that you miss the diagnosis of SBO in 25%!)
    - It may be difficult to distinguish small bowel obstruction (SBO) from colonic obstruction (CO).

	SBO	CO
o Air in the rectum	Yes	No
o Dilation of both small and large intestinal	No	Yes (if ileocecal valve is incompetent)

  - o It may be difficult to distinguish small bowel obstruction (SBO) from ileus (SBI):
    - SBO
      - Dilated small bowel, air-fluid levels, no gas in colon

354

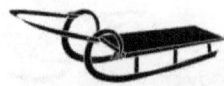

- o CT site, cause 95% for high grade sens 90-95%, spec 96%
- o Cut-off (transition) point ("beak" sign)
- o CT
  - – Whirl sign
  - – Beak sign
  - – Target sign
  - – Pneumatosis
  - – Thick bowel wall
- o CT scanning
  - – Performance characteristics (for high-grade SBO)
    - ▪ Sensitivity, 90% to 95%
    - ▪ Specificity, 96%
  - – May give the etiology, such as internal hernia, volvulus, strangulation, tremor, gallstone
  - – Please see Sleisenger and Fordtran's Gastrointestinal and Liver Disease. 9th Edition. Saunders/Elsevier, Philadelphia, 2010, Box 123-2, page 2158.

- • Give the clinical diagnostic advantage of CT enteroclysis vs CT scanning for SBO.
  - o Diagnostic accuracy for SBO
  - o CT, ~50%
  - o CT enteroclysis, ~100%
  - o Oral contrast reaching cecum within 4 to 24 hours has a 96% sensitivity and specificity that the SBO will not require surgery
  - o MRI with gadolinium enhancement, or PET (positron emission tomography) are useful if the SBO is caused by a tumour, distinguishing a benign from a malignant lesion.
  - o Strangulation (ischemia) in obstruction

"Play a crucial role in finding your own humility and humanity."
Grandad

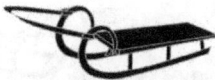

Postoperative Ileus

➢ Definition

- o "The contents of the small intestine are acutely unable to transit through because of impairment neural or muscular inadequacy", or "the inhibition of propulsive intestinal motor activity in the absence of a mechanical obstruction".

➢ Causes/associations

- Give pathophysiological causes of postoperative ileus.

  - o Neural pathways and neural inhibitors
    - – ↑ sympathetic inhibitory activity
    - – ↓ cholinergic activity (possibly due to ↑ VIP, ↑ neuropeptide Y, ↑ NO, ↑ CRF (corticotropin-releasing factor)
    - – Reflex motor inhibition from splanchnic afferents

  - o Inflammation (handing bowel)
    - – ↑ activity of iNOS (inducible nitric oxide synthase) and ↑ COX (cyclooxygenase)-2
    - – ↑ release of submucosal mast cells, monocytes, neutrophils
    - – ↑ proinflammatory cytokines (IL-1β, IL-6, TNF-α)
    - – ↑ MCP-1 (monocyte chemotactic protein-1)
    - – ↑ ICAM-1 (intercellular adhesion molecule-1)
    - – ↑ activity of α2- adrenoceptors

  - o Fluid overload

  - o Drugs
    - – Anaesthetics (epidural, versus general)
    - – Opiods

➢ Treatment/prevention

- Give factors/approaches that have been shown to enhance recovery from postoperative ileus.

  - o Surgery
    - – Thoracic epidural local anesthetics
    - – Intravenous or wound local anesthetics
    - – Goal-directed fluid therapy and avoiding fluid excess
    - – Laparoscopic surgery
    - – Avoid NG tubes

  - o Patient
    - – Laxatives
    - – Peripheral opiod antagonists
    - – Early oral feeding
    - – Chewing gum
    - – Minimize opiod use

Adapted from: Kehlet, H. *Nat Clin Pract Gastroenterol Hepatol* 2008;5:pg 552-8.

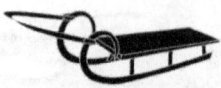

Chronic Intestinal Pseudo-Obstruction (CIPO)

➢ Definition

○ "A chronic neuromuscular disorder that can induce the small intestine alone, the colon alone, or other regions of the gastrointestinal tract in combination......." (Sleisenger and Fordtran's Gastrointestinal and Liver Disease. 9th Edition. Saunders/Elsevier, Philadelphia, 2010, page 2121 and 2124).

➢ Causes

Please see Sleisenger and Fordtran's Gastrointestinal and Liver Disease. 9th Edition. Saunders/Elsevier, Philadelphia, 2010, Table 120.1, page 2124, "Factors that Contribute to Ileus". Also, please see Sleisenger and Fordtran's Gastrointestinal and Liver Disease. 9th Edition. Saunders/Elsevier, Philadelphia, 2010, Table 119.1, page 2106, "Causes of Intestinal Obstruction", as well as Sleisenger and Fordtran's Gastrointestinal and Liver Disease. 9th Edition. Saunders/Elsevier, Philadelphia, 2010, Table 120.5, page 2128, "Conditions Commonly Associated with Acute Colonic Pseudo-obstruction".

➢ Familial

○ Familial visceral myopathies
MNGIE (megachondrial neurogastro intestinal enteropathy)
   – Type 1 to 3

○ Familial visceral neuropathies
   – Primary-degeneration of myenteric plexus
      • Secondary
      • Collagen vascular disease sclera, dermato, SLE
      • Neuromuscular disease
      • Infection
      • Endocrine
        - Diabetes
        - Hypothyroid
        - Parathyroid disease

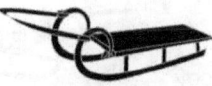

➢ Manometry

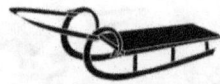

Intussusception

➢ Definition: "Intussusception is the imagination of a proximal segment of bowel (intussusceptum) into an adjacent distal segment (intussuscipiens" (Sleisenger and Fordtran's Gastrointestinal and Liver Disease. 10th Edition. Saunders/Elsevier, Philadelphia, 2016, page 2163).

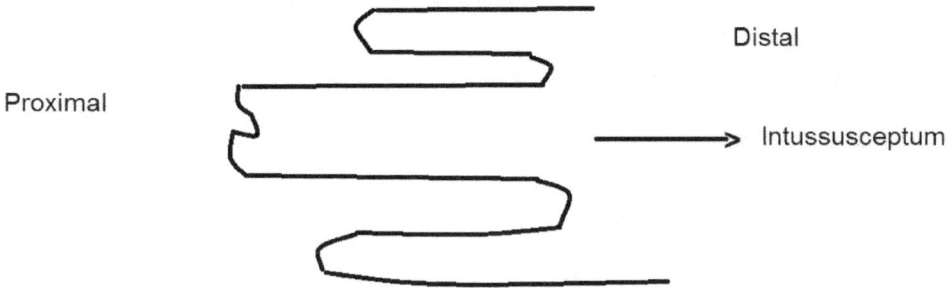

➢ Causes

  o Children   – Idiopathic

  o Adults   – Small intestine, benign tumours
                   – Colon (ileocolic, colocolic), adenocarcinoma

➢ Diagnostic imaging

  o Abdominal ultrasound, accuracy > 90%

  o CT scanning
       – "double bowel" (intussusceptum and intussuscipiens)
       – Concentration rings
       – Low density fat between intussuscipiens

Gallstone Ileus

Large gallstone enters the duodenum through a cholecystoduodenal fistula, and blocks the bowel in the ileum (60%), jejunum or stomach (both 15%), or colon.

CLINICAL GEM

     In the patient with suspected SBO, the presence of pneumobilia raises the possibility of a gallstone ileus. Remember that because only ~10% of gallstones have enough calcification to be seen on abdominal films, the absence of seeing a gallstone does not exclude the possibility of gallstone ileus as a cause of SBO.

359

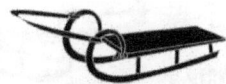

Volvulus of the Small Bowel

- ➢ Definition
  - o Small bowel obstruction (SBO) in neonate is due to "inadequate counter clockwise rotation of the mid gut loop around the SMA" (superior mesenteric artery) (Sleisenger and Fordtran's Gastrointestinal and Liver Disease. 9th Edition. Saunders/Elsevier, Philadelphia, 2010, page 2116).
  - o Positioning
    - – Small bowel to right of midline
    - – Colon, to left of midline
    - – Cecum, midline

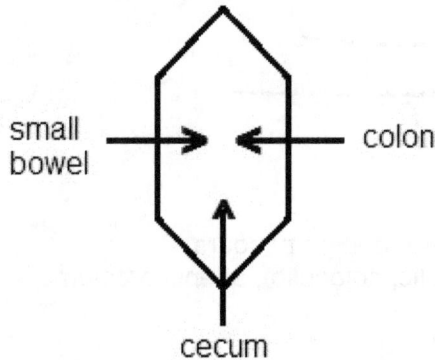

"Motivation is what gets you started.
Habit is what keeps you going."

Jim Rohn

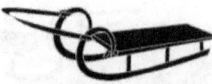

INTESTINAL ISCHEMIA

- The diagnosis of mesenteric ischemia and ischemic colitis may be missed until late, when the bowel is necrotic or perforates.
  - Prognosis once intestinal infarction has occurred
    - Mortality rate ~80%
- To encourage us all to have this diagnostic possibility at the front of our mind, this topic is often tested.
- In the MCQ stem, look for
  - Several abdominal pain with minimal findings on abdomen examination
  - Risk factors for low flow, thrombosis or embolism causing mesenteric ischemia
    - Atrial fibrillation
    - Athrosclerosis
    - Vasculitis
    - Drugs, such as
      - Digitalis
      - Cocaine
      - 5-HT3 antagonists / 5-HT4 agonists
      - Vasopressors
      - Octreotide

Acute Mesenteric Ischemia (AMI)

➢ Types

- Arterial
  - **SMAE** (SMA embolus; 50%)
    - Thrombus in SMA distal to the takeoff of the ileocolic artery is minor, proximal is major
    - If no peritonitis, consider TTT (transcatheter thrombolytic therapy)
  - **NOMI** (non-occlusive mesenteric ischemia; 25%)
    - Splanchnic vasoconstriction
    - Seen in hypoperfusion (shock, MI, CCF, arrhythmia, digitalis); CABG; chronic renal failure, hemodialysis, peritoral dialysis
    - Treat with infusion of papaverine
  - **SMAT** (SMA thrombosis; 10%)
    - Occurs in area of narrowing from atherosclerosis
    - May occur on top of CMI (chronic mesenteric ischemia)
    - Important to distinguish between acute versus chronic thrombosis: "the absence of collateral vessels or the presence of collaterals with inadequate filling of the SMA indicates an acute occlusion and demands prompt intervention" (Sleisenger and Fordtran's Gastrointestinal and Liver Disease. 9th Edition. Saunders/Elsevier, Philadelphia, 2010, page 2035), i.e., SMA infusion of papaverine followed by surgery for peritoneal signs
  - FSI (focal segmental ischemia; 5%)
  - Note: approximate frequency of causes of AMI are given in brackets

361

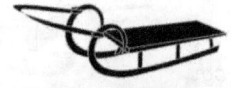

- o Mesenteric Venous Thrombosis (MVT, 10%)

Types of Emboli	Site of Supply from Branches of SMA
o Major (proximal to origin of ileocolic artery)	– MCA (middle colic artery) • Transverse colon – RCA (right colic artery) • Distal ascending colon
o Minor (distal to origin of ileocolic artery)	– Ileocolic • Terminal ileum, cecum, plus proximal ascending colon

- Give the anastomatic circulation between the CA (celiac axis) and the SMA (superior mesenteric artery), and between the SMA and the IMA (inferior mesenteric artery).

CA ↔ SMA	SMA ↔ IMA
o Superior pancreaticoduodenal artery (comes off CA)	– Margina artery of Drummond
o Inferior pancreaticoduodenal artery (comes off SMA)	– Central ananstomatic artery – Arc of Riolan

- o The central anastomatic artery or the arc of Roilan may be called the "meandering artery" when SMA or IMA are obstructed.

➢ Pathophysiology

- Give the mechanism of tissue injury which occurs with reperfusion following a period of ischemia.
  - o During ischemia, the enzyme XDH (xanthine dehydrogenase) becomes XO (xanthine oxidase)
  - o During reperfusion, XO produces reactive oxygen radicles
  - o Reactive oxygen radicals cause
    - – ↑ permeability of microvessels
    - – ↑ necrosis of epithelial cells
    - – ↑ LT (leukotriene) B4 release
    - – ↑ PAF (platelet-activating factor)
  - o LTB4 and PAF → neutrophil adherence/migration → ↑ proteases → ↑ damage to endothelium

➢ Clinical
  - o Severe abdominal pain out of keeping with minimal findings on abdominal examination
  - o When the findings are present (distention, guarding; rebound, ↓ bowel sounds), the bowel wall is probably necrotic/infarcted, and surgery is urgent.

362

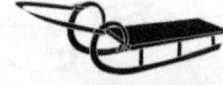

➢ Causes/associations

• Give factors which are associated with ↑ risk of AMI (acute myenteric ischemia) in young persons.
  o Vasoactive drugs (e.g., amphetamine, phenylephrine)
  o Cocaine use
  o Thrombophilia

➢ Laboratory
  o ↑ LDH
  o Metabolic acidosis
  o ↑ WBC, "shift to the left"
  o Diagnostic imaging (please see later details)
    – Abdominal film thumb printing
    – CT
    – Colonoscopy

➢ Diagnostic Imaging
  o CT or CTA (CT angiography) changes in the early stages of AMI are not specific, except for the findings
    – Air in the wall of the bowel or in the portal circulation
    – Thrombi in the mesenteric vessels
    – Acute infarction of other organs from emboli
  o Performance characteristics of CT scan for occlusive AMI (not NOMI)
    – Sensitivity, 92%
    – Specificity, 100%
  o CT angiography may be diagnostic when CT is not
  o Performance characteristics of selective mesenteric angiography for AMI
    – Sensitivity, 90% to 100%
    – Specificity, 100%
  o Criteria for angiographic diagnosis of NOMI
    – Narrowed origin of branches of SMA
    – Irregular intestinal branches
    – Arcades
      ▪ Spasm
    – Intramural vessels
      ▪ ↓ filling

CLINICAL ALERT
  o Normal diagnostic imaging does not exclude AMI, unless angiography has been done and is normal.
  o Prognosis once intestinal infarction has occurred: the mortality rate is ~80%

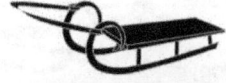

Mastering the Boards: Gastroenterology   A.B.R. Thomson

- Give the findings suggestive of acute MVT on CT scanning and on selective mesenteric arteriography.

  - CT (MRI or abdominal ultrasound)
    - Bowel wall
      - Thick
      - Enhanced
    - SMV
      - Dilated
      - Thrombus (lucency) in lumen of the vein
      - Wall of vein shows ↑ density
    - Collaterals
      - Dilated

  - Selective mesenteric arteriography of acute superior mesenteric venous thrombosis
    - SMV
      - Thrombus in lumen
      - No visualization of SMV or portal vein
      - Slow/no filling of mesenteric veins
    - SMA
      - Spasm
      - Arterial arcades slow to empty
      - Blush

Clinical Curiosities

- The sensitivity of plain films of the abdomen for AMI is only 30%, until infarction occurs.

- Abdominal pain out of proportion to the physical findings is usually common in AMI, except for AMI due to NOMI, in which case there may be little or no pain in ~25% of sufferers.

- Give the limitation of ultrasound studies, including Duplex and Doppler flowmetry, in diagnosing AMI.
  - The peripheral portion of vessels is not seen
  - Reliable diagnosis of AMI due to NOMI not possible
  - Just because blood flow is reduced does not prove ischemia, since even total occlusions may not be causing symptoms when collaterals have developed.

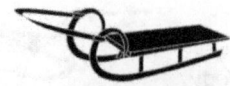

Mastering the Boards: Gastroenterology   A.B.R. Thomson

PROTEIN-LOSING ENTEROPATHY

- Give causes of protein-losing enteropathy.

    - Increased lymphatic pressure
        - Congestive heart failure
        - Constrictive pericarditis
        - Primary, secondary lymphangiectasia

    - Ulcerating intestinal disease
        - IBD (Crohn disease, ulcerative colitis)
        - Colon cancer

    - "Leaky gut"
        - Celiac disease
        - Small intestinal bacterial overgrowth
        - Whipple disease
        - Vasculitides

"Don't overlook medication compliance of patient,
even when in hospital."

Dr. Joel Hurnitz

365

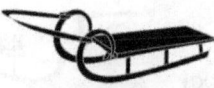

INTESTINAL ADAPTATION

Clinical Challenge

Ileal resection increases gastric acid secretion, as well as speeds up the rate of gastric emptying and small intestinal transit.

- Give the ileal-specific GI peptides which are lost with a distal small bowel resection, and which may cause increased gastric secretion by way of reducing some of the inhibition of gastric secretion caused by these peptides.
  - The presence of unabsorbed fat and carbohydrates in the ileum release the GI peptides GLP, PYY (peptide YY) and neurotensin.
  - These peptides normally inhibit gastric acid secretion
  - Reducing some of this inhibition on gastric secretion will lead to reduced acid secretion.

Clinical Alert

A patient with an extensive ileal resection develops unexplained neurological symptoms/signs (e.g., nystagmus, opthalmoplegia, ataxia, confusion, inappropriate behavior).

- Give the pathophysiology of the likely diagnosis.
  - The patient likely has D-lactic acidosis (not L-lactic acidosis) due to the spillage of large amounts of unabsorbed carbohydrate into the colon.
  - The polysaccharides are metabolized to SCFA (shot chain fatty acids), which acidify the stool.
  - This acidity reduces the growth of the usual Bacteriodes, and increases the growth of gram-positive anaerobes.
  - These gram-positive anaerobes produce ↑ D-lactate, which accumulates in the body because it is not metabolized by the usual L-lactate dehydrogenase.
  - The mortality rate and TPN-dependence rates after an extensive small bowel resection resulting in SBS (short bowel syndrome) are approximately 3% and 10% per year, respectively.

- Give the complications of cholestyramine therapy given to a patient with ileal resection (>100 cm).
  - Possible deficiency of fat-soluble vitamins when used long-term
  - Worsening of steatorrhea due to cholestyramine—associated bile salt deficiency

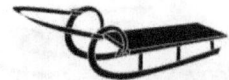

- Give the dietary therapy during the intestinal adaptive phases which occur after extensive small intestinal resection in the patient with Crohn disease who develops short bowel syndrome.

  o Acute phase
    - Starts immediately after intestinal resection
    - Lasts less than 4 weeks
    - Infusion therapy using Ringer's solution, glucose and amino acid solutions, substitution of water soluble vitamins and trace elements
    - Start parenteral nutrition

  o Adaptation phase
    - Lasts from less than 4 weeks to 2 years
    - Maximal stimulation of intestinal adaptation is achieved by gradually increasing intestinal nutrient exposure
    - Oral/enteral nutrition with gradually increasing nutrient loads: isosmolar salt–glucose-solutions, tea, carbohydrate solutions, medium chain triglycerides, amino acids
    - Predominantly long chain triglycerides, free fatty acids, small amounts of medium chain triglycerides in patients with preserved colon; saccharose, maltose, glutamine, pectin; addition of vitamins and minerals as needed, in particular calcium

  o Maintenance phase
    - Permanent dietetic treatment must be individualized
    - Frequent small meals, high fat diet, small amounts of medium chain triglycerides in patients with preserved colon; fluids can usually be taken with meals, addition of vitamins and minerals as needed, in particular calcium
    - Avoidance of nutrients rich in oxalate if distal small intestinal resection
    - Effective therapy of acute exacerbations and optimal maintenance therapy of Crohn disease are of pivotal importance.

OBSCURE GI BLEEDING (OGIB)

➤ Pathology

• Give the common sites of obscure GI bleeding from the small bowel.

  o Arteriovenous Malformations (AVMs)
    - Jejunum-36%
    - Ileum-34%
    - Jejunum and ileum-30%

  o Polyps
    - Jejunum-70% (36% in proximal jejunum)
    - Ileum-30% (16% in terminal ileum)

➤ Diagnostic imaging/endoscopy

• Give diagnostic methods for determining the cause of obscure GI bleeding.

  o Endoscopy
    - Second-look EGD/colonoscopy
    - Capsule endoscopy (CE)
    - Double balloon enteroscopy (DBE)
    - Push enteroscopy (PE)
    - Intraoperative endoscopy
    - Repeat endoscopy
    - Repeat colonoscopy

  o Small bowel contrast X-ray
    - Small bowel single contrast
    - Small bowel double contrast (enteroclysis)

  o CT/MRI
    - CT angiography
    - CT/MRI enterography
    - CT-enterocylsis

  o Angiography
    - In the presence or absence of acute bleeding

  o Scintigraphy
    - Erythrocyte scintigraphy (RBC scan)
    - Meckel's scintigraphy

Abbreviations: CE, capsule endoscopy; DBE, double balloon enteroscopy; EGD, esophagogastroduodenoscopy; PE, push enteroscopy

Adapted from: Heil U. and Jung M. *Best Pract Res Clin Gastroenterol* 2007;21(3): pg. 402.

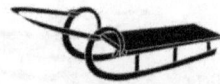

- o **Second Look EGD**
  - – In persons with Obscure GI bleeding (OGIB), 35-75% of the causes are revealed by second-look EGD, and 6% by second-leak colonoscopy (Leighton 09)
  - – Small bowel lesions account for only 5% of OGIB, and most of these (70%) are vascular lesions (Cellier C. *Best Pract Res Clin Gastroenterol* 2008:329-40).
  - – Most of the lesions diagnosed by push enterstomy in persons with OGIB are within the reach of standard EGD.

- o **Capsule Endoscopy**
  - – The diagnostic yield of capsule endoscopy (CE) in the patient with OGIB ranges from 38-83% (Rondonotti E, et al. *World J Gastroenterol* 2007:6140-9).
  - – CE is more likely to give a positive yield when there has been more than one episode of bleeding, the bleeding is overt rather than occult (60% vs 46%), CE is performed within 2 weeks of the bleeding episode (91% vs 34%), the bleeding has occurred over more than the 6 months, and the bleeding has resulted in the hemoglobin concentration being < 10 g/dl (Carey EJ, et al. *Am J Gastroenterol* 2007;102:89-95).
  - – The false negative rate for CE is 19% for tumours, and 11% overall.
  - – CE cannot be performed in persons with a structure or obstruction, since this would require that the capsule be removed surgically.

- • Give accepted indications for the use of capsule endoscopy (CE).
  - o Occult gastrointestinal bleeding
  - o Suspected Crohn disease (unless stricture may be present)
  - o Suspected small bowel tumour
  - o Surveillance of inherited polyposis syndromes
  - o Evaluation of drug induced small bowel injury
  - o Partially responsive celiac disease

Adapted from: Eliakim, R. *Curr Opin Gastroenterol* 2008(2): g. 161.

- o **Double Balloon Enteroscopy** (DBE)
  - – Double balloon enteroscopy (DBE) is superior to single balloon enteroscopy (SBE). DBE can be performed in an oral/antegrade, or anal/ retrograde manner.
  - – Approximate depth of endoscopic penetration of small bowel
    - ▪ Push enteroscopy   90-150 cm
    - ▪ Ileoscopy   50-80 cm
    - ▪ DBE,
      - - Oral   240-360 cm
      - - Rectal   102-140 cm

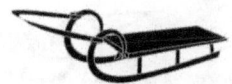

- DBE has a diagnostic yield of 60-80% in persons with OGIB suspected to be from the small intestine, with therapeutic intervention being possible in 40-73%.
- Meta-analysis has shown comparable diagnostic yield for DBE and CE (57-60%), with therapeutic potential with DBE (Pasha SF, et al. *Clin Gastroenterol* Heptaol 2008:671-6.; Chen X, et al. *World J Gastroenterol* 2007;13:4372-8.).
- The rate of complete enteroscopy is three times higher with double than with single balloon enteroscopy (66% vs 22%) (May et al., 2010; 105: 575-81).

o **Nuclear Meducine Scans**
  - Meckel scan for a Meckel diverticulum is performed with technetium 99 m pertechnetate, and has a sensitivity of 64-100% for bleeding from ectopic gastric mucosa.
  - A false negative Meckel scan may be the result of
    • A recent barium X-ray obscuring the area of uptake,
    • Too small a diverticulum, too small a vascular supply to the diverticulum,
    • Too rapid bleeding from the diverticulum washing out the technetium.
  - The technetium 99 m labeled RBC scan can show slow bleeding, (0.1-0.4 ml/min), whereas angiography needs higher rates of bleeding (>0.5 ml/ min) in order to be positive
    • With active bleeding, the bleeding site may be localized in 50-75% of patients, but the sensitivity rate falls below 50% with slower rates of bleeding.

o **Angiography**
  - An angiography suggests angioectasia from a vascular tuft or slow filling of a vein.
  - Therapeutic embolization may be performed with gelfoam or coils
  - Pipaverine may be infused at the time of angiography.

o **CT Enterography** CTE)
  - Oral contract is given by mouth and by nasojejunal tube for CT enterocyclis
  - The diagnostic yield of CTE in OGIB is 45% (Huprich JE, et al. *Radiology* 2008:562-71.)
  - May be useful to distinguish fibrostenotic from inflammatoryCrohn disease (Paulsen SR, et al. *Radiol Clin North Am* 2007:303-15.; Horsthuis K, et al. *Radiology* 2008:64-79.).

Abbreviations: CE, capsule endoscopy; CTE, CT enterography; DBE, double balloon enteroscopy; HHT, hereditary hemorrhagic telegangiectasia; OGIB, obscure GI bleeding; SBE, single balloon enteroscopy

370

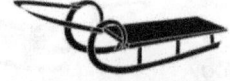

➢ Differential diagnosis

• Give differential diagnoses of bleeding from the upper and from the lower GI tract in persons suffering from HIV/AIDS, excluding non-AIDS-related diagnoses.

Infection	Esophagus	Stomach	Small bowel	Colon
o Candida	+			
o Cytomegalovirus	+	+	+	+
o Herpes simplex	+			
o Idiopathic ulcer	+			+
o Cryptosporidiosis		+	+	
o Salmonella sp.			+	
o Entamoeba histolytica				+
o Campylbacter				+
o Clostridium difficile				+
o Shigella sp				+
o Kaposi sarcoma		+	+	+
o Lymphoma		+	+	+

Adapted from: Wilcox, C. Mel. *Sleisenger & Fordtran's gastrointestinal and liver disease: Pathophysiology/Diagnosis/Management* 2006: pg. 676; and 10th edition, 2016, box 34-5, page 550.

371

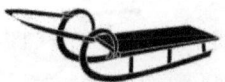

Mastering the Boards: Gastroenterology A.B.R. Thomson

- Compare and contrast the endoscopic findings and treatment of portal hypertensive gastropathy (PHG) and gastric antral vascular ectasia (GAVE).

Feature findings	PHG	GAVE
o Site	Fundus	Antrum
o Mosaic pattern	Yes	No
o Red colour signs	Yes	Yes
o Findings on gastric mucosal biopsy		
- Thrombi	No	+++
- Spindle cell proliferation	Sparse	++
- Fibrohyalinosis	No	+++
➢ Management	o ↓ portal hypertension	o Estrogens
	o β adrenergic blockers	o Antrectomy
	o TIPS	o Endoscopic laser therapy
	o Liver transplantation	o Liver transplantation

*Note: Gastric vascular ectasia (GVE) may occur anywhere in the stomach, not just in the asntrum, so do not distinguish GAVE/EVE from PHG just on the site of localization

➢ Treatment
  o Endoscopic therapy for AVMs (AV malformations, angiodysplasia, angioectasia, angioma, venous ectasia)
    – <10% of persons with angioectasia never bleed; 50% will never rebleed.
  o Cessation rates from AVM using push enteroscopy (PE), 57-85%
  o One year after double-balloon enteroscopy for AVM, about half are bleeding-free; other studies have shown rebleeding rates ranging from 20-63%

Printed with permission: Feagins LA, and Kane SV. *Am J Gastroenterol* 2009;104:770.

➢ Prognosis
  o Small bowel vascular lesions have a potential for recurrence after endoscopic therapy.
  o Long-term recurrence varies between 10 and 50%
  o Independent rebleeding risk factors are
    – Higher number of lesions
    – Associated valvular/arrhythmic cardiac disease.

Source: Samaha E, et al. Am J Gastroenterol 2012; 107: 240-246.

 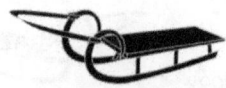

MISCELLANEOUS

Scleroderma (aka SSC [systemic sclerosis])

➢ Types

- o Limited (limited to skin)
- o Diffuse
  - – Involvement of stomach and small bowel in 40%
  - – Wide-necked intestinal and colonic diverticular
  - – Also may involve esophagus and stomach

➢ Diagnostic Imaging

● Give the diagnostic imaging findings in scleroderma of the GI tract.

- o Stomach   - ↓ rate of emptying

- o Small bowel   - Dilation
                    - Closely packed valvulae conniventes →
                      looks like an "accordion"

- o Colon   - Wide-mouthed diverticula

"Let's see if there is mechanistic information that
we can tease out."

Grandad

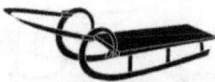

Dermatomyositis/Polymyositis

- o Involvement of GI tract in 50%
- o STE
    - – Esophagus
        - • Involvement of upper skeletal muscles → transfer dysphagia
    - – Small bowel
        - • Megaduodenum
        - • ↓ transit
- ➢ Histopathology
    - o Visceral myopathy
        - – Smooth muscle
        - – Atrophy, fibrosis

Systemic Lupus Erythematosus (SLE)

- ➢ Histopathology
    - o Ischemia → visceral myopathy
        - – Dysphagia
        - – Diarrhea
    - o Lupus enteritis
        - – Vasculitis of small blood vessels of small intestine

Paraneoplastic Visceral Neuropathies

- ➢ Definition
    - o A visceral neuropathy caused by "…. autoimmune processes triggered by the cancer and directed against antigens [onconeural antigens] common to both the cancer and the nervous system (Feldman M., et al. Sleisenger and Fordtran's Gastrointestinal and Liver Disease. 9th Edition. Saunders/Elsevier, Philadelphia, 2010, page 2137).
    - o Diffuse lymphocytic (CD3+, CD4, CD8) infiltration of the myenteric plexus.

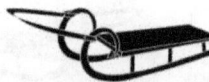

Myotonic Dystrophy

    o   Nerve as well as predominant smooth muscle dysfunction → dysmotility

---

SO YOU WANT TO BE A GASTROENTEROLOGIST!

- Give the common tumours and antibodies to onconeural antigens, seen in paraneoplastic visceral neuropathies (PVN).

  o The commonest tumour associated with PVN is SCLC (small cell lung cancer); also associated are thymoma, gynecological and breast tumours, colorectal cancer, as well as HL (Hodgkin lymphoma) and MM (multiple myeloma).

  o The commonest antibodies are
    - Hu-Ab
    - Cv2-Ab
    - nAchR

Duchenne Muscular Dystrophy (DMD)

➤ Genetic abnormalities

    o   Mutation in the gene for dystrophin → ↑ cell muscle membrane leakiness → muscle necrosis → fat and fibrosis replace muscle

    o   Dysphagia, gastroparesis

Amyloidosis

➤ Definition

    o   "….. mixed group of disorders characterized by extracellular deposits of abnormal protein fibrils with a β-sheet fibrillar structure" (Sleisenger and Fordtran's Gastrointestinal and Liver Disease. 10th Edition. Saunders/Elsevier, Philadelphia, 2016, page 2189).

➤ Types

    o   AL, primary

    o   AA, secondary to
        - Crohn disease
        - ankylosing spondylitis
        - PBC
        - Rheumatoid arthritis

    o   AB2MG, hemodialysis-related

    o   ATTR, hereditary

    o   Senile

    o   Localized

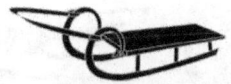

➢ Histopathology

    ○ Amyloid is deposit in-muscle fibres, which become replaced by amyloid → myopathy
        – Close to neural tissue causing presume atrophy → neuropathy
        – Vasculature → ischemia, infarction

Hereditary Hemorrhage Telangiectasia (HHT; aka Osler-Weber-Rendu syndrome)

➢ Pathogenesis

    ○ Defective endoglin and ALK genes which determine properties of endothelial cells during angiogenesis

    ○ Contractile elements of vessel: defect in muscle and elastic tissue

    ○ High output cardiac failure

➢ Causes/associations

    ○ Aortic aneurysm

    ○ Renal cell cancer

    ○ ↑ risk in pregnancy

➢ Treatment

    ○ Bevacizumab (humanized endothelial growth factor antagonist)

Neurofibromatosis

• Give the forms of involvement of the GI tract in neurofibromatosis.

    ○ The forms of intestinal involvement in neurofibromatosis include
        – Mucosa – ganglioneuromatosis submucosal and myenteric plexus – hyperplasia
        – GIST tumours
        – Carcinoid of the periampullary region of the duodenum

376

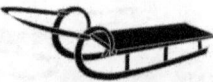

ABBREVIATIONS

5-ASA	Acetylsalicylic acid
6-MMP	6-methyl mercaptopurine
6-TGN	6-thio guanine nucleotides
AAD	Antibiotic-associated diarrhea
Ach	Acetylcholine
AIH	Autoimmune hepatitis
ALCA	Anti-laminaribioside carbohydrate antibodies
AM	Apical membrane
AMCA	Anti-mannobioside carbohydrate antibodies
AMI	Acute Mesenteric Ischemia
APA	Anti-pituitary antibodies
ASCA	Anti-Saccharomyces cerevisiae antibody
ASCT	Autologous stem cell transplantation
AUWI	Area under wash in
AUWO	Area under washout
AVMs	AV malformations
AZA	Azathioprine
BA	Bile acid
BBM	Brush border membrane of ileocyte
BCG	Bacilli Calmette-Guerin
BLM	Basolateral membrane of ileocyte
BP	Blood pressure
BRIC	Benign recurrent intrahepatic cholestasis
BS	Blood sugar
BSEP	Bile salt export protein
CA	Celiac axis
CA	Cholic acid
Ca^{2+}_i	Intracellular calcium
CBC	Complete blood count
CCFC	Crohn and Colitis Foundation
CCK	Cholecystokinin

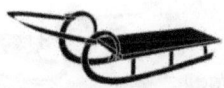

CD	Celiac disease
CD	Crohn disease
CDA	Cladribine
CDAI	Crohn disease activity index
CDCA	Chenodeoxycholic acid
CE	Capsule endoscopy
CFTR1	Cystic fibrosis transmembrane conductance regulator
CIPO	Chronic intestinal pseudo-obstruction
CM	Canalicular membrane
CMV	Cytomegalovirus
CNS	Central nervous system
CRP	C-reactive protein
CTE	CT enterography
CVID	Chronic variable immunodeficiency
CVS	Cardiovascular syndrome
CyA	Cyclosporin A
DBE	Double balloon enteroscopy
DCA	Deoxycholic acid
DEXA	DEXA scan for bone mineral density
DH	Dermatitis herpetiformis
D-IBS	Diarrhea predominant IBS
DM	Diabetes mellitus
DMD	Duchenne muscular dystrophy
DMPM	Dermatomyositis/polymyositis
DPG	Deamidated gliadin peptide
DRA	Down-regulated adenoma
DRE	Digital rectal examination
EAEC	Enteroaggregative escherichia coli
EAggEC	Enteroaggregative E. coli
EATL	Early aberrant T cell lymphoma
EBV	Ebstein Barr virus

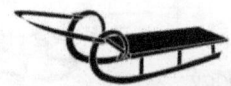

EGD	Esophagogastroduodenoscopy
EGF	Epidemal growth factor
EHC	Enterohepatic absorption of bile acids
EHEC	Enterohemorrhagic escherichia
EIEC	Enteroinvasive escherichia coli
AKAP	A kinase-anchoring proteins
EMA	Endomyseal antibody
ENaC	Epithelial sodium channel
ENS	Enteric nervous system
EPEC	Enteropathogenic E. coli
ESR	Erythrocyte sedimentation rate
ETEC	Enterotoxigenic escherichia coli
EUA	Examination under general anaesthesia
EUS	Endoscopic ultrasound
FA	Folic acid
FAP	Familial adenomatous polyposis
FMF	Familial Mediterranean fever
G	Gastrin
GABA	Gamma -amino butyric acid
GALT	Gut-associated lymphoid tissue
GCS	Glucoscorticosteroids
GFD	Gluten-free diet
GGTP	Gamma glutamyl transpeptidase
GI	Gastrointestinal
GIP	Gastric inhibitory peptide
GIST	Gastrointestinal stromal tumour
GKAP	G kinase-anchoring proteins
GSE	Gluten sensitive enteropathy
HAHAs	Human antihuman antibodies
HAPC	High-amplitude propagated contractions
HBV	Hepatitis B virus

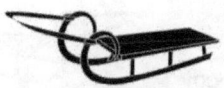

HCV	Hepatitis C virus
HF	Heart failure
HGPRT	Hypoxanthine-guanine phosphoribosyltransferase
HHT	Hereditary hemorrhagic telegangiectasia
HIV	Human immunodeficiency syndromes
HL	Hodgkin lymphoma
HLA	Human leukocyte antigen
HNPCC	Hereditary non-polyposis colorectal cancer
HSV	Herpes Simplex virus
HZV	Herpes Zoster virus
IBD	Inflammatory bowel disease
IBS	Irritable bowel syndrome
IBS-D	Predominant irritable bowel syndrome
ICC	Intestinal Cells of Cajal
ICC-DMP	Intestinal Cells of Cajal -deep muscle plexus
ICC-IM	Intestinal Cells of Cajal - intramuscular plexus
ICC-MY	Intestinal Cells of Cajal - myenteric plexus; pacemaker cells
IDMC	Interdigestive motor cycle
IEL	Intraepithelial T-cells lymphocytes
IFN	Interferon
IFX	Infliximab failures
IL	Interleukin
IM	Intramuscular
iNOS	Inducible nitric oxide synthase
IPSID	Immunoproliferative small intestinal disease
JP	Juvenile Polyposis
LACA	Low-amplitude contractile activity
LCA	Lithocholic acid
LE	Liver enzymes
LP	Lamina propria
LT	Leukotriene

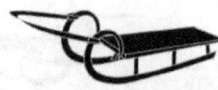

A.B.R. Thomson

LHD	Limited human data
M	Motilin
MAC	Mycobacterium-avium complex infection
MAd CAM	Mucosal addressin cell adhesion molecule
MCA	Middle colic artery
MD	Myotonia dystrophy
MDCT-E	Multidetector CT enteroclysis
MM	Multiple myeloma
MM	Muscularis mucosae
MMR	Measles, Mumps, Rubella
MP	Mercaptopurine
MRP_2	Multidrug resistance-associated protein-2
MS	Multiple sclerosis
MTOR	Mammalian target of rapamycin
MTX	Methotrexate
MVT	Mesenteric venous thrombosis
N	Neurotensin
NET	Neuroendocrine tumour
NGS	Non-celiac gluten sensitivity
NHL	Non Hodgkins lymphoma
NNT	Number needed to treat
NO	Nitric oxide
NOD2	Nucleotide Oligomerization Domain 2
NOMI	Non-occlusive mesenteric ischemia
NRCD	Non-responsive CD
NSAIDs	Non-steroidal anti-inflammatory drugs
NTCP	Sodium-taurocholate cotransporting polypeptide
OCA	Oral contraceptive agent
OCIF	Osteoclastogenesis inhibitory factor
OGIB	Obscure GI bleeding
OPG	Osteoprotegerin

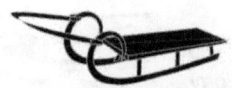

OR	Odds ratio
PAF	Platelet-activating factor
pANCA	Perinuclear anti-neutrophil cytoplasmic antibodies
PAT1	Putative anion transporter 1
PBC	Primary biliary cirrhosis
PE	Push enteroscopy
PET	Positron emission tomography
PF	Perianal fistulae
PHM	Peptide histidine methionine
PINES	Paracrine, immunologic, neural, and endocrine systems
PJS	Peutz-Jeghers syndrome
PKA	Protein kinase A
PKC	Protein kinase C
PMN	Polymorphonuclear
PSC	Primary sclerosing cholangitis
PTLD	Post-transplant lymphoproliferative disorder
PVN	Paraneoplastic visceral neuropathies
RA	Rheumatoid arthritis
RCA	Right colic artery
RCD	Refractory celiac disease
S	Secretin
SBBO	Small bowel bacterial overgrowth syndrome
SBE	Single balloon enteroscopy
SBO	Small bowel obstruction
SCFA	Short-chain fatty acids
SCLC	Small cell lung cancer
SERT	Serotonin reuptake transporter
SIBO	Small intestinal bacterial overgrowth syndrome
SLE	Systemic lupus erythematosus
SM	Sinusoidal membrane
SMA	Superior mesenteric artery

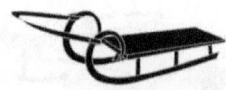

SP	Substance P
SS	Somatostatin
SSC	Systemic sclerosis
TB	Tuberculosis
TCR	T-cell receptor
TD	Travellers' diarrhea
TFM	Tumour-free margins
TG	Therapeutic gain
TGF	Transforming growth factor
TJs	Tight junctions
TLR	Toll-like receptors
TNF	Tumour-necrosis factor-α
TNM	Tumour, node (regional lymph node)
TPN	Total parental nutrition
tTG	Tissue transglutamase
UC	Ulcerative colitis
UDCA	Ursodeoxycholic acid
UGIS-SBFT	Upper GI series with a small intestinal follow-through
VIP	Vasoactive intestinal peptide
XDH	Xanthine dehydrogenase
XO	Xanthine oxidase
ZOT	Zonula occludens toxin

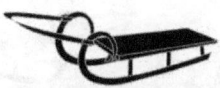

COLON

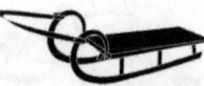

TABLE OF CONTENTS

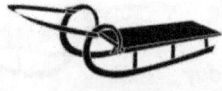

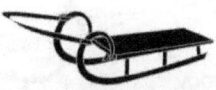

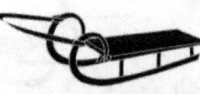

COLONIC MOTILITY

- o Rhythmic myoelectric activity from layer of middle of circular smooth muscle
    - – MPOs (myenteric potential oscillations)
        - ▪ ↓ 10-12 per minute
        - ▪ ↓ arise from myenteric plexus
        - ▪ MPO-related contractions summate to result in longer and stronger contractions
    - – Slow waves
        - ▪ Arise from submucosal border of inner circular muscle
        - ▪ 2-4 per minute

- o Unlike small intestine where slow waves propagate predominantly aboard (down the colon, way from the mouth and towards the anus), in the colon slow waves propagate over short distances both up and down the colon.

➢ Colonic and Rectal Motor Patterns

- o Non-propagating
    - – Random
    - – Segmenting and mixing
    - – 2-4 cpm (cycles per minute)

- o Propagating
    - – Summation of MPOs (myenteric potential oscillations)
    - – Aka high-amplitude propagating sequences, or HAPCs (high-amplitude propagating contractions)

- o Rectal motor complex (RMC, aka PRMA [periodic rectal motor activity])

➢ Interstitial cells of Cajal (ICC)

- o ICC MP
    - – Myenteric plexus
        - ▪ Pacemakers for rapid oscillations in MPOs of circular and longitudinal muscle

- o ICC SM
    - – Submucosal plexus
        - ▪ Pacemakers for high amplitude, slow waves

- o ICC IM
    - – Intramuscular, between circular and longitudinal muscles
        - ▪ Integrate pacemaker activity and neuronal inputs to smooth muscle

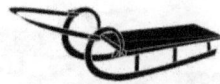

Enteric Neuron System (ENS)

- o Nerve cell Bodies

- Give the location of the nerve cell bodies which occur in plexuses in the various histological layers of the colon.

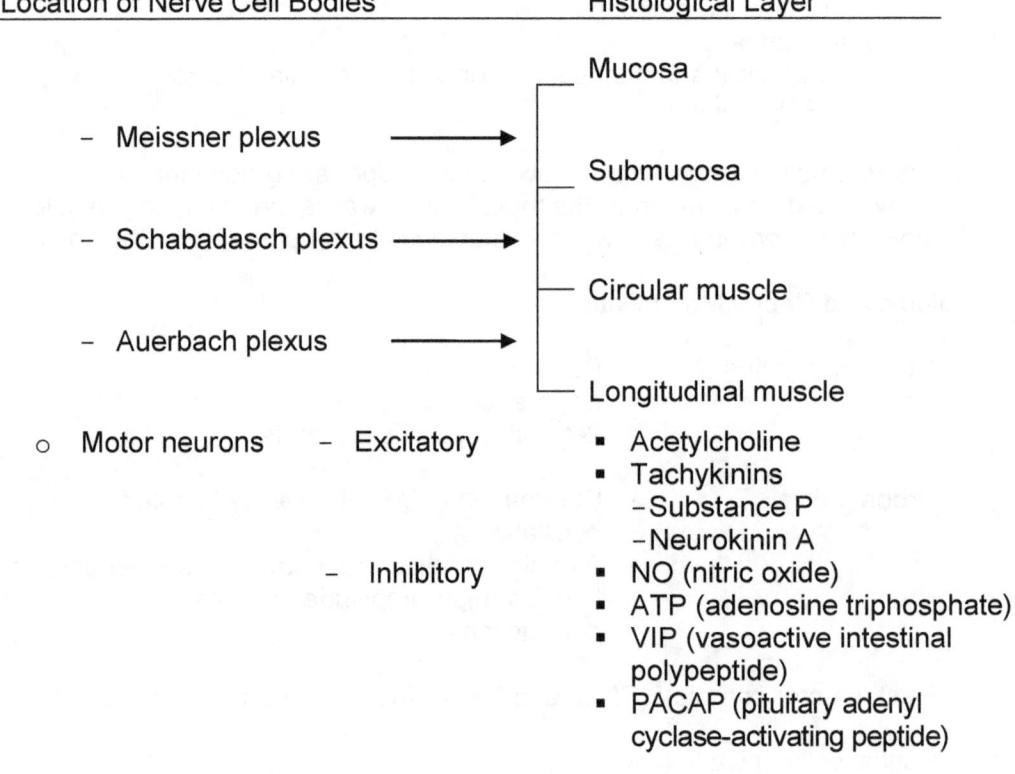

Location of Nerve Cell Bodies	Histological Layer
	Mucosa
– Meissner plexus ⟶	Submucosa
– Schabadasch plexus ⟶	Circular muscle
– Auerbach plexus ⟶	Longitudinal muscle

- o Motor neurons – Excitatory
  - ▪ Acetylcholine
  - ▪ Tachykinins
    - – Substance P
    - – Neurokinin A
  - – Inhibitory
  - ▪ NO (nitric oxide)
  - ▪ ATP (adenosine triphosphate)
  - ▪ VIP (vasoactive intestinal polypeptide)
  - ▪ PACAP (pituitary adenyl cyclase-activating peptide)

- o Colonic stimulus → activation of IPANS (intrinsic primary afferent neurons) → excitation of
  - – Ascending excitatory nerves, proximal contraction
  - – Descending inhibitory nerves, distal relaxation

- o Parasympathetic innervation
  - – ↓ muscle activity
  - – ↓ blood flow
  - – ↓ secretion
  - – ↑ contraction of IC (ileocecal) function and IAS (internal anal sphincter)

IAS Inhibitory Innervation	EAS Stimulatory Innervation
– Lumbar sympathetic	▪ Pudendal nerve
– Sacral parasympathetic	

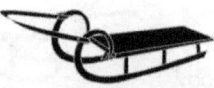

IRRITABLE BOWEL SYNDROME (IBS)

➢ Definition

- o IBS is defined as "... the presence of abdominal discomfort or pain associated with disturbed defecation" (Sleisenger and Fordtran's Gastrointestinal and Liver Disease. 10th Edition. Saunders/Elsevier, Philadelphia, 2016, page 2139).

- o There are several criteria used to define the disease, such as the Manning, Krius or Rome (I, II, III, IV) criteria.

- o Performance characteristics of Rome I
    - – Sensitivity, 71%
    - – Specificity, 85%

➢ Epidemiology

- o Incidence depends on criteria used for diagnosis; using Manning criteria, $6700/10^5$ person-years (!)

- o Upon with definition or criteria used, the prevalence varies (~10% or more, females > males)

- o Prevalence increases with age, although it has often been suggested that IBS is a disorder of women age 20 to 40 years

- o At any point in time, the community prevalence is
    - – IBS-D (diarrhea predominant), 6%
    - – IBS-C (constipation predominant), 5%
    - – IBS-M (mixed: alternating diarrhea and constipation), 5%

➢ Pathophysiology (proposed)

- • Give proposed **pathophysiological causes** of IBS.

    - o Genetic
        - – ↑ concordance in monozygotic is dizygotic twins
        - – SCN5A (sodium channel) mutation
        - – Clustering of IBS in monozygotic twins

    - o CNS, ENS
        - – Sensitization in dorsal horn of spinal column
        - – Mid-cingular cortex alterations on PET scans in response to rectal distention
        - – Putative neurotransmitters
            - ▪ Serotonin (5 HT)
            - ▪ Neurokinins
            - ▪ CGRP (calcitonin gene-related peptide)
                - – NMDA receptor
                    - ▪ Modulates central neuronal excitability

391

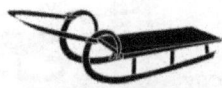

- o Diet
  - – Wheat, lactose, fructose, sorbitol
  - – Food-exclusion diets may be successful, especially when IBS-sufferer has a positive IgG antibody response to the food
  - – Exclusion of gluten from diet may be useful in some persons (NCGS; non-celiac gluten sensitivity)

- o GI tract
  - – Motility
    - ▪ HAPCs (high-amplitude propagated contractions):
      - – ↓ in IBS-C
      - – ↑ in IBS-D
    - ▪ ↑ gastrocolic reflex
    - ▪ Transit
      - – ↑ in IBS-D
      - – ↓ in IBS-C
    - ▪ ↑ frequency and duration of jejunal contractions
  - – Visceral hypersensitivity
    - ▪ Dysfunction
      - – IBS-D ↑ sympathetic adrenergic dysfunction
      - – IBS-C ↑ vagal dysfunction
    - ▪ Abnormal sensation
      - – Spinal cord (dorsal horn)
      - – CNS
    - ▪ Abnormal receptors
      - – TRPV1 (transient receptor potential vailloid -1)
      - – NMDA (N-methyl-D-aspartate)
      - – PARs (proteinase-activated and serine proteases receptors)
  - – Altered microbiotica
    - ▪ Microbiotica – increased risk of IBS after enteric infection, abnormalities in fecal microbiotica
    - ▪ The fecal microbiota is altered in IBS patients, as compared with healthy persons
    - ▪ A proportion of IBS patients have associated small intestinal bacterial overgrowth (SIBO). Eradication of the SIBO may improve IBS symptoms

- o Immunity/ Inflammation
  - – Innate immunity – increased numbers or altered functions of innate immunity cells (innate cells, monocytes/monocytes/macrophages, CD3+ or CD4+ T cells, CD8+ T cells, or B-cells in the small and/or large intestine, and in the blood).

392

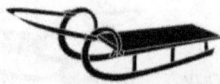

- o Nervous system
  - – Psychological factors
    - Depression, anxiety, somatization
    - Abuse sexual, physical, emotional
    - Childhood stress
  - – Psychological difference between consultors and non-consultors
  - – Hypervigilance (↑ attention to pain)
    - Central dysregulation
    - PET scanning changes in ACC (anterior cingulate cortex) activity with
    - Rectal distention
  - – Hyperanalgesia and/ or the cognitive process of hypervigilance towards adverse events occurring in the viscera alters the perception towards, for example, pain or distention.
  - – Neuroimmune interactions – increased number of sensory nerve fibres expressing the capsaicin receptor TRPV1

- o Permeability/ Cytokines
  - – Intestinal permeability – decreased expression in the jejunum of the tight junction protein ZO1 (aka zonula occludins protein)
  - – ↑ intestinal permeability
  - – ↑ intestinal IL-1b
  - – ↑ enterochromaffin cells
  - – ↑ serotonin blood levels after food
  - – The severity of IBS is associated with both enhanced colonic permeability and increased mucosal mast cells.
  - – Altered permeability suggesting alterations in TJs (tight junctions)
  - – Rational for FODMAPs
    - Luminal acting antibiotics (rifaximin 550 mg tid)

- Give examples of pathophysiological changes found in IBS which suggest an organic etiology.

  - o Chromogranins and secretogranins
    - – Chromogranins (Cg) and secretogranins (Sg) are expressed and secreted by cells of the enteric, endocrine, and immune system, and may reflect activity of these systems.
    - – Irritable bowel syndrome (IBS) patients demonstrate higher levels of fecal chromogranins A (CgA), secretogranins II (Sg II), and Sg III but lower levels of CgB than healthy individuals.
    - – Fecal levels of Sg II, Sg III, and CgB than healthy individuals.
    - – Increased fecal levels of granins were associated with faster colonic transit, increased average stool frequency, and more severe abdominal pain in IBS.

393

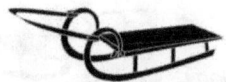

- o Inflammatory cells
  - Increased colonic mucosal inflammatory cellularity has been reported in post-infectious IBS (PI-IBS) and with less consistency in non-PI-IBS.
  - ↑ T cells in post-infectious (PI) IBS
- o Cytokines
  - Elevated basal and stimulated cytokine levels in the blood have been reported in some but not all IBS studies.
  - Interleukin-10 (IL-10) mRNA expression in the sigmoid colon mucosa is decreased in female irritable bowel syndrome (IBS) patients compared with female controls.
  - Cytokine levels in the blood do not correlate to their respective expression levels in the sigmoid colon mucosa in IBS.
  - Levels of cytokines and CRF- and NK - related neuropeptides and cell counts are not significantly elevated in non-PI-IBS and thus, do not support that colonic mucosal inflammation consistently has a primary role in these patients.
- o Neurokinin-1 receptor
  - Neurokinin (NK)-1 receptor expression in the sigmoid colon mucosa is decreased in female IBS patients compared with female controls, but again there is no difference in males.
- o CRF R
  - Corticotropin releasing factor 1 receptor (CRF R) mRNA is expressed at levels below usual detection limits in most non-post-infectious IBS (non-PI-IBS) patients and healthy controls.

Source: Chang L, et al. Am J Gastroenterol 2012; 107: 262-272; Ohman L, et al. Am J Gastroenterol 2012; 107: 440-447.

- Give observations which suggest that inflammation may play a role in the pathophysiology of post-infectious IBS.
  - o ↑ mast cells in muscularis externa
  - o ↑ TNF-α
  - o ↑ SIBO (mall intestinal bacterial overgrowth)
  - o ↑ lymphocytes around myenteric plexus
  - o ↑ neuron degeneration
  - o Post-infection IBS
    - ↑ permeability
    - ↑ enterochromaffin cells
    - ↑ CD3, CD4, and CD8 T cells
    - ↑ macrophages

Please see Sleisenger and Fordtran's Gastrointestinal and Liver Disease. 9th Edition. Saunders/Elsevier, Philadelphia, 2010, Table 118.4, page 2101.

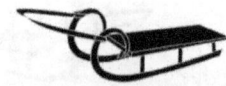

> Clinical

- o Approximately 78% of IBS patients of all subtypes fluctuate between the extremes of loose/watery stools and hard/lumpy stools.

- o IBS drugs might produce better outcomes.

- o In IBS-D, pain is associated with the passage of a loose/watery stool.

- o In IBS-C, pain increases with distention from cumulative days without a stool.

Source: Palsson OS, el al. Am J Gastroenterol 2012; 107: 286-295.

- o There is an association of IBS with other disorders
  - – Intestinal
    - ▪ GERD
    - ▪ Crohn disease, 33%
    - ▪ Ulcerative colitis, 42%
    - ▪ Enteric infection
  - – Intestinal surgery

	IBS	Control
▪ Cholecystomies	12%	4%
▪ Hysterectomies	33%	17%
▪ Appendectomies	21%	12%

  - – Extraintestinal
    - ▪ Headache
    - ▪ Backache
    - ▪ Poor-sleep
    - ▪ Fatigue
    - ▪ Joint aches and pains

- o If abdominal tenderness is found on physical examination, check for
  - – Abdominal wall tenderness (Carnett test)
  - – Painful rib syndrome

- o IBS may be chronic, and if these sufferers develop alarm symptoms, they should be appropriately investigated as for a non-IBS person.

Please see Sleisenger and Fordtran's Gastrointestinal and Liver Disease. 9th Edition. Saunders/Elsevier, Philadelphia, 2010, Box 122-2, page 2148.

> Clinical course

- o A person's IBS subgroup of IBS may change over a year:
  - – IBS-D → IBS-C ⎤ < 1/3
  - – IBS-C → IBS-D ⎦
  - – IBS-M → IBS-DOR-C ⎤ > 75%
  - – IBS-DOR-C → IBS-M ⎦

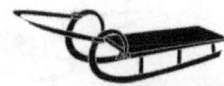

- o About 1/3 of IBS patients lose their symptoms per year
- o ↑ risk of developing ischemic colitis ($43/10^5$ person-years)
- o ↓ health-related quality of life
- o ↑ risk of abdominal surgery (gallbladder, appendix, uterus)

➢ Diagnosis

- Give the **ROME IV criteria** for IBS.
  - o Symptom onset at least 6 months prior to the diagnosis
  - o Recurrent abdominal pain or discomfort for at least 3 days of the month in the last 3 months
  - o Association with at least 2 of the following:
    - – Improvement with defecation
    - – Onset associated with change in stool frequency
    - – Onset associated with change in stool form

Printed with permission : Longstreth GF, Thompson WG, Chey WD, et al. *Gastroenterology* 2006;130(5):1480-1491.

- o Note:
  - – Relapsing symptoms
  - – The diagnostic criteria define the symptoms, and vice versa

- Pain from injury to the viscera in the abdomen often presents as referred pain. In the following pathologies, give the origin of the disorder and the site to which the pain is referred.
  - o Biliary colic – To right shoulder or scapula
  - o Renal colic – To groin
  - o Appendicitis – Epigastric to RLQ (right paracolic gutter)
  - o Pancreatitis – To the back
  - o Perforated ulcer – To RLQ Ruptured aortic aneurysm- back or flank

Adapted from: Connor BA. *Clin Infect Dis* 2005;41suppl 8:S577-86.; and Spiller RC. *Gastroenterology* 2003;124(6):1662-1671.

➢ Treatment

The MCQ stem may suggest IBS, but IBS symptoms may masquerade in several treatable conditions

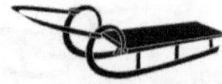

- ❖ Treat associated conditions
- • Give treatable conditions which may mimic IBS.
  - o Celiac disease
  - o Lactose intolerance
  - o Gluten intolerance (different from celiac disease)
  - o SIBO (small intestinal bacterial overgrowth)
  - o Cholerrheic diarrhea (bile salt wastage)
  - o Microscopic colitis (collagenous colitis and lymphocystic colitis)

- ❖ Establish good physician-patient relationship
- • Give guidelines to enhance the physician-patient relationship.
  - o Listen actively
    - – Focus on the patient's world (i.e., "Sit where the patient sits")
    - – Allow the patient to tell his/her story without interruption
    - – Seek to understand the symptom experience within a biopsychosocial context
  - o Identify and respond to the patient's concerns and expectations
    - – What do you think is going on?
    - – What are your worries and concerns?
    - – What are your expectations from me?
  - o Validate the patient and illness
    - – Acknowledge the pain
    - – Acknowledge the impact of the illness
    - – Provide a physiologic explanation of the symptoms
  - o Set realistic and consistent limits when ordering tests
    - – "Don't just do something, stand there"
    - – Order tests on the basis of objective data rather than pain severity
  - o Psychosocial assessment
    - – Why is the patient coming now?
    - – Is there a history of traumatic life events?
    - – What is the impact of the pain on quality of life?
    - – What is the role of family or culture?
    - – What are the patient's psychosocial resources?
  - o Help the patient take on responsibility for the care
    - – Involve patient in treatment options
    - – "How are you managing with your pain?" rather than "How is your pain?"
  - o Provide some continuity of care (along with primary care provider)

Printed with permission: Drossman D. *Clin Gastroenterol Hepatol* 2008;6:980.

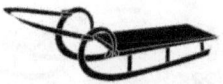

❖ Consider the Menu of medications
- o Amitryptyline
- o Anticholinergics
- o Bulking agents – Psyllium, methylcellulose, fibre
- o CFTR stimulants
- o Chloride – Channel agonists
- o Cholinergics – Neostigmine, bethanechol
- o Colchicine
- o Desipramine
- o Doxepin
- o 5HT4 agonist
- o Lubricant – Mineral oil
- o Motilin agonist
- o Osmotic laxatives – M of M, lactulose, PEG, sorbitol, mannitol
- o Peppermint oil
- o Prokinetics – Dopamine
- o Prostaglandins
- o Stimulant laxatives – Senna, Bisacodyl, castor oil
- o TCAs, SSRIs
- o Trimipramine

Abbreviation: IBC-C, constipation-predominant IBS

Adapted from: Connor BA. *Clin Infect Dis* 2005;41 suppl 8:S577-86.; and Spiller RC. *Gastroenterology* 2003;124(6):1662-1671.

Specific Symptoms

Pain

- o Present for ≥ 3 mon, with onset of ≥ 6 mon before diagnosis of:
  - – Continuous or nearly continuous abdominal pain; and
  - – No or only occasional relationship of pain with physiologic events (e.g., eating, defecation, or menses); and
  - – Some loss of daily functioning; and
  - – The pain is not feigned (e.g., malingering); and
  - – Insufficient symptoms to meet criteria for another disorder of gastrointestinal function that would explain the pain

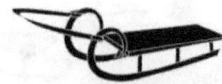

- Give categories/classes of drugs used for pain in functional GI disorders.

Category	Examples/Typical Doses	Comments
o Opiate analgesics	– Hydrocodone 5-10mg QID	Avoid if possible; chronic use should be monitored by pain management physician
o Central opiate agonists	– Tramadol 50mg TID-QID	May cause GI side effects: nausea, vomiting, constipation
o NSAIDS	– Ibuprofen 400mg QID	Beware dyspepsia, ulcer not significant
o Tricyclics SSRI/SNRI	– Paroxetine 20mg daily Duloxetine 30-60mg daily	Good choices if coexisting panic disorder or depression
o Anticonvulsants	– Gabapentin 300mg TID – Pregabalin 50-100mg TID	Sleepiness a problem with higher doses

Printed with permission: Schiller LR. *2008 ACG What's new in GI pharmacology course book*: pg. 34.

Note that some of these agents used to treat abdominal pain in IBS may worsen constipation.

Psychosocial

- o Useful psychological therapy includes
    - – Cognitive behavioural therapy
    - – Dynamic psychotherapy, and
    - – Hypnotherapy
- o Hypnotheapy
    - – Gut-directed hypnotherapy done in highly specialized research centres is an effective treatment alternative for patients with refractory irritable bowel syndrome (IBS), but the effectiveness is lower when the therapy is given outside.
    - – The effectiveness of gut-directed hypnotherapy is superior to the available pharmacological treatment options for IBS.

Please also see: Thompson WG. Chapter 64. In: Therapeutic Choices. Grey J, Ed. 6th Edition, Canadian Pharmacists Association: Ottawa, ON, 2011, Table 4: Drugs used for the Management of Irritable Bowel Syndrome, page 864.

Diarrhea

- o Anti-laxatives
- o Bile salt binders
- o Peptobismal

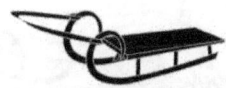

Constipation

- o Please see later section on treatment of idiopathic constipation, not distinct from treatment of IBS-C (constipation predominant IBS)

- o Traditionally, constipation has been classified into normal transit, slow transit, and functional defecatory disorders.
  - – This is not an ideal approach, since the changes in slow transit do not necessarily reflect problems with motor function, and colonic tone and compliance (presence-volume relationships) were not taken into account.
  - – A new mechanistic classification is suggested based on
    - ▪ Fasting phasic activity and tone
    - ▪ Phasic activity and tonic postprandial high amplitude contractions, and responses.

Bloating and Gas

- o Pancreatic enzymes: uncertain efficacy for gas

- o Diet
  - – Eat small, non-fatty meals slowly (reduce aerophagia)
  - – Reduce poorly digested carbohydrates (beans, legumes etc)
  - – Avoid carbohydrate beverages
  - – Take liquids at end rather than during a meal
  - – Avoid chewing gum or chewing tobacco
  - – Treat underlying conditions e.g., celiac disease, IBS, bacterial overgrowth, heightened emotional awareness
  - – Reduce surface tension
    - ▪ Simethicone
    - ▪ Activated charcoal
    - ▪ Bismuth subsalicylate
  - – FODMAP diets under study

- o Antibiotics
  - – Meta-analysis and systemic review show that rifampicin is more effective than placebo for global IBS syndrome improvement and bloating. Adverse effects were similar among patients in the two groups.
  - – Rifaximin increases IBS symptom improvement from 20% with placebo, to about 40%
  - – Probiotics, and antibiotics
    - ▪ For benefit, NNT=4
    - ▪ Systematic Review: many sub-optimal study designs; 2 high quality studies suggested that only Bifidobacter infantis 35,624 showed benefit in IBS.

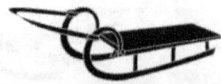

- o Treat associated conditions
  - – GERD
    - • There is a large overlap between IBS and GERD, with gastroesophageal reflux-type symptoms found in 27% to 42% of IBS sufferers, depending upon whether the Manning or the Rome II criteria respectively were used to diagnose IBS. The pooled or for GERD with versus without IBS was 4.17 (95% CI = 2.85-6.09)
  - – Diverticulitis
    - • Persons with IBS (particularly diarrhea-predominant or mixed diarrhea/constipation) may have diverticulitis (9% of males and 17% of females with IBS), but the presence of IBS is not associated with an increased risk of diverticulitis.
  - – Treat gastroparesis
  - – For lactose intolerance: Lactase
  - – For legume-rich meals α-galactosidase
  - – Modify gut flora
    - • Antibiotics
    - • Probiotics
    - • Prebiotics
  - – Treat associated constipation
  - – Visceral hypersensitivity (↑ perception): TCAP, SSRIs, SNRIs

Adapted from: Farthing, Michael J.G. Tropical *Sleisenger & Fordtran's gastrointestinal and liver disease: Pathophysiology/ Diagnosis/Management* 2006: pg 2308.

- • Give claimed benefits for using 5-ASA (Mesalazine) for IBS.
  - o Clinical
    - – Observational data suggests clinical benefits of mesalazine
    - – Randomized, placebo controlled pilot study in IBS patients from Italy showed clinical benefit
  - o Compared to placebo
    - – Mesalazine ↓ mast cell infiltration
    - – ↓ mast cell histamine release
    - – ↓ abdominal pain intensity scores
    - – ↑ general well being

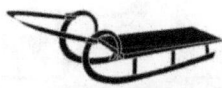

IBS in Pregnancy

- Give a summary of drugs commonly used for irritable bowel syndrome and diarrhea during pregnancy.

Drug	Pregnancy Use Category	Usual Dosage	Additional Comments
o Tegaserod	B	6 mg twice daily	Limited data; should be considered only when other measures fail to control constipation – predominant irritable bowel syndrome
o Loperamide	B	2-4 mg daily or after each unformed stool	Antidiarrheal agent of choice during pregnancy
o Diphenoxylate with atropine sulphate	C	1-2 tablets four times daily	Should be avoided during pregnancy. Contains 2.5 mg diphenoxylate plus 0.025 mg atropine per tablet
o Dicycloverine (dicyclomine)	B	10-20 mg four times daily	Should be reserved for women with refractory symptoms
o Hyoscyamine	C	0.125-0.250 mg every 6 hr as needed	Should be reserved for women with refractory symptoms
o Tricyclic antidepressants	C/D	Dose differs according to retail brand	Questionable safety in pregnancy; use should be limited to the severely symptomatic

Printed with permission: Thukral, Chandrashekhar., and Wolf, Jacqueline L. *Nat Clin Pract Gastroenterol Hepatol* 2006; 3(5): pg. 261.

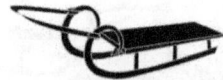

ANORECTAL AND PERIANAL DISEASE

➢ Anatomy of the Anal Region

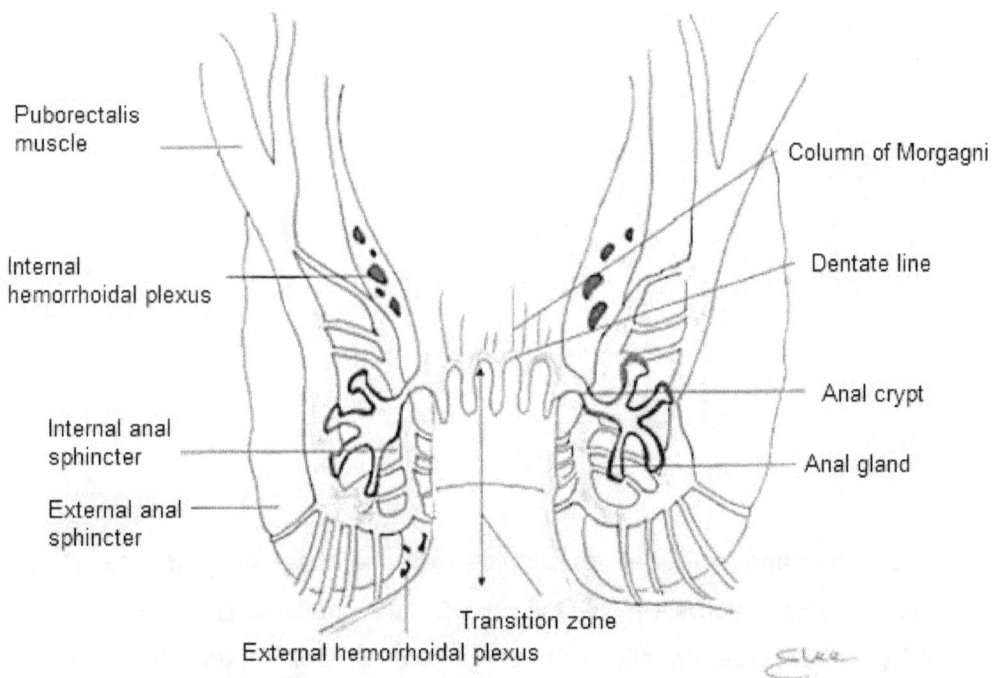

Puborectalis muscle

Internal hemorrhoidal plexus

Internal anal sphincter

External anal sphincter

Column of Morgagni

Dentate line

Anal crypt

Anal gland

Transition zone

External hemorrhoidal plexus

Adapted from: Sleisenger and Fordtran's Gastrointestinal and Liver Disease. 8th Edition. Saunders/Elsevier, Philadelphia, 2016, Figure 129-1, page 2317.

• Disorders of the Anal Canal

Anorectal ring/sling of puborectalis

Sympathetic and Parasympathetic

Somatic innervation

Columns of Morgagni

Dentate line
Columnar transitional zone
Squamous mucosa
(no hair!)

Anal verge/orifice

403

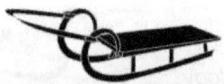

Approximate normal diameters of large bowel

Site	Diameter (cm)
Rectosigmoid, descending	< 6.5
Ascending	8
Cecum	12

supralevator ②

ischial ③   levator ani muscle

intersphincter ①   Internal anal sphincter

External anal sphincter

ANUS

- o Infection in anal crypts at dentate line → rectal abscess → fistulas
- o May be gross/microscopic CD in anal canal → perianal disease
- o Why do CD fistula usually not become red – E. Coli bacteroids (anaerobic) do not cause skin damage, as with Staphylococcus or Streptococcus
- o When you bear down, the anal sphincter relaxes
- o Bowel rest and diversion colostomy for watering can CD perineum
- o No effect on inflammation but ↑ throughout – so easier for patient (patient comfort) and ↓ protein loss
- o Recurrence of CD after or – 10% per year → ~100% in 10 yrs!

"A pessimist see the difficulty in every opportunity; and optimist sees the opportunity in every difficulty."

Sir Winston Churchill

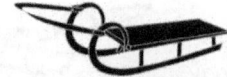

Rectal Pain "Proctalgia"

- o Solitary rectal ulcer syndrome (SRUS)
- o Proctalgia fugax (spasm in levator ani?)
- o Intermittent severe rectal pain at night, no Δ BM
- o Itch
    - – Perianal redness
        - ▪ Pinworms (tap test)
        - ▪ Yeast infection – cream
        - ▪ Cancer
        - ▪ Soaps, detergents, dyes underclothes

Anal Fissure

- o Definition
    - - A longitudinal cut in the anoderm
- o Position
    - - Mid posterior, 90%
    - - Anterior, 10%
- o Constipation → stretch strains spasm – fissure?
- o Anal area "Animus"
- o Sharp pain in anus

A 78 year old female with severe, poorly controlled Parkinson's disease is admitted to a geriatric unit. She has decompensated over the holidays with dysphagia. A gastroscopy was unremarkable. Plans are underway regarding a percutaneous gastrostomy for feeding. In the interim, you are called due sudden onset rectal pain and bleeding. On examination you diagnose an acute anal fissure, in the posterior midline (6 o'clock position).

- • Give other causes of bright red rectal bleeding that this patient is specifically at risk for in relation to her underlying disease process (Parkinson disease).

- o Internal hemorrhoid
- o Stercoral (ischemic) ulcer
- o Solitary rectal ulcer syndrome

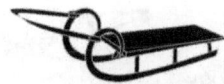

- Give risk factors that this patient has for developing an anal fissure.
    - Age
    - Immobility
    - Constipation
    - Parkinson's Disease related decreased colonic activity
    - Antiparkinsonian drugs L-DOPA, anticholinergics (cogentin)
    - Dehydration/electrolyte imbalance
    - Fecal incontinence (overflow diarrhea)
    - Manual stool extraction
    - Enemas

Fistula-in-Ano
- Definition: "…… a tunnel that connects an internal opening, usually at an anal crypt at the base of the columns of Morgagni, with an external opening, usually on the anal skin" (Sleisenger and Fordtran's Gastrointestinal and Liver Disease. 10th Edition. Saunders/Elsevier, Philadelphia, 2016, page 2326).

Abscess of Anal Region

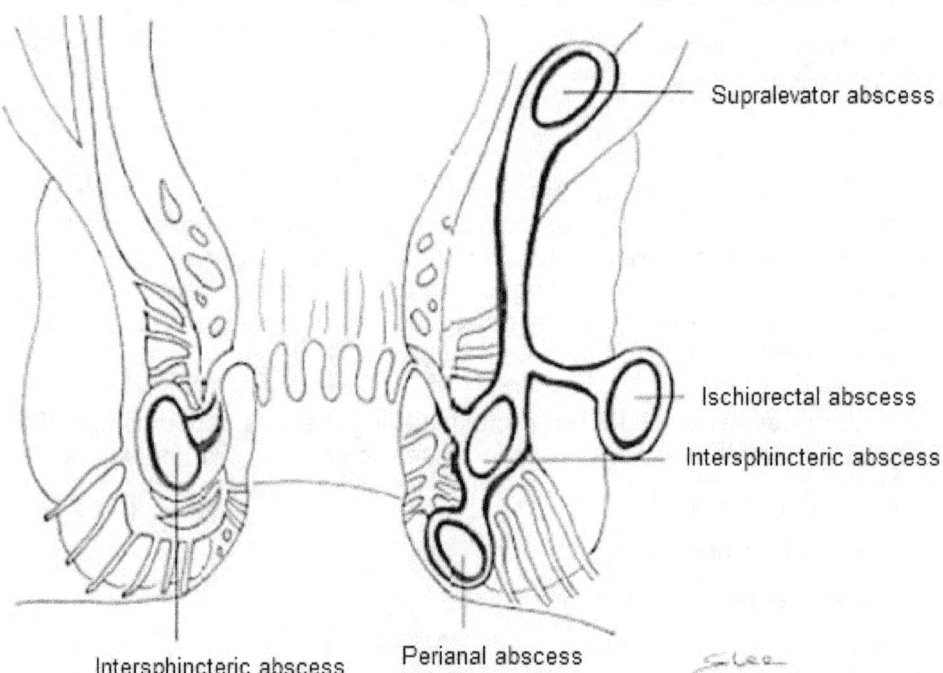

Adapted from: Feldman M., et al. Sleisenger and Fordtran's Gastrointestinal and Liver Disease. 8th Edition. Saunders/Elsevier, Philadelphia, 2006, Figure 122-3, page 2843.

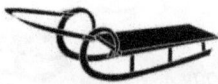

- Give causes of anorectal disease in patients with AIDS (not including non AIDS specific conditions).

  More frequent conditions are marked with and asterix (*)

  o Infections
    - Bacteria
      - Chlamydia trachomatis*
      - Lymphogranuloma venereum
      - Neisseria gonorrhoeae*
      - Shigella flexneri
      - Mycobacterium tuberculosis
    - Viruses
      - Herpes simplex*
      - Cytomegalovirus*
    - Protozoa
      - Entamoeba histolytica
      - Leishmania donovani
    - Fungi
      - Candida albicans
      - Histoplasma capsulatum

  o Neoplasms
    - Lymphoma*
    - Kaposi sarcoma
    - Condyloma acuminatum
    - Squamous cell carcinoma (HPV)
    - Cloacogenic carcinoma

  o Other
    - Idiopathic ulcers*
    - Perirectal abscess
    - Fistula*

Abbreviations: AIDS, acquired immunodeficiency syndrome. HPV, human papillomia virus

"We don't see things the way they are.
We see them the way WE are."

Talmud

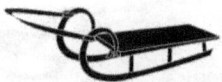

Sexual Transmitted Conditions

- Give symptoms, investigations and treatment of sexually transmitted infections (STI) of the anorectal region.

STI	Symptoms	Investigations	Treatment
o Gonorrhea	- Pruritus ani - Mucopurulent anal discharge - Rectal pain - Tenesmus - Bleeding	▪ Culture and/or NAAT ▪ Anoscopy; rectal friability, erythema, ulceration and mucus	- Ceftriaxone (250 mg intramuscularly) - Doxycycline (100 mg orally twice daily) for 1 week
o HSV	- Vesicular lesions - Anal pain - Tenesmus - Discharge - Viremic symptoms - Lymphadenopath - Pruritus ani - Mucoid and/or bloody diarrhea - Psychogenic constipation - Sacral paraesthesia - Impotence	▪ Viral culture and/or NAAT ▪ Anoscopy; perianal vesicles, rectal ulcers, rectal inflammation	- Acyclovir (200 mg orally five times daily) for 5 days
o Amebiasis	- Bloody diarrhea	▪ Microscopy of stool ▪ Anoscopy; friable rectal mucosa, shallow ulcers with exudates and ring of erythema	- Metroidazole (500-750 mg orally three times daily) for 5-10 days
o Shigellosis	- Abdominal cramps - Fever - Bloody diarrhea	▪ Stool culture	- Trimethoprimsulfa methoxazole (double strength) orally twice daily for 7 days - Tetracycline 1.5 g once and ampicillin 500 mg orally four times daily for 7 days

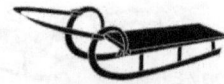

STI	Symptoms	Investigations	Treatment
o Non LGV chlamydia	- Commonly asymptomatic but can involve pruritus ani, mucoid discharge, perianal pain	• NAAT	- Doxycycline (100 mg orally twice daily) for 1 week
o LGV chlamydia	- Purulent anal discharge - Pain - Tenesmus - Fever - Malaise - Genital ulcers/papules - Lymphadenopathy (buboes)	• NAAT • Anoscopy; friable, ulcerated rectal mucosa with or without rectal mass	- Doxycycline (100 mg orally twice daily) for 3 week
o Primary syphilis	- Anorectal chancres - Anal pain - Discharge - Tenesmus - Itching - Bleeding - Mucus membrane lesions - Maculopapular rash	• Dark field microscopy • Serology tests (e.g.,RPR, TPPA, TPHA)	- Procaine penicillin (750 mg intramuscularly once daily) for 10 days or benzothine penicillin (2.4 g intramuscularly once) or - Doxycycline (100 mg orally twice daily) for 14 days
o Secondary syphilis	- Snail track ulcers - Perianal condylomata lata	• Dark field microscopy • Serology tests (e.g.,RPR, TPPA, TPHA) • Anoscopy; painful anal ulcer	- Procaine penicillin (750 mg intramuscularly once daily) for 10 days or benzothine penicillin (2.4 g intramuscularly once) or - Doxycycline (100 mg orally twice daily) for 14 days

Abbreviations: HSV, Herpes simplex virus; LGV, lymphogranuloma venereum; NAAT, nucleic acid amplification testing; RPR, rapid plasma regain test; STI, sexually transmitted infection; TPHA, treponema pallidum hemagglutination assay; TPPA, treponema pallidum particle agglutination

Printed with permission: Siew C. Ng & Brian Gazzard. *Nat Rev Gastroenterol. Hepato* 2009;6:592-607, Table 1, page 594.

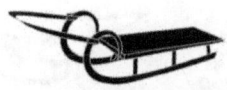

Hemorrhoids

➢ Definition
  o Dilated vascular channels

➢ Endoscopy
  o Position
    – 3, 7, 11 o'clock positions
  o Surface
    – Internal
      ▪ Above dentate line
      ▪ Covered by columnar or transitional mucosa
    – External
      ▪ Below dentate line
      ▪ Covered by squamous mucosa

➢ Treatment

• Give the medical and surgical treatment of chronic internal hemorrhoids.
  o Treat underlying associated conditions
    – Cleaning/nipping
      ▪ Sitz baths
      ▪ Paper
      ▪ Perfume
      ▪ Colouring
      ▪ No soap near perineum
      ▪ Hot water may make itch worse (histamine release)
      ▪ Gloves, cut nails
    – Diarrhea/constipation, prolapse, bleeding, deficient intake of fibre and fluids
  o Supportive therapy
    – Avoid straining and limit time on commode
  o Pharmacological
    – Barrier creams: zinc oxide, lanolin (limit contact of stool and mucus with sensitive anoderm)
    – Stool softeners, bulk, sitz bath, diet, fluids
    – Topical nitroglycerin(0.2% t.i.d paste or ointment)
      ▪ Hypotension, headache, flushing
    – Diltiazem (calcium channel blocker [CCB]) cream (2%, t.i.d), or Anusol HC/Anusol with lidocaine
      ▪ Flushing, headache, hypotension, bradycardia
    – Botulin toxin injection into the sphincter ("breaks the cycle")
      ▪ Fecal incontinence, flatus incontinence (7%); effect wears off

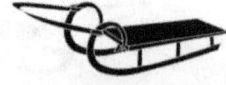

- Surgical
  - Repair fissures to limit further trauma
  - Hypertrophic squamous epithelium: "extra skin" like a callus on top of your hemorrhoid
  - Lateral sphincterotomy
    - Fecal incontinence
    - Recurrence (10%)
  - Surgery – rubber band ligation, injection sclerotherapy, surgical excision, PPH-stapled hemorrhoidopexy
  - Diverting colostomy

Adapted from: *Sleisenger & Fordtran's Gastrointestinal and Liver Disease: Pathophysiology/Diagnosis/Management*, 10th Edition, 2016: pg. 2323.

Solitary Rectal Ulcer Syndrome (SRUS)

➢ Pathogenesis

  - "occult or overt rectal prolapse with paradoxical contraction of the pelvic floor during defecation...." (Feldman M., et al. Sleisenger and Fordtran's Gastrointestinal and Liver Disease. 9th Edition. Saunders/Elsevier, Philadelphia, 2010, page 2080).

  - Usual site of prolapse of rectal mucosa is anterior wall of the rectum, 7 cm to 10 cm above the verge the anus.

➢ Endoscopy

  - Single or multiple ulcers, or polypoid lesion

➢ Histopathology

  - Lamina propria replaced by fibromuscular tissue

  - Muscularis mucosa hypertrophied, with muscle fibres extending towards the lumen

"Treat a man as he is and he will remain as he is.
Treat a man as he can and should be and
he will become as he can and should be."

Stephen R. Covey

DEFECATION

➤ Anatomy

- Give the anatomical structures and the mechanisms by which they contribute to normal fecal continence.
  - o Nerves – pudenal nerve/sacral segments S2 – S4/brain
    - The pudenal nerve has both afferent and efferent limbs, sensing stool entry into the rectum and delivering the impulse through the sacral nerves, spinal cord, to the brain.
    - The efferent limb carries the sensation of distension which causes central pathways to send signals via the afferent limb to allow for conscious contraction of external sphincter to maintain continence.
  - o Muscles
    - Internal anal sphincter (IAS)
    - External anal sphincter (EAS)
    - Levator ani complex:
      - The internal anal sphincter is tonically contracted providing continence at rest.
      - When stool enters the rectum the IAS relaxes, however, continence is maintained if consciously desired by contraction of the EAS.
      - The IAS returns to resting tone, the rectum demonstrates compliance allowing intrarectal pressure to decrease and the urge to defecate to pass.
      - The levator ani muscles provide additional support to the EAS. As well, they form a sling around the anal canal, forming an acute angle during rest, creating a mechanical barrier for continence. Inability to distend without substantial rise in pressure thus not overwhelming resting anal tone.
    - Rectum - reservoir

Abbreviations: EAS, external anal sphincter; IAS, internal anal sphincter

Adapted from: Schiller LR. *Sleisenger & Fordtran's Gastrointestinal and Liver Disease: Pathophysiology/Diagnosis/Management* 2006: pg. 200-201.

➤ Physiology

- Give the physiology of fecal incontinence and defecation.
  - o Muscle Sequences with Defecation
    - Colonic motility advances stool into rectum
    - Sit on toilet
      - Perineum (anorectal junction) descends
      - ↑ ARA (anorectal angle)

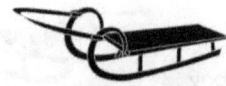

- o Conscious decision to follow the "urge to purge"
  - – Relax EAS
  - – Relax puborectalis ↑ ARA even more
  - – Levator ani contracts
    - ▪ Perineum descends more
  - – Stool is "funneled" into anal canal
  - – Beginning one hour before defecation, there is
    - ▪ ↑ colonic phasic and tonic activity (gastrocolonic response)
    - ▪ ↑ frequency of propagating pressure waves (which represents the preparatory phase to defecation)
    - ▪ This gastrocolonic response occurs with 300 kcal, especially from fat, and may result from the food-induced effects on 5-HT3 receptors on vagal afferent
    - ▪ These propagating waves push stool into the rectum, and
      - – Stimulate sacral spinal efferent mechanoreceptors
      - – Activate an enteric descending inhibitory reflex (DIR)
  - – The DIR causes transient
    - ▪ ↓ IAS pressure
    - ▪ ↑ EAS pressure
  - – The mechanoreceptors cause the defecatory urge, and defecation can be postponed with
    - ▪ Receptive rectal accommodation (↑ rectal volume, with no ↑, intrarectal pressure, mediated by inhibitory nerves
    - ▪ Voluntary suppression of the defecatory urge
    - ▪ ↓ gastric emptying
    - ▪ ↓ small bowel transit
    - ▪ ↓ colonic transit (by ↓ proximal colonic propagating pressure waves)
- o Straining
  - – ↑ perineal descent
  - – ↑ ARA
  - – Ingestion, digestion and absorption of food
  - – MMCs more food to ileocecal valve
  - – Monophasic, ileal propagating pressure plus inhibition of phase contractions of the ileocecal junction, pumps chime into the cecum within 90 mm of a meal
  - – Cecal filling triggers proximal colonic propagating contractions
  - – MPOs and slow waves in colon
    - ▪ Non propagating waves mix stool
    - ▪ Excitatory motor neurons cause MPOs to summate and lead to HAPCS (high-amplitude propagating contractions)
  - – The HAPC overcomes the RMC (rectal motor complex)
  - – The rectum fills, and dilates to accommodate the stool bolus

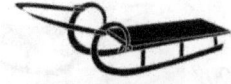

- Stretching of the rectal wall
  - Simultaneously activates an enteric descending inhibitory reflex to relax the IAS
  - Extrinsic reflex pathway to contract EAS
- As the rectum distends further, the signal of discomfort and the need to defecate is transmitted centrally.

○ If defecation is not to be postponed, then there is
- ↓ IAS pressure
- Stool moves into upper anal canal
- Anorectal junction descends with sitting
- Rectum descends further with straining
- Sitting and straining increase cause ↑ anorectal angle
- Puborectalis relaxed with ↑ anorectal angle
- Levator ani muscles contract
- Perineum descends
- Stool moves further into anal canal
- Voluntary ↓ EAS pressure
- Successful expulsion of stool

Fecal Incontinence (FI)

➤ Definition
  ○ The recurrent uncontrolled passage of fecal material for at least one month duration
  ○ Subtypes
    - Passive – involuntary release of stool or flatus
    - Urge – release of fecal contents despite voluntary attempts to retain contents
    - Seepage – leakage of small amounts of stool following an evacuation

➤ Causes/associations

• Give causes of fecal incontinence.

Note: Ensure the patient does not have constipation/fecal impaction leading to fecal incontinence.

  ○ Rectum
    - Congenital abnormalities of the anorectum
    - Fistula
    - Rectal prolapse
    - Anorectal trauma
    - Fissure – treatment (Botoxin)
    - Childbirth injury
    - Surgery (including hemorrhoidectomy)
    - Sequelae of anorectal infections
    - Crohn disease

414

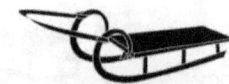

- o Central nervous system processes
  - – Dementia
  - – Encopresis (childhood)
  - – Mental retardation
  - – Stroke
  - – Brain tumour
- o Spinal cord injury
  - – Multiple sclerosis
  - – Tabes dorsalis
  - – Cauda equina lesions
- o Pudendal nerve damage
  - – Polyneuropathies
  - – Diabetes mellitus
  - – Shy-Drager syndrome
  - – Toxic neuropathy
  - – Traumatic neuropathy
  - – Perineal descent syndrome
- o Pelvic dyssynergy

Printed with permission: *Sleisenger & Fordtran's gastrointestinal and liver disease: Pathophysiology/Diagnosis/Management, 10th Edition,* 2016, pg. 253.

- Give the likely diagnosis and the characteristic findings on anorectal monometry.
  - o She likely has pelvic dyssynergy (aka functional anorectal outlet obstruction).
  - o Normally, when straining down, as if to have a bowel movement (valsalva maneuver), the pressure measured from the rectal lead on manometry increases, and the pressure from the lead in the anus relaxes.
  - o With pelvic dyssynergy, with straining, there is a paradoxical increase in the pressure in the anus (failure of relaxation).

- Give risk factors for the development of **incontinence post-partum**.
  - o Vaginal delivery
  - o Instrumental delivery
  - o Emergency cesarean section
  - o Epidural anesthesia
  - o Perineal laceration

Printed with permission: Quigley EMM. *Best Pract Res Clin Gastroenterol* 2007; 21(5): pg. 885.

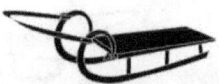

- Give tests/procedures which are useful to investigate the patient with fecal incontinence.

➢ Clinical
  ○ History, physical examination
    – Value of rectal examination in the person with fecal incontinence
      ▪ Perianal sensation
      ▪ Sphincter tone at rest and with voluntary contraction of perineum
      ▪ Length of anal canal
      ▪ Anorectal angle
      ▪ Perianal descent (normally 1.5-3.0 cm)
  ○ Mucosa
    – Endoscopy and biopsy
  ○ Muscle
    – Structure
      ▪ EUS
      ▪ MRI/ CT
    – Function
      ▪ Colon transit study
      ▪ Contraction pressure: pellet retention test
      ▪ Expulsion pressure: balloon expulsion test
      ▪ Co-ordination: anorectal manometry "defecography"
  ○ Nerve
    – Pundendal nerve terminal latency
  ○ Diagnosis
    – US, CT, MRI, EUA, DRE, EUS (transrectal)

Abbreviations: DRE, digital rectal examination; EUS, endoscopic ultrasound

Adapted from: Sleisenger and Fordtran's Gastrointestinal and Liver Disease. 10th Edition. Saunders/Elsevier, Philadelphia, 2016, Table 18-2, page 261.

➢ Treatment

- Give medical and surgical treatments of fecal incontinence.
  ○ Treat underlying cause (s)
  ○ Supportive therapy (the patient)
    – Education/counselling/habit training
    – Trained defecation
    – Diet (fibre; lactose, fructose, reduce caffeine intake)
    – Incontinence pad
    – Perianal hygiene/skin care

416

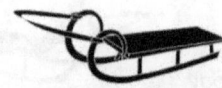

- o Pharmacological (the stool)
  - – Fibre/psyllium
    - ▪ Psyllium has been shown in a RCT to reduce the number of episodes of fecal incontinence by 50%; uncontrolled studies suggest a benefit for cholestyramine or amitriptyline.
  - – Loperamide
  - – Lomotil
  - – Codeine
  - – Cholestyramine/colestipol
  - – Estrogen
  - – Phenylephrine
  - – Sodium valproate
- o Biofeedback therapy
  - – Anal sphincter muscle strengthening
  - – Rectal sensory conditioning
  - – Recto-anal coordination training
  - – The operant conditioning techniques of biofeedback training using visual, auditory or verbal feedback, are meant to improve the strength of the anal sphincter muscles, anorectal sensory perception, and coordination of anal sphincter, gluteal and abdominal muscles following rectal balloon dilation or voluntary squeeze
  - – Both biofeedback training and Kegal exercises each produce a 50% reduction in fecal incontinence.
    - ▪ One study has shown superior improvement with biofeedback as compared to exercises, on a per protocol but not an intention-to-treat basis.
    - ▪ Another study showed 77% of persons with fecal incontinence showing improvement with biofeedback versus 40% treated with Kegal exercises and with 66% versus 48%, respectively, being totally content.
  - – Biofeedback is also of benefit in persons with solitary rectal ulcer syndrome
  - – 5 out of 10 studies of biofeedback therapy (neuromuscular training) have shown a significant benefit over placebo

Sleisenger & Fordtran's gastrointestinal and liver disease: Pathophysiology/Diagnosis/Management 10th Edition, 2016, Table 18-3, pg 2674.

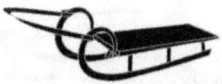

- o RCTs have shown a benefit for sacral nerve stimulation for fecal incontinence when the anal sphincter is intact
- o Perianal
  - – Anal plugs
  - – Pessary
  - – Kegal exercises
  - – Sphincter bulking (collagen, silicone)
  - – Anal electrical stimulation
  - – Injection sclerotherapy
  - – Sacral nerve stimulation (requires an intact anal sphincter)
- o Surgery
  - – Artificial anal sphincter
  - – Sphincteroplasty
  - – Anterior repair (rectocele)
  - – Gracilis/gluteus muscle transposition +/- stimulation
  - – Colostomy
  - – Pelvic reconstruction
  - – Options: rubber band ligation
  - – Surgical excision
  - – PPH-Stapled Hemorrhoidopexy
  - – The Malone procedure (antegrade continent enema procedure – cecostomy or appendicostomy for antegrade washing of the colon) gives a 61% success rate for fecal incontinence over 39 months

Adapted from: Schiller L. *Sleisenger & Fordtran's gastrointestinal and liver disease: Pathophysiology/Diagnosis/Management* 2006: pg. 207; please also see 10th Edition, 2016, Table 18-5, pg 267.

"The difference between how a person treats the powerless versus the powerful is as good a measure of human character as I know."

Robert Sutton

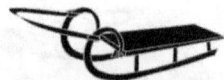

MALAKOPLAKIA

- ➢ Definition
  - o The presence of yellowish, friable mucosal lesions arising from the pigment is lipofuscin within macrophages.

- ➢ Causes/associations
  - o More common in persons exposed to chemotherapy, immunosuppression for organ transplantation, or with AIDS.
  - o The focal form (as compared to the diffuse or isolated [to the rectosigmoid area] form) may be associated with adenomatous polyps or CRC.

- • In the context of malakoplakia, give the meaning of von Hansemann cells, and Michaelis-Gutmann bodies.
  - o Von Hansemann cells
    - – Coliform bacteria in the cytoplasm of macrophages in the colonic mucosal biopsies
  - o Michaelis-Gutmann bodies
    - – Laminated intracytoplasmic inclusion bodies

- ➢ Histopathology

- • Give histological features associated with colonic **malakoplakia**, and indicate (*) which feature is considered to be diagnostic.
  - o Macrophages
    - – Sheets of large, pale macrophages
    - – Cytoplasm may contain coliform bacteria
  - o Inclusion bodies*
    - – In cytoplasm
    - – Laminated

- ➢ Treatment
  - o Dealing with associated risk factors
    - – Antibiotics (ciprofloxacin, or trimethoprim-sulfamethoxazole),
    - – Surgery for complications (such as bleeding or obstructing strictures)

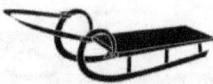

CHRONIC IDEOPATHIC CONSTIPATION (CIC)

➢ Pathophysiology

o Slow proximal colonic transit put normal distal transit suggests slow transit constipation. Normal proximal colonic transit but slow distal transit suggests pelvic dyssynergy or anorectal dysfunction

o Only slow transit constipation will respond to subtotal colectomy with ileorectal anastomosis

o With dilation of both the colon and rectum, as well as normal anal sphincter function proctocolorectomy and an ileoanal anastamosis may be suitable; if anal sphincter function is abnormal, an ileostomy needs to be performed

Please see: Chaun H. Chapter 56. In: Therapeutic Choices. Grey J, Ed. 6th Edition, Canadian Pharmacists Association: Ottawa, ON, 2011, Table 3: Constipation, page 741-745.

➢ Causes/associations

• Give the causes/associations of constipation in each category.

❖ Neurogenic

o Central
  – Multiple sclerosis
  – Parkinson disease
  – Cerebral infarction (CVA; stroke)
  – Medullary trauma

o Spinal
  – Cognitive challenge
  – Dementia
  – Meningocele
  – Spinal cord lesions (trauma, tumour)
  – Cauda equina lesions

o Gut
  – Autonomic neuropathy (paraneoplastic, pseudoobstruction, diabetes)
  – Aganglionosis: congenital (Hirschsprung's) or acquired
  – Cathartic colon (laxative abuse)
  – Narcotic bowel syndrome
  – In a young person, suspect Hirschprung disease (abnormal embryological migration of neural crest cells) when rectal manometry shows
    ▪ ↑ rectal pressure, plus
    ▪ ↑ anal pressure (failure of relaxation)

420

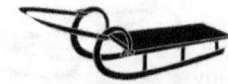

- ❖ Drug-associated
  - o Analgesic: narcotics e.g., opiates ("cathartic colon"), non-narcotics
  - o Antacid (aluminum)
  - o Anticholinergics (dopaminergics)
  - o Anti-Parkinson drugs
  - o Antipsychotics
  - o Antidepressants (tricyclics, but not SSRIs – serotonin reuptake inhibitors)
  - o Antidiarrheals
  - o Antihypertensives (calcium channel blockers, clonidine)
  - o Antiseizure medications
  - o Bile acid sequestrants
  - o Chemotherapeutic agents
  - o Nutrient supplements: calcium, iron
  - o 5-HT3 antagonists
  - o Somatostatin analogs

- ❖ Metabolic
  - o Diabetes mellitus
  - o Glucagonoma
  - o Hypothyroidism
  - o Hypoparathyroidism
  - o Hypopituitarism (panhypopituitarism)
  - o Hypocalcemia
  - o Hypomagnesium
  - o Hypokalemia
  - o Heavy metal poisoning
  - o Pregnancy
  - o Progesterone level cyclic fluctuation (just before menses)
  - o Porphyria
  - o Low intake of water
  - o Outlet obstruction (dyssynergy)

- ❖ Pelvic dyssynergy
  - o Obstetrical trauma

Printed with permission: Müller-Lissner S. *Best Pract Res Clin Gastroenterol* 2007; 21(3): pg. 475.

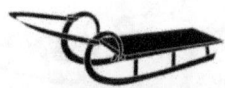

- Give the affected structure and pathophysiology of disorders causing functional anorectal outlet obstruction.

Affected Structure	Pathophysiology
o Internal sphincter – Hirschsprung disease	– No relaxation
o External sphincter – Pelvic floor dyssynergia ('anismus')	– Paradoxical contraction
o Pelvic floor – Pelvic floor descent	– Loss of pressure
o Rectal wall – Intussusception	– Luminal obstruction
o Rectal wall – Anterior, rectocele	– Loss of pressure

Printed with permission: Müller-Lissner S. *Best Pract Res Clin Gastroenterol* 2007; 21(3): pg. 474.

➢ Clinical

- Rome III diagnostic criteria for **functional constipation**, using Criteria fulfilled for the last 3 months with symptom onset at least 6 months before diagnosis. This definition will be revised Rome IV.

  o Must include two or more of the following:
  - Straining during at least 25% of defecations
  - Lumpy or hard stools in at least 25% of defecations
  - Sensation of incomplete evacuation for at least 25% of defecations
  - Sensation of anorectal obstruction/blockage for at least 25% of defecation
  - Manual maneuvers to facilitate at least 25% of defecations (e.g., digital evacuation, support of the pelvic floor)
  - Fewer than three defecations per week

  o Loose stools are rarely present without the use of laxatives

  o There are insufficient criteria for irritable bowel syndrome I(BS).

Source: Longstreth GF, et al. *Gastroenterology* 2006; 130: 1480-9, Table 1.

  o Rome III diagnostic criteria for **functional defecation** disorders using criteria fulfilled for the last 3 months with symptom onset at least 6 months before diagnosis. This definition will be revised in Rome IV.
  - The patient must satisfy diagnostic criteria for functional constipation
  - During repeated attempts to defecate must have at least two of the following
    ▪ Evidence of impaired evacuation, based on balloon expulsion test or imaging
    ▪ Inappropriate contraction of the pelvic floor muscles (i.e., anal sphincter or puborectalis) or < 20% relaxation of basal resting sphincter pressure by manometry, imaging, or EMG
    ▪ Inadequate propulsive forces assessed by manometry or imaging

Source: Bharucha AE, et al. *Gastroenterology* 2006; 130: 1510-8, Table 2.

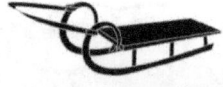

Chronic Idiopathic Constipation (CIC): **American College of Gastroenterology Monograph**

Ford AC, et al. Am J Gastroenterology 2014; 109 Suppl 1:S2-26.

➢ Definition
  o Rome IV defines functional constipation as: the presence of ≥ 2 of:
    – Straining during at least 25 % of defecations
    – Lumpy or hard stools in at least 25 % of defecations
    – Sensation of incomplete evacuation for at least 25 % of defecations
    – Sensation of anorectal obstruction/blockage for ≥ 25 % of defecations
    – Manual maneuvers to facilitate at least 25 % of defecations (e.g., digital evacuation, support of the pelvic floor)
    – Fewer than three defecations per week

These criteria should be fulfilled for the past 3 months with symptom onset at least 6 months before diagnosis.

	NNT
o Medications	
– Soluble fibre, psyllium	2
– Sodium pico sulfates, bisacodyl	3
– Polyethylene glycol	3 / 4
– Lubiprostone	4
– 5-HT4 agonist	6
– Linaclotide	6

  o Biofeedback for pelvic floor dysynergia-proven effective

• Give the **investigations** which are appropriate for the investigation of persons with constipation.
  o History and physical– social, laxative and drug use, psychological assessment, stool chart; full examination including digital rectal exam (DRE)
  o Laboratory tests
    – CBC
    – HG A, C
    – TSH
    – Electrolytes
    – Mg^{2+}
    – Ca^{2+}
  o Colonoscopy, defecating proctogram (defecogram), colonic transit study, EUS, colonic manometry
  o Diagnostic imaging
  o 3 views of the abdomen
  o Manometry, anorectal manometry
  o Functional testing, balloon expulsion

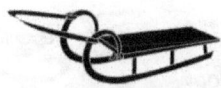

➢ Treatment

❖ Non-pharmaceutical

- Give non-pharmacological treatments of constipation.
  - ○ Treat underlying conditions
  - ○ Bowel management programs, including fibre
  - ○ Psychological management
  - ○ Avoid constipating medications
  - ○ Exercise
  - ○ Adequate water intake
  - ○ Dietary measures
  - ○ Biofeedback (pelvic floor retraining)
  - ○ Total colectomy with ileorectal anastomosis

  - ○ Note:
    - – There is no proven benefit of fibre to treat constipation, but fibre supplement up to 30 gm per day may be offered on a person-by-person basis.
    - – In the absence of dehydration, ↑ water intake does not help constipation

❖ Pharmacological
  - ○ There is a long menu of choices to treat CIC (chronic idiopathic constipation). Expensive new agents have been developed, but these do not necessarily perform any better than polyethylene glycol, sodium, picosulfate, bisacodyl or lactulose.
  - ○ The NNTs (number needed to treat) to prevent one patient failing to respond to therapy was between 3 and 6. Scan these relative risks (RR) from RCTs reporting old laxatives or new pharmaceuticals versus placebo:

	RR	95% CI
○ Older osmotic and stimulant laxatives	0.52	0.46-0.60
○ Newer pharmaceuticals with a big price tag		
– Prucalopride	0.82	0.76-0.88
– Lubiprostone	0.67	0.56-0.80
– Linaclotide	0.84	0.80-0.87

  - ○ Note that none of these newer agents were studied against the older laxatives.

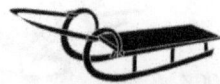

- Because of the possible heterogeneity of the studies and the variable placebo response rates, the values of the RR or the NNTs (if they had been reported) could not be directly compared. However, the osmotic and stimulant laxatives were certainly not "poor second cousins"

- It has been suggested that long-term use of the anthraquinone (e.g., cascara, senna) and bisacodyl laxatives may cause changes in the colon on diagnostic imaging (barium studies), and on histopathology.

- "there is no evidence that currently used laxatives can produce "carthartic colon" (Sleisenger and Fordtran's Gastrointestinal and Liver Disease. 9th Edition. Saunders/Elsevier, Philadelphia, 2010, page 2246).

- Brown discoloration of the mucosa may occur in ~70% of chronic users of cascara or senna laxatives (melanosis coli).

SO YOU WANT TO BE A GASTROENTEROLOGIST!

- Give the **manometric changes** in the colon which occur with severe slow-transit constipation.
  - ↓ high-amplitude of propagating pressure waves
  - ↑ frequency of low-amplitude antegrade and retrograde propagating sequences
  - ↓ nighttime suppression of propagating sequences
  - ↓ colonic response to a high-calorie meal

- Give the approximate frequency of 5 undesirable outcomes after colectomy for chronic constipation.

Undesirable Outcomes	Approximate Frequency (%)
Abdominal pain	40
Small bowel obstruction	15
Reoperation	10
Fecal incontinence	10
Diarrhea	10
Recurrent constipation	10
Stoma dysfunction	5

Printed with permission: Müller-Lissner S. *Best Pract Res Clin Gastroenterol* 2007; 21(3): pg. 476.

425

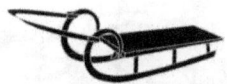

Mastering the Boards: Gastroenterology   A.B.R. Thomson

Constipation in Pregnancy

- Give causes of **constipation in pregnancy**.
  - Hormonal – slow transit
  - Mechanical
  - Medications
  - Lifestyle
    - Reduced exercise
    - Dietary changes
  - Pre-existing disease:
    - Chronic slow-transit constipation
    - Irritable bowel syndrome
    - Congenital or acquired megacolon
    - Chronic idiopathic intestinal pseudo-obstruction

Adapted from: Quigley EMM. *Best Pract Res Clin Gastroenterol* 2007;21(5): pg. 882.; and Cullen G, and O'Donoghue D. *Best Pract Res Clin Gastroenterol* 2007; 21(5): pg. 810.

- Give the **FDA category*** of laxatives in pregnancy.

Safe (B)	Caution (C)	Unsafe (D)
○ Lactulose	– Saline osmotic laxatives	-Anthraquinones
○ Glycerine		-5HT4 agonists
○ Polyethylene glycol (PEG)	– Castor oil	-Prostaglandins (misoprostol)
○ Bulking agents	– Senna	
○ Bisacodyl	– Docusate sodium	

* While the FDA category of pharmaceutical agents is no longer widely used, some physicians find the use of these categories useful.

Adapted from: Cullen G, and O'Donoghue D. *Best Pract Res Clin Gastroenterol* 2007; 21(5): pg. 815.; and Thukral C, and Wolf JL. *Nat Clin Pract Gastroenterol Hepatol* 2006; 3(5): pg. 260.; Printed with permission: Kane SV. *AGA Institute 2007 Spring Postgraduate Course Syllabus:*511.

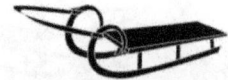

ULCERATIVE COLITIS (UC)

➤ Demography
  - o Incidence $8/10^5$ person-years
  - o Prevalence $150/10^5$

Approximate figures, USA, Canada and Europe

➤ Genetics
  - o ~ 15% of UC patients have affected family member, often first-degree relative
  - o 3x ↑ risk among first degree relatives of Jewish patients
  - o For first degree relatives, high concordance for
    - – Type of IBD (UC, not Crohn disease)
    - – Extraintestinal manifestations

● Give genetic mutations which are associated with UC.
  - o Multiple susceptibility genes, especially on chromosome 12

  C3435T polymorphism for MDR1 (multidrug resistance 1) gene

Gene	Chromosome
IL-23R	1p31
MST1	3p21
IL-12B (aka p40)	5q33
NKX 2-3	10q24
STAT3	17q21

➤ Pathophysiology
  - o Microbiome

● Give the changes in the GI **microbiome** which are observed in UC.
  - o ↓ biodiversity by 30% to 50% due to
    - – ↓ Firmicutes (e.g., Streptococcaceae and Lactobacillales)
    - – ↓ Bacteroides
    - – ↑ Proteobacteria (e.g., E. Coli)
    - – ↑ Actinobacteria

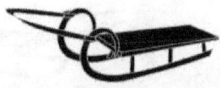

- o Immunity

- Give aspects of altered humoral, cellular and adaptive immunity which are involved in the immunopathogenesis of UC.

- Humoral Immunity
  - o ↑ plasma cells producing IgG1 and IgG3 antibodies food, bacteria and self (autoantibodies, including a 40 kDa autoantigen to normal colonic epithelium)
  - o pANCA in ~ 75% of UC patients (IgG1 anti-50kDa nuclear envelop protein in myeloid cells), and may be a marker for more aggressive disease.
  - o Antibodies to bacterial antigens
    - Anti-CBir 1 (antibody to flagellin from Clostridium species), in 6% of UC patients, and is a marker for development of pouchitis
    - Anti-PMOc (outer membrane porin C of E. Coli)

- Cellular Immunity
  - o Innate immunity
    - Bacteria produce immune response in monocytes, macrophage and dendritic cells
    - Involves PPRs (pattern-recognition receptors, e.g., TLRs [toll-like receptors], NLRs [NOD-like receptors])
    - Activation of TLRs and NLRs activates NF-kB (nuclear factor kB)
    - NF-kB increases transcription of genes coding for proinflammatory cytokines (e.g., IL-1, -6, -8, TNF), chemokines, adhesion molecules and costimulatory molecules
    - NF-kB increases maturation of dendritic cells, which enhances further antigen presentation
  - o Adaptive Immunity
    - LP (lamina propria) lymphocytes express α4β7, a surface adhesion molecule which attracts CD4+ and CD8+ T cells
    - IELs (intraepithelial lymphocytes) is normal or ↓ MUC
    - ↑ production of
      - Monocytes (in circulation)
      - Macrophage (in mucosa)
      - Granulocytes
    - Both Th1 and Th2 response, as well as Treg, NKT and Th17
    - Th1
      - Differentiation of T cells into Th1 pathway is stimulated by IL-12
      - Production of IL-2 and IFN (interferon)-γ
    - Th2
      - ↑ IL-4, -5, -10, -13 → enhance the humoral immune response

428

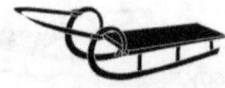

- Treg
  - Produce IL-10 and TGF-β
  - Inflammation
- NK T cells (natural killer) T cells produce IL-5 and -13, which are cytotoxic to colonic epithelium
- Th17 produce IL-6 and -17
- Functions of IL-17
  - Proinflammatory
  - Stimulates
    - T cell activation
    - Macrophages
    - Fibroblasts
    - Epithelial cells
  - T17 inhibited by Th1, Th2 cells stimulated by IL-6, -12, -23R, and TGF-β
- ↑ mucosal cytokines → ↑ release of metalloproteinase from fibroblasts
- ↑ mucosal content of active macrophage and neutrophils release
  - Leukotrienes
  - NO (nitric oxide)
  - ROS (reactive oxygen species)
  - PAF (platelet-activating factor)

➢ Clinical

  o Severe first attack leading to colectomy, 10%

  o Chronic continuous UC, 10%

  o Intermittent flares, 80%

  o Risk of colectomy, ~ 1% to 2% per year (24% at 10 years, 30% at 25 years)

  o The longer the remission, the longer the patient with UC is likely to remain in remission

  o Patient with UC of rectum or rectum plus sigmoid has a 1% to 3% risk of extension for each year of disease (e.g., 10% to 3% at 10 years)

  o Even patients with proven IBS need a screening colonoscopy for colorectal cancer at age 50, or earlier depending upon the family history

Please see: Sleisenger and Fordtran's Gastrointestinal and Liver Disease. 10th Edition. Saunders/Elsevier, Philadelphia, 2016, Table 116-3, page 2037.

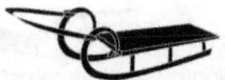

- Give extracolonic manifestations of IBD.
  - o CNS
    - – Depression
  - o Malignancy
    - – Colorectal cancer, small bowel adenocarcinoma
    - – Lymphoma
    - – Hepatosplenic lymphoma
    - – Cholangiocarcinoma
  - o Musculoskeletal
    - – Peripheral arthropathy
    - – Ankylosing spondylitis
    - – Sacroiliitis
    - – Clubbing
    - – Avascular necrosis (osteonecrosis)
    - – Osteopenia, osteoporosis
    - – Osteomalacia
  - o Ophthalmologic
    - – Uveitis/iritis
    - – Episcleritis
    - – Scleritis
    - – Conjunctivitis
    - – Retinal vascular disease
    - – Cataracts
    - – Glaucoma (may be related to steroid use)
  - o Dermatologic
    - – Erythema nodosum
    - – Pyoderma gangrenosum
    - – Angular stomatitis
    - – Aphthous stomatitis
    - – Pyostomatitis vegetans
    - – Psoriasis
    - – Metastatic Crohn
    - – Sweet syndrome

    > - Give which extracolonic manifestations of UC do not improve with colectomy.
    >   - o Skin   – Pyoderma gangrenosum
    >   - o Spine   – Ankylosing cholangitis
    >   - o Biliary tree – Primary sclerosing cholangitis

  - o Hematologic
    - – Iron deficiency anemia
    - – Autoimmune hemolytic anemia
    - – Anemia of chronic disease
    - – Leukocytosis or thrombocytosis
    - – Leukopenia or thrombocytopenia
    - – Hypercoagulable state

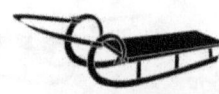

- o Hepatobiliary
  - Drugs (e.g., azathioprine, methotrexate, α-TNF, salazopyrin)
  - Metastatic malignancy
  - Granulomatous autoimmune hepatitis
  - Primary biliary cholangitis (PBC)
  - Liver abscess
  - Hepatic amyloidosis
  - Hepatic granulomas
  - Steatosis, (NAFLD, NASH)

- o Blood vessels
  - Portal vein thrombosis
  - Budd-chiari syndrome

- o Biliary
  - Primary sclerosing cholangitis (PSC – see Hepatobiliary section for discussion of secondary sclerosing cholangitis [SSC])
  - Cholangiocarcinoma
  - Gallstones

- o Genitourinary
  - Renal calculi
  - Amyloid
  - Interstitial nephritis
  - Fistulae

- o Nutrition/growth defects

- o Psychological

- o Obstetrical/Gynecological
  - Infertility
  - Low birth weight
  - Preterm delivery
  - Teratogenicity (drug effects, e.g., MTX, thalidomide)
  - Amenorrhea
  - Vaginal fistulae

Adapted from: Sleisenger and Fordtran's Gastrointestinal and Liver Disease. 10th Edition. Saunders/Elsevier, Philadelphia, 2016, Box 116-10, page 2058.

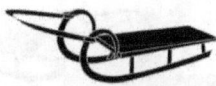

Mastering the Boards: Gastroenterology   A.B.R. Thomson

> ➤ Endoscopy

There are endoscopic scoring systems to determine the severity of UC.

Useful background: Mayo Score for mucosal severity in ulcerative colitis

Mayo Index	0	1	2	3
o Stool frequency	Normal	1-2/day >normal	3-4/day >normal	5/day >normal
o Rectal Bleeding	None	Streaks	Obvious	Mostly blood
o Mucosa	Normal	Mild friability	Moderate friability	Spontaneous bleeding
o Physician's global assessment	Normal	Mild	Moderate	Severe

- Give the **endoscopic differentiation** between UC and Crohn colitis, in terms of distribution, inflammation, ulceration, and appearance of colonic lumen.

Variable	Ulcerative Colitis	Crohn Disease (Colon)
o Distribution	– Diffuse inflammation – Extends proximally in continuity from the anorectal junction	▪ Rectal sparing ▪ "skip" lesions
o Inflammation	– Diffuse erythema – Loss of vascular markings with – Mucosal granularity or friability	▪ Focal /asymmetric, "cobblestoning" ▪ Granularity and friability
o Ulceration	– Small ulcers in a diffusely inflamed mucosa; deep, ragged ulcers in severe disease	▪ Aphthoid ulcers ▪ Linear/serpiginous ulceration ▪ Intervening mucosa is often normal
o Colonic lumen	– Narrowed in long-standing chronic disease – Strictures are rare	▪ Strictures are common

Adapted from: Sleisenger and Fordtran's Gastrointestinal and Liver Disease. 10th Edition. Saunders/Elsevier, Philadelphia, 2016, Table 116-3, pg 2037.

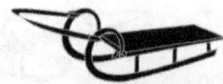

> Histopathology

  o ½ to ¾ of persons with UC on the left side have inflammation in the cecum and around the appendix

  o Characteristics of chronic quiescent UC
    - Mucosa
      ▪ Paneth cell metaplasia distal to hepatic flexure
      ▪ Drop out of cells
      ▪ Distortion of architecture of glands
        - Branching
        - Shortening
        - Separation
    - Crypt abscesses
    - Muscularis mucosa
      - Hypertrophy
        ▪ Neurons
      - Hyperplasia
        ▪ Muscle

- Give the biopsy features of **acute self-limiting colitis** (AC) which help to distinguish it from chronic idiopathic ulcerative colitis (UC).

  o Crypts are straight, parallel, close

  o PML are abundant, and scattered in the lamina propria (LP)

  o No lymphoplasmacytosis at base of crypts

  o Large, bulging, cystic dilation with a "necklace" of cells around any crypt abscess

Abbreviations: AC, acute self-limiting colitis; LP, lamina propria; PML, polymorphonuclear leucocytes; UC, ulcerative colitis

"Buzzwords" which suggest whether IBD is ulcerative colitis (UC) or Crohn Colitis (CD)

UC	CD
o Crypt abscess	o Granulomas
	o Perianal and disease
	o Rectal sparing
	o Skip lesions
	o Fistulae

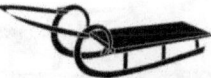

UC-associated Arthropathy

➢ Clinical

• Give features which help to distinguish between type 1 and 2 peripheral arthropathy in UC.

Feature	Type 1	Type 2
o # of joints	< 5 (pauciarticular)	> 5 (polyarticular)
o Symmetrical	No	Yes
o Type of joints	Large	Small
o Association with active UC	Yes	No
o Duration of attacks (median)	5 wk	3 yr

Adapted from: Sleisenger and Fordtran's Gastrointestinal and Liver Disease. 10th Edition. Saunders/Elsevier, Philadelphia, 2016, Table 116-8, pg 2059.

➢ Laboratory

o Serological tests are seldom performed to distinguish between ulcerative colitis (UC) and Crohn disease (CD). Yet they frequently make an appearance on MCQs and smoking has a different effect in UC and CD.

	UC	CD
– ASCA	Positive in 10%	Positive 60%
– p-ANCA	Positive in 75%	Positive in 10%
– Smoking	Helps UC	Worsen CD

• Give the sensitivity, specificity, PPV and NPV of the serological markers ASCA and pANCA in persons with Crohn disease (CD) and ulcerative colitis (UC).

Marker	Diagnosis	Sensitivity (%)	Specificity (%)	PPV (%)	NPV (%)
o ASCA	CD	50-65	70-85	80	64
o pANCA	UC	65-80	70-85	64	80

Abbreviations: NPV, negative predictive value; PPV, positive predictive value

Adapted from: Targan SR. *AGA Institute PostGraduate Course book.* pg. 47.

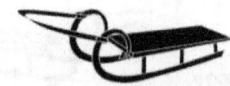

> Differential

- Give conditions that cause "colitis" and may **mimic** ideopathic UC.

❖ Infection
  o Viral
    – Cytomegalovirus (CMV)
    – Herpes (HSV)
  o Bacterial
    – Clostridium difficile
    – Salmonella species
    – Shigella species
    – Yersinia enterocolitica
    – Campylobacter jejuni
    – Vibrio perahaemolyticus
    – Aeromonas hydrophila
    – Neisseria gonorrhoeae
    – Listeria monocytogenes
    – Chlamydia trachomatis
    – Syphilis
    – Staphylococcus aureus
    – Escherichia coli 0157:H9
  o Protozoan
    – Amebiasis (amoeba histolytica)
    – Balantidiasis
    – Schistosomiasis
  o Fungal
    – Histoplasmosis
    – Candidiasis

❖ Iatrogenic (drugs)
  o Enemas
  o Laxatives
  o Oral contraceptive agents (OCA)
  o Ergotamine
  o Amphetamines
  o Phenylephrine
  o Cocaine
  o Nonsteroidal anti-inflammatory drugs (NSAIDs)
  o Penicillamine
  o Gold
  o Methyldopa

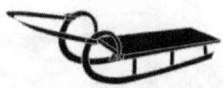

Abbreviations: CMV, cytomegalovirus; HSV, herpes simplex virus; OCA, oral contraceptive agent

Adapted from: Sleisenger and Fordtran's Gastrointestinal and Liver Disease. 10th Edition. Saunders/Elsevier, Philadelphia, 2016, Box 116-1, pg 2037.

> Treatment

- Give the treatment goals of IBD patients.
  - o Induce and maintain clinical symptoms, laboratory abnormalities, as well as endoscopic and histological changes ("deep healing" of mucosa)
  - o Optimizing quality of life
  - o Rapidly relieve symptoms
  - o Avoid surgery
  - o Avoid hospitalization

- Mild UC
  - o Confirm diagnosis
  - o Exclude precipitants
    - Non-compliance with maintenance therapy
    - Drug (e.g., 5-ASA, NSAIDs)
    - Interferon (e.g., C.difficile)
    - Pregnancy
    - Stop
    - Smoking
  - o Patient education
  - o 5-ASA or sulfasalazine, or
    - PO or PR (enema or suppository) depending on extent of disease
  - o Prepare for possible future use of immune suppression, or biological
  - o Sample meta-analyses of efficacy of 5-ASA in UC (vs placebo)

	OR
– 5-ASA suppositories/enemas	
▪ Achieving remission distal colitis	7.4
▪ Maintaining remission	16.2
	RR
– po-5-ASA less likely to fail in	
▪ Achieving remission	0.79
▪ Maintaining remission	0.65
	OR
– ↓ risk of CRC	0.51
– ↑ risk of renal toxicity	2.48

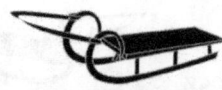

  o Is there a "better" 5-ASA product?

Product	Comparator	Outcome	Stats
– Mesalamine	Sulfasalazine	Induction of remission	Trend
– Balsalazine	Mesalamine (5-ASA)	Induction of remission	RR 1.30

  - It is likely that all mesalamine preparations are similarly effective, but
    there have been few head-to-head trials.

Curiously, in about 3% of persons treated with 5-ASA the mesalamine is
stopped; future use of 5-ASA in these persons should be curtained.

- Ulcerative proctitis (UP)
  o Inflammation of distal 15 cm of colon
  o Present in 30% of UC patients at diagnosis
  o Proximal spread (proctosigmoiditis – distal UC (distal to splenic plexus
    pancolitis) 50% in 10 years.

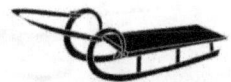

Mastering the Boards: Gastroenterology   A.B.R. Thomson

- Rectal (topical) therapy
  - 5-ASA suppositories (coat 10 cm of distal bowel)
    - 1 gm PR at bedtime each day for 4 weeks, then taper (q 2 days for 2 weeks then q 3 days for 3 weeks)
    - Remission 93%
    - Maintenance 75% (after 1 attack, consider stopped remission therapy after 3 weeks, and wait to see what is he pattern of the patient's UP, i.e., few recurrences (retract for 3 weeks), or frequent recurrences → maintenance Rx
  - 5-ASA enemas (coat up to splenic flexure)
    - 4 gm at bedtime
    - Consider combing with 5-ASA po for greater effect

		Remission
	5-ASA Enemas	5-ASA Enema and po 5-ASA
4 weeks	34%	44%
8 weeks	43%	64%

  - Steroid enemas/foams
    - Interior to 5-ASA
    - Low systemic absorption, few AEs
    - Never use long-term
  - Budesonide enemas
    - Low systemic absorption
    - Use for failure of 5-ASA enemas

- Oral therapy
  - Use if patient cannot tolerate PR Rx
  - Response PO < PR
  - PO steroids not used for maintenance (including budesonide)
  - Response usually seen in 4 weeks, then taper

- Proctocolitis, left-sided colitis or pancolitis
  - Mild-to-moderate activity
    - To achieve remission 5-ASA containing drugs
    - Sulfasalazine 500 mg, tab II-III qid for 3 months
    - Asacol 400 mg po, tabs II-III qid for 3 month
    - Mesalamin or vs placebo 0.79
    - Other 5-ASA 500 mg po tab II-III qid for 3 months (salofalk, mesasal, pentasa, lialda, dipentum, colazal, apriso)
      - Annual relapse on 5-ASA 20%; not on 5-ASA 80%

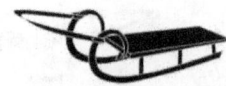

- Trend for greater benefit of mesalamine vs sulfasalazine
- Mucosal healing rates at 6 week 4.8 g/day, 80% 2.4 g/day, 68%
- To maintain remission 50 mg po tab II bid
- If patient does not go into remission in 4 weeks, stop 5-ASA and start prednisone po

- Corticosteroids
  - Prednisone 5 mg po tab 8/day in am or 4 weeks clinical important begin slow taper by eliminating one 5 mg tab each week (e.g., 40 mg for 4 weeks – 35 mg for 1 week, 30 mg or 1 week, 25 mg for 1 week .... STOP)
  - If rectal complaints are prominent, may co-therapy with steroid or 5-ASA enemas
  - If symptoms do not improve, stop improving or worsen after ~2 weeks of prednisone 40 mg po per day, then increase dose to maximum of 12 tabs (60 mg) per day.
  - If no response,
    - Do not continue increasing oral dose of prednisone
    - Begin IV steroids
    - Consider starting AZA (azathioprine) or po 6-MP
  - If patient was on 5-ASA when prednisone started, 5-ASA may be stopped.
  - To emphasize the learning point-do not use steroids in any form for maintenance therapy.
  - Once taper of prednisone is nearing completion and patient is in remission, restart 5-ASA po.
- The immunosuppressants (azathioprine, 6-MP) and biologics (anti-TNF-α drugs) are generally considered in UC patients if they are steroid
  - Refractory or steroid-dependent
- Steroids-responsive disease: "meaningful clinical response to high dose glucocorticoids (prednisone 40 to 60 mg/day or equivalent) within 30 days for oral therapy or 7 to 100 days for IV therapy".
- Steroids-refractory disease: "lack of meaningful clinical response to glucocorticoids up to doses of prednisone 40 to 60 mg/day (or equivalent within 30 days for oral therapy or 7 to 10 days [*] for IV therapy".
- Steroid-dependent disease – "patients [initially] respond to glucocorticoids, but experience a dose of clinical response when glucocorticoids are tapered to less than 10 to 30 mg/day, or rapidly relapse once glucocorticosteroids are stopped".

From: Cohen RD and Stein AC, UpToDate April 2012.

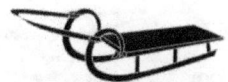

Mastering the Boards: Gastroenterology   A.B.R. Thomson

*Note:

- o When prednisone 40 mg to 60 mg po per day is not providing a satisfactory response, switch to methylprednisolone 40 mg to 60 mg IV per day.

- o In the context of severe UC, the patients is considered to be steroids-refractory after 3 to 5 days of IV glucocorticosteroids, and "bridge therapy" with infliximab or cyclosporine plus azathioprine needs to be started.

- o If the UC patient is considered to be steroid-dependent, introduce immunosuppression, and if severe disease and cyclosporine fails or is contraindicated, start infliximab.

- o Azathioprine (AZA) and 6-MP in UC
    - Limited data for efficacy in UC maintenance, except for benefit for patient successfully treated with IV/PO cyclosporine for severe attack
    - Mesalamine enhances TPMT and increases 6-TGN
    - Uses is for
        - Steroid non-response (seen in ~16% of UC patients)
        - Steroids-dependence: ≥ 4 months of continuous steroids to control symptoms (22%)
        - Frequent relapses (≥ 3 flares per year, despite 5-ASA

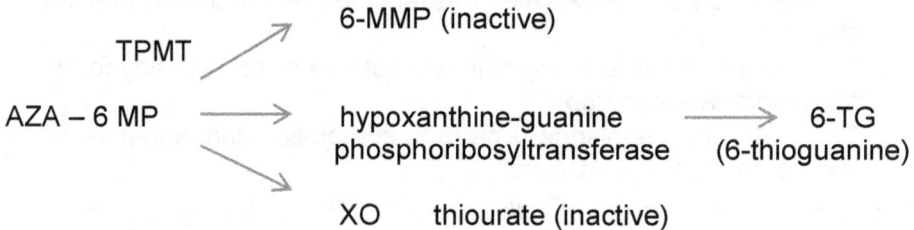

    - Mechanism of action
        - ↓ synthesis of purine, DNA, RNA
        - ↓ proliferation of T and B lymphocytes

    ↑ TPMT → ↓ 6-TG

    ↓ TPMT → ↑ 6-TG (↑ AEs from immunosuppression) low TPMT in 11% of people, negligible TPMP in 0.3%

    - Dosage
        - AZA 2.5 mg/kg per day, continued indefinitely in UC patients who have achieved remission.
        - Dosage conversion of AZA to 6-MP ~50%
        - Allopurinol blocks xo; when ↓ XO; more 6-M is converted to 6-TG, so dose of 6-TG needs to be decreased.
        - Dose reduction or discontinuing AZA may be necessary if there develops bone marrow suppression (2%) or abnormal liver tests (0.5%).
        - Steroid-nonrespondent, adding AZA ↑ likelihood of response ~50%

440

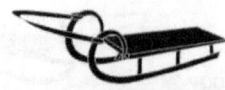

- If UC patient is steroid-dependent, adding AZA decreases steroid requirement by ~70%.
- Maintenance: AZA vs PL, RR of relapse – 0.4 to 0.6 absolute risk reduction of relapse -23%; NNT ~5
- 3 months for therapeutic effect to be achieved
- AZA po = IV effectiveness

	WBC, x 10 (g)/L	Platelets, x 10(g)/L	ALT Transaminases
▪ Reduce AZA	< 4	<120	Normal
▪ Stop AZA	< 3	<80	> 50% of ULN (upper limit of normal)
			↑ bilirubin (cholestasis)

Note: If jaundice develops while on AZA, the AZA should be stopped, and not restarted

- There is no therapeutic benefit of continuing 5-ASA with AZA when the AZA is used for 5-ASA failures
- Some patients may be continued on 5ASA while on AZA because 5-ASA → ↑ TG concentrations, and using the 5-ASA may allow the dose of AZA to be reduced.

o Need for colectomy after failure to respond to IV-steroids for severe UC

	Anti-αTNF	PL (placebo)	TG
– Within 3 months	30%	66%	36%
– Within 3 years	50%	76%	26%

o Biologicals
- Adalimmumab (ADAL, i.e., 160 mm at week 0, 80, mg at week 2, 40 mg every second week)

	ADAL	PL (placebo)	TG
▪ Inducing remission, wk 8	17%	9%	8%
▪ Maintaining remission, wk 52	17%	9%	8%

There is a greater response in ADAL naiive than in "switch (infliximab → adalimumab) UC patients

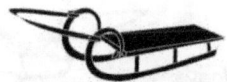

Patients who are hypersensitive to AZA, or cannot tolerate AZA for any reason, are able to tolerate 6-MP.

- Give the reason why 6-MP may be used by persons intolerant or hypersensitive to AZA.
    - When AZA is metabolized to 6-MP, the nitromidazole part of the AZA is lost.
    - The hypersensitivity reactionists AZA are partly to the nitromidazole moiety.
    - Only some of such persons who are switched from AZA to 6-MP are able to tolerate 6-MP, presumably because there are additional unknown reasons to intolerance besides nitromidazole.

- Give the generally accepted indications for performing a CT scan or MRI of the abdomen and pelvis in the patient with IBD (UC or Crohn disease).
    - Penetration
    - Abscess
    - Fistula
    - Perforation
    - Obstruction
    - Megacolon
    - Non-IBD conditions
        - Renal calculi
        - Cholecystitis
        - Diverticulitis

- Give the indications for the use of infliximab in persons with UC.
    - Induction of remission in adults and children who are outpatients with moderately to severely active disease who have failed therapy with and are treated concomitantly with aminosalicylates, corticosteroids, or immunomodulators
    - Maintenance of remission after infliximab for induction therapy
    - Hospitalized patients with severe UC
    - Steroid-sparing
    - Extraintestinal manifestations of UC
        - Spondyloarthropathy
        - Pyoderma gangrenosum
    - Unresponsive iritis/uveitis

Adapted from: Sandborn W. *AGA Institute PostGraduate Course book* 2007;138.

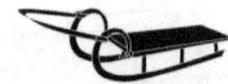

Severe Acute UC

- Give the clinical factors upon which basis the patient is judged to have severe UC include

  - \> 6 BM per day

  - Bleeding

  - Fever

  - HR/PR > 90 bpm

  - ESR > 30 mm/h

  - Anemia

> Note:
> - The Toronto Guidelines for the diagnosis of acute severe ulcerative colitis include hypotension and CRP (C-reactive protein)

"Why should I know this?" If the patient has severe UC, their treatment moves beyond outpatient care with 5-ASA/sulfasalazine + immunosuppressants (azathioprine or 6-MP). Such patients with severe UC require

- Admission to hospital
  - To monitor response, i.e., daily history and physical examination
  - To prepare patient for possible biologics or colectomy
  - To monitor development of megacolon (transverse colon > 6 cm)
  - Begin venous thromboembolism prophylaxis care of mental health
  - To monitor closely for possible development of toxic megacolon
  - Ostomy nurse consultation
  - Daily stool charting
- Continue po food/fluid intake if tolerated
- Peripheral nutrition if po intake inadequate
- If after 3 to 5 days of trend of symptoms to remission suggested, then
  - Consult surgical service (colorectal, or very expressed general surgeon), to assess patient and follow, or
  - Prepare patient or
    - Recue therapy – cyclosporine – serum creatinine, magnesium, cholesterol concentrations
  - For anti-TNF-α exclude TB
    - Tuberculin test
    - Chest X-ray
    Immunizations HAV, HBV, HZV, HPV, annual flu, pneumococcus
- If starting on cyclosporine for "rescue therapy" ("rescue from needing a colectomy on this admission) after IV steroid failure.
  - Cyclosporine 2 mg/kg per day by continuous infusion for 7 to 10 days adjust dose to maintain trough level at 150 to 250 nanogram/mL
  - Check serum creatinine and avoid use if high; check magnesium and cholesterol and avoid use if low
  - Dose IV at 2 mg/kg, PO at 4 mg/mL

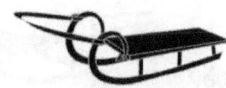

- Aim for trough concentration of 200 to 400 ng/mL
- For long-term use, prophylaxis with trimethoprim-sulfamethoxazole against Pneumocystis carinii is necessary
- Start azathioprine 2.5 mg/kg per day when cyclosporine started or after 7 to 10 days if patient has responded, or if patient responds to IV cyclosporine within 7 to 10 days, then
  - Switch to oral cyclosporine 8 mg/kg per day (same trough level of 150 to 250 nanagram/mL) for 3 months.
  - Begin azathioprine po 2.5 mg/kg per day, to be used as continuous maintenance therapy.
  - Begin PCP (pneumocystitis carini) pneumonia prophylaxis
- If patient fails to responds to IV cyclosporine for 7 to 10 days, then options are
  - Cross-over rescue therapy to infliximab, or colectomy
- If staring on infliximab rescue therapy
  - Infliximab 5 mg/kg on day 0, 14 and 42 (2 and 6 weeks)
  - May consider adding azathioprine 2.5 mg/kg per day to improve response (long colectomy-free survival)

o Prepare for possible use of immune suppression, or biologicals

o Prepare for possible need for colectomy

o Avoid barium enema study
  - MRI may be used to access disease severity

o Avoid colonoscopy; unprepared sigmoidoscopy may be safe to confirm diagnosis
  - IV steroids ~ ¾ respond

o ¼ non-responders
  - Cyclosporine ~ ¾ respond
  - Infliximab ~ ¾

o Infliximab for UC (8 weeks)
  - Response ~ 2/3
  - Remission ~ 1/3
  - Durability of remission (54 weeks)
    - Response ~ ½
    - Remission ~ 1/3

o For severe UC
  - Colectomy was avoided at 3 months in ~ 2/3, and 1/2 at 3 years
  - Long-term studies not available
  - Suggest using "bridge therapy" with cyclosporine IV → po plus AZA in severe UC or anti-TNF plus AZA

o There is no role for po antibiotics in the context of treatment UC, except in the context of the patient with severe (± toxic megacolon)

444

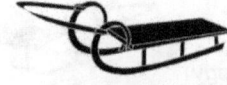

- Once the patient is "out of the word" with regards to going into remission after a severe attack, there is a high risk of another severe recurrence needing colectomy for example if sequence is severe colitis → steroid failure → cyclosporine or infliximab-failure switched to infliximab or cyclosporine

  Rate of colectomy-free survival:

3 months	6 months	12 months
61%	53%	41%

- The outcome from colectomy is superior if performed electively.
- View rescue therapy as a means to compare the patient for elective colectomy.
- If colectomy not performed, then
  - Maintain patient on AZA/6-MP
  - Assess for screening/surveillance for development of dysplasia/CRC (colorectal cancer)
- Severe/fulminant colitis
  - > 10 bloody BMs per day
  - Pain, fever, anemia, tachycardia
  - Systemic steroids
    - Hydrocortisone 100 mg IV q 8 h, or
    - Methylprednisolone 20 mg IV q 8 h
    - No evidence of benefit from high doses: if no response in 3 to 5 days, prepare for use of cyclosporine, anti-TNF therapy colectomy
    - Abdominal film for assessment of transverse colon size (< 6 cm)

- Give predictive factors for non-adherence to therapeutic recommendations in patients with UC.
  - Patient
    - Depressed
    - New patient status
    - Male gender
    - Single status
    - Younger age
    - Full-time employment
    - Patient agreeableness
    - Education level

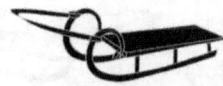

- o Drug
  - Three times daily dosing
  - Four or more concomitant medications
  - Immunomodulator use (if required for remission)
  - Previous adverse events attributed to medication
- o Disease
  - Left-sided disease
  - Lower disease duration
  - Recent disease course
- o MD-patient relationship

Adapted from: Hawthorne, A.B., Rubin, G., and Ghosh S. *Aliment Pharmacol Ther* 2008; 27: pg 1159.

- ➤ Potentially modifiable risk factors
  - o Cost of co pay and other barriers to refilling medications
  - o Treatable depression
  - o Physician- patient relationship
  - o Dosing regimen

Printed with permission: Higgins PD, Rubin DT, Kaulback K, et al. Aliment Pharmacol Ther. Systematic Review: Adherence to 5- ASA, flares and costs in UC. *Journal Compilation* 2009;29:255.

Note:
- o In the patient with severe colitis, avoid doing barium enema (with or without contrast) or colonoscopy, for fear of causing megacolon, including toxic severe UC (because of transmural thickness of CD and the often associated fibrosis, megacolon is much less common in the patient with CD unless there is a fibrotic stricture or cancer).
- o Beware
  - If the MCQ describes the patient with longstanding UC, and the biopsy is reported as showing dysplasia, then the action they wish is for you to refer the patient for a possible colectomy.

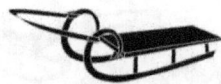

Steroid Resistance

- Give molecular mechanisms of steroid resistance.

    o Abnormalities in absorption/metabolism (liver disease)

    o Altered number of GCS receptors, or altered numbers of isoforms (α, β, δ)

    o Altered affinity of GCS for GCS receptors

    o Reduced affinity of the GCS receptor ligands to bind to DNA

    o Altered expression of transcription factors (AP-1, NF-k B) and/or cytokines (IL-2, IL-4, p38 activated MAP kinase)

    o Genetic factors (primary steroid resistance, MDR-1 [P-glycoprotein 170], HLA class II allele DRB1*0103)

Adapted from: Farrell RJ, and Kelleher D. *J Endocrinol* 2003; 178(3): 339-46.

- Give clinical causes of "steroid resistance" in patients with "colitis" (factors causing persistence of symptoms).

    o Infection – C. difficile, CMV

    o NSAIDs

    o Smoking discontinuation

    o Drug interactions

    o UC with CD-like features – discontinuous disease, superficial fissuring ulcers, aphthous ulcers, ileal involvement, involvement of the upper GI tract, granulomas

    o CD with UC-like features – pancolitis, superficial colitis

    o Other forms of "colitis" that may mimic UC

    o Development of colorectal cancer (CRC)

"With self-discipline most anything is possible."

Theodore Roosevelt

447

 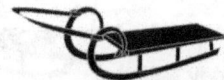

- Give a clinical strategy for dealing with steroid resistance in patients with IBD, in whom the above factors causing persistence of symptoms have been excluded.
  - Adjust dose, change to IV
  - Higher dose of 5-ASA (controversial), or 5-ASA enemas
  - Cyclosporine
  - Azathioprine, 6-MP
  - Methotrexate
  - Biologics – anti TNF
  - Probiotics
  - Fish oil, nicotine patch
  - Colectomy

Adapted from: Mayer LF. *AGA Institute post graduate course book* 2007. pg. 109.

Surgery for UC
  - Infliximab used for severe acute UC – in 3 months, 2/3 still have colon (colectomy-free)
  - R. colon, report of hyperplastic polyp → suspect that it is really a SSA
  - Inflammation may be transmural in severe acute UC
  - Obstruction in UC is usually from tumour
  - Toxic megacolon
    - Mucus fistula – rectum brought to skin, in case the anastomosis breaks, the leak is not into the peritoneum
    - Pressure from stool bacteria, gas
  - For toxic megacolon
    - Remove colon initially leave rectum with mucus fistula (90% of patients have resolution of rectal colitis – if left in place, do surveillance for CRC
  - Anastomoses
    - If rectal sparing involvement → ileoanal anstamosis (IAA)
    - If rectal sparing → ileorectal anastomosis (IRA) (end-to-end, or end-to-side)
  - Proctocolectomy – colectomy plus removal of sphincter
  - Colectomy, just the colon
  - Proctocolectomy, rectum, colon

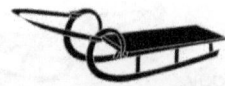

- Proctocolectomy, especially in older persons
    - Sexual dysfunction
    - Bladder emptying problems
- 9% of IAA require dysfunctioning ileostomy (taking out the IAA pouch is a BIG procedure), or medical treatment
- "snare polypectomy with electrocautery is the best method for small polyps"
- Jumbo bx instrument is rounded, so gives bigger bx volume compared to standard by instrument, but join width is almost the same
- Interval CRC rate 4%
    - Not known what is risk of CRC if with some interval adenomatous tissue is left behind after polypectomy

- Give "**alternative therapies**" for UC and CD.

    - UC
        - Phosphatidyl choline
        - Curcumin (phytochemical in tumeric)
        - Hypnosis
        - Granulocyte/monocyte apheresis
        - Probiotics

    - CD
        - Omega-3 fatty acids (DHA - and EPA-containing fish oil)
        - AST-120 oral spherical absorption carbon (for fistulae)
        - IL-12/IL-23 (ustekinumab)
        - Naltrexone
        - Probiotics
        - 4.0 to 4.8 gm/day of 5-ASA po (dose difference depends upon product choosen) for 4 weeks, then with clinical improvement reduce dose by one tablet every 3 days until maintenance dose of 2.0 to 2.4 g PO /day
        - May use both PO plus PR 5-ASA for distal disease

SO YOU WANT TO BE AN IBD-ologist!

The **thiazolidinediones** (such as rosiglitazone) are used in patients with diabetes to control their hyperglycemia. There is not an increased risk of diabetes in UC, and the hyperglycemia noted in some UC patients on glucocorticosteroids is reversible.

- Give the mechanism thought to explain why rosiglitazone (a thiazolidinedione [thio]) was shown in limited preliminary studies to be useful in mild-moderate active UC.

    - Thio → ↑ PPAR (peroxisome proliferator-activated receptors [or ligands]) → ↓ proinflammatory cytokines.

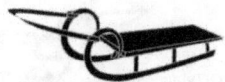

Pyoderma Gangrenosum (PG)

➢ Definition

  o An ulcerative skin condition associated with accumulation of neutrophils in the skin lesions.

➢ Treatment

● Pharmacological

  o Use a combination of topical and systemic therapy
    – Moist dressing
      ▪ Zinc oxide, petrolatum to protect surrounding skin and prevent pathergy (worsening of lesions at sites of trauma)

  o Local
    – Glucocorticosteroids
      ▪ Superpotent topical steroids for 1 to 2 times per day, 2 to 3 weeks
    – Calcineurin inhibitor (cyclosporine, tacrolimus, 0.3%)

  o Systemic
    – Dapsone 50 to 200 mg per day
    – Minocycline
    – Steroids
    – Cyclosporine 4 to 5 mg/kg per day, slow taper
    – Infliximab 5 mg/kg, single dose
    – Adjunct therapy with
      ▪ Azathioprine
      ▪ Methotrexate 10 mg to 30 mg per week
      ▪ Mycophenolate
      ▪ Mofetil 2 g to 3 g per day
    – IVIG IV immunoglobulin
    – Alkylating agents
      ▪ Cyclophosphamide 500 mg/m^2, IV, once per month or 6 months
      ▪ Chlorambucil 2 mg to 4 mg per day ($\pm$ prednisone)

  o May be severe

  o May be out of proportion to size/appearance of PG lesion

● Hyperbaric O_2

● Surgical

  o Skin
    – Careful debridement
    – Skin flaps
    – Skin grafts
    – Bioengineered keratinocyte autografts

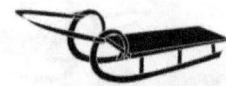

- o Consider subcuticular stitiches
- o Colon
  - – PG does not follow the activity of UC, so colectomy does not usually impair PG

- Associated conditions
  - o IBD (UC, CD)
  - o Arthritis
  - o Hematologic malignancy
  - o Prognosis
    - – Overall, all treatments
    - – Remission
      - ▪ 6 month 68%
      - ▪ 12 months 95%

- Give indications and one major contraindication for the use of dapsone in gastroenterology.
  - o Indication
    - – DH (dermatitis herpetiformis)
    - – PG (pyoderma gangrenosa
    - – Leprosy
  - o Contraindication
    - – G-6-PD (glucose-6-phosphhate dehydrogenase) deficiency

xxxxxxxxxxxxxxxxxxxxxxxxxxxxxxxxxxxxxxxxxxxxxxxxxx

SO YOU WANT TO BE A GASTROENTEROLOGIST!

A patient with severe UC has a proctocolectomy with temporary ileostomy. The patient has mild distal leg pyoderma gangrenosa (PG), responding to local therapy including topical tacrolimus.

- When the patient develops ileostomy dysfunction and you examine the stoma, give what you are specifically looking for with regards to the stoma?

  - o Pyoderma gangrenosa (PG) may involve the stoma after a patient with UC has a proctocolectomy.

  - o The PG is treated in the usual manner with local therapy, which may be possible given its location, as well as with the extensive list of systemic options, noted above.

451

 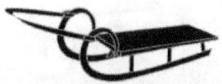

Ileal Pouch Anal Anastomosis

Pouchitis

➤ Demography

  o The likelihood of developing chronic pouchitis in a UC patient having an IAPP is over 80% if serological testing shows high levels of pANCA (Fleshner P, et al. *Clin Gastroenterol Hepatol* 2008:561-8.)

  o Complications may develop in the pouch after proctocolectomy and IPAA (ileal pouch-anal anastomosis)

  o Prevalence
    – When IPAA is done for UC
      ▪ Year 1 ~ 20%
      ▪ Year 5 ~ 50%
    – When done for FAP
      ▪ < 1%

➤ Pathophysiology

  o Microbiota in pouchitis (unique pattern)
    – ↑ Clostridium perfringens
    – ↓ Streptococcus sp (species)
    – Unchanged Fusobacteria

  o It is unknown why the prelavence of pouchitis is very much more common after IPAA for UC than for FAP

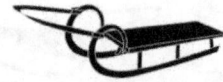

➤ Causes/associations

• Give factors which contribute to the wide variation in the prevalence biopsy-proven pouchitis.

  o Variation in reported values or prevalence depend upon severity and time span.

Clinical severity	Months after IPAA		
	6	12	48
– Mild	21	26	39
– Severe	9	11	14

  – Extensive colitis pre IPAA
  – Use of steroids pre IPAA
  – Use of NSAIDs
  – PSC (primary sclerosing cholangitis)
  – Serology
    ▪ NOD_2/CARD 15 gene mutations (60% vs 5% asymptomatic NOD_2/CAR15-negative UC patients post IPAA
    ▪ pANCA (perinuclear cytoplasmic antibody) positive (higher risk with higher pANCA titre)

• Give predictive factors for the development of pouchitis.

  o Positive association
    – Extraintestinal manifestations
    – Primary sclerosing cholangitis
    – Antineutrophil cytoplasmic antibody with a perinuclear staining pattern (p-ANCA)
    – Extent of pre-operative UC

  o Negative association
    – Smoking

Printed with permission: Gionchetti P, et al. *Best Pract Res Clin Gastroenterol* 2004;18(5): pg 995.

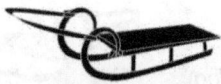

➢ Clinical

• Give the features which distinguish acute and chronic pouchitis after IPAA (ileal pouch anal anastomosis) for UC.

Feature	Acute	Chronic
o Incidence (% per year)	~ 4	▪ 3
o Risk factors	– Pre-operative use of steroids – Smoking	▪ Pre-operative thrombocytosis ▪ Extraintestinal associations ▪ ↑ length of follow-up
o Serology		▪ Low pANCA plus anti-CBir 1 ▪ High pANCA
o Clinical course	– Recurrent episodes of pouchitis, 50% – Chronic symptoms (> 4 weeks), 10% to 20%	

• A patient has an ileoanal pouch (IAPP) after proctocolectomy for UC. Give 8 differential diagnoses for late pouch-related symptoms.
  o Poor reservoir capacity
  o Adhesions
  o Stricture
  o Abscess
  o Cuffitis
  o Pouchitis
  o Irritable pouch syndrome

454

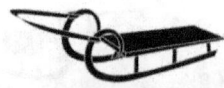

➢ Causes/associations

- Give factors which contribute to the wide variation in the prevalence biopsy-proven pouchitis.

  o Variation in reported values or prevalence depend upon severity and time span.

Clinical severity	Months after IPAA		
	6	12	48
– Mild	21	26	39
– Severe	9	11	14

  - Extensive colitis pre IPAA
  - Use of steroids pre IPAA
  - Use of NSAIDs
  - PSC (primary sclerosing cholangitis)
  - Serology
    - NOD$_2$/CARD 15 gene mutations (60% vs 5% asymptomatic NOD$_2$/CAR15-negative UC patients post IPAA
    - pANCA (perinuclear cytoplasmic antibody) positive (higher risk with higher pANCA titre)

- Give predictive factors for the development of pouchitis.

  o Positive association
    - Extraintestinal manifestations
    - Primary sclerosing cholangitis
    - Antineutrophil cytoplasmic antibody with a perinuclear staining pattern (p-ANCA)
    - Extent of pre-operative UC

  o Negative association
    - Smoking

Printed with permission: Gionchetti P, et al. *Best Pract Res Clin Gastroenterol* 2004;18(5): pg 995.

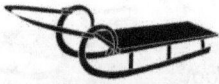

- o Pouchitis with IPAA for UC has numerous complications.
- o If the pouchitis is severe or if mucosal biopsies show persistent atrophy, surveillance must be annually; otherwise, sigmoidoscopic surveillance with multiple biopsies should be performed q 3 years to q 5 years.
- o If UC patients have had a colectomy, have an ileostomy and the rectum remains in place, sigmoidoscopic surveillance with multiple biopsies should be performed q 3 years to 5 years.

➤ Clinical

- Give the features which distinguish acute and chronic pouchitis after IPAA (ileal pouch anal anastomosis) for UC.

Feature	Acute	Chronic
o Incidence (% per year)	~ 4	▪ 3
o Risk factors	– Pre-operative use of steroids – Smoking	▪ Pre-operative thrombocytosis ▪ Extraintestinal associations ▪ ↑ length of follow-up
o Serology		▪ Low pANCA plus anti-CBir 1 ▪ High pANCA
o Clinical course	– Recurrent episodes of pouchitis, 50% – Chronic symptoms (> 4 weeks), 10% to 20%	

- A patient has an ileoanal pouch (IAPP) after proctocolectomy for UC. Give 8 differential diagnoses for late pouch-related symptoms.
  - o Poor reservoir capacity
  - o Adhesions
  - o Stricture
  - o Abscess
  - o Cuffitis
  - o Pouchitis
  - o Irritable pouch syndrome

454

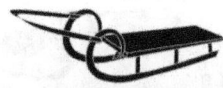

- Crohn disease
- NSAID-induced damage (especially with isolated afferent limb ulcers)
- Pelvic floor dysfunction
- Late anastomotic leak
- Small intestinal bacterial overgrowth syndrome (SIBO)
- Malignancy (squamous cell cancer) of anus, small bowel cancer
- Unmasked celiac disease
- Unrelated conditions, including infections

> Pathology
- Multiple biopsies must be taken from the mucosa of the reservoir (pouch) – suggestion, 6
- Abnormalities present in 95%
- Inflammation degree
  - Mild, 56%
  - Chronic, 39%
- Partial colonic metaplasia
  - 35% to 96%

Cancer Surveillance in IPAA Pouch

- Partial colonic metaplasia in 35% to 96%
- Mucosal atrophy and dysplasia may develop
- Dysplasia/cancer is more common if there is a remnant rectal cuff
- Perform sigmoidoscopy with multiple biopsies q 3 yr
- If biopsies show atrophy → sigmoidoscopy plus multiple biopsies q 1 yr

> Treatment
- Antibiotics
  - Ciprofloxacin 500 mg bid, for 7 days
  - Metronidazole 500 mg to 1 gm po bid, for 7 days
  - Because of AEs of 33% vs 0% for cipro', use as second choice for when cipro' fails)
  - For the 50% of patients with recurrent episodes of pouchitis, use the antibiotic to which they previously responded
  - For those who have frequent recurrent symptoms or chronic symptoms and maintenance therapy is considered, use lowest useful dose of cipro' or metronidazole, or rifaximin (useful in 65% of chronic pouchitis patients, but not useful to induce remission), or use probiotic maintenance (please

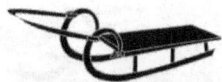

see below)
- Persons who fail to respond to one antibiotic for pouchitis may respond to two antibiotics
- Some persons with IAPP require chronic continuous antibiotics to maintain remission (antibiotic-dependent chronic pouchitis)
- For antibiotic-dependent chronic pouchitis, one option is to alternate 3 or 4 antibiotics every week

- o Steroids
  - Budesonide 9 mg po per day for 8 weeks
  - Used for pouchitis patients who fail treatment with antibiotics
  - Budesonide suppositories or enemas may also be therapeutically effective
  - The efficacy of budesonide enemas is comparable with metronidazole tablets
  - Glucocorticoid enemas or tablets may also be useful

- o Treatment results of probiotics (PRO; VSL #3, 3 g/day) in pouch + IPAA

	Pro	PL
– Development of pouchitis after IPAA	10%	40%
– Maintenance of remission induced by antibiotics	85%	6%

Abbreviations: PL, placebo; Pro, probiotic

- o Probiotics
  - VSL#3
    - Continuously for maintaining remission (85% remission at 1 year versus 6% to 15% for placebo)
  - The 9 month relapse rate of pouchitis when using VSL #3 is 15%, vs 100% for placebo

- o Mesalamine enemas
  - Topical or oral mesalamine, or anti-TNF therapy, may also be effective for pouchitis

- o Infliximab
  - For refractory pouchitis, or pouchitis associated with fistulae
  - May be useful for maintenance

- o Immuno-suppressants
  - Azathioprine, 6-MP for maintenance

Probiotics and Pouchitis

- Give postulated mechanisms of action of probiotics (mostly animal studies).

456

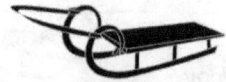

- o ↓ pathogenic organism growth, binding or invasion of epithelium (↑ temporary colonization of probiotic species)

- o ↓ intestinal permeability (↑ TJ [tight junction] function)

- o ↑ anti-inflammatory cytokines (e.g., IL-10, TGF-B), and ↓ pro-inflammatory TNF

- o ↑ expression of receptors for opiods and cannabinoids on intestinal epithelial cells (↓ pain threshold and ↓ pain perception)

- o ↑ apoptosis mediated by an EGFR (epidermal growth factor receptor) – dependent mechanism

There are several circumstances in which probiotics might be of therapeutic benefit, but there is wide variable in the results of clinical trials of probiotics in IBD.

- • Give possible explanations for the high variability of clinical response to "probiotics".

  - o There are many different microorganisms in various probiotic preparations, for example, from pasteurization.

  - o The ratio (combination) of microorganisms may be as important as their numbers.

  - o Some of the microorganisms in various probiotics
    - – May be dead (loss of viability)
    - – May be destroyed in gastric acid fail to colonize the lumen microbiota

  - o Characteristics of patients

  - o Duration of studies

  - o Assessed endpoints

- • Give the use of probiotics in UC and in other GI disorders.

- ➢ UC acute mild-to-moderate disease activity

		VSL #3	PL
o Induction of remission	o 6 weeks	33%	10%
	o 12 weeks	43%	16%
	VSL #3 + 5-ASA	5-ASA (balsalazide)
o Maintenance of remission	73%	21%

- ➢ Mixed results

  - o AAD (antibiotic-associated diarrhea)

457

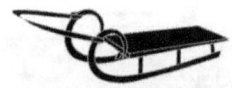

- Saccharomyces boulardi, or Hansen CBS 5926: ↓ risk of developing AAD, RR 0.58 (↓ risk by 42%, NNT 13)
- Lactobacillus: ↓ risk of developing AAD, RR 0.64 (↓ risk by 36%)

o Infectious diarrhea, including rotavirus (minimum of 10 billion colony-forming units for first 2 days overall results) probiotics
- ↓ duration of diarrhea by 17 to 30 hours

o Risk of Travellers' diarrhea: probiotics
- ↓ risk RR 0.85

o IBS probiotics may be helpful to ↓ bloating, ↓ flatulence, ↓ pain

o Allergic disease

o Crohn disease
- Induction of remission
- Maintenance of remission
- Prevention of post-surgical recurrence

o SIBO (small intestine bacterial overgrowth)

o Lactose intolerance

o Hepatic encephalopathy

o Pancreatitis

o Prevention of hospital acquired C. difficile infections

o Diverticular colitis
- Limited data for VSL #3 plus beclomethasone po

o Collagenous colitis

o Severe constipation

Dysplasia in IBD

➢ Terminology

o DALM (dysplasia-associated lesion or mass) is raised, and comes in several shapes: plaque, polyp, mass, stricture

o About half of patients with UC plus a DALM with high-grade dysplasia already have colon cancer

o In UC plus low-grade dysplasia (LGD) on biopsy, the risk of future development of colon cancer is 1% to 3% per person per yea after diagnosis of LGD

o Multifocal LGD has an even higher risk of colon cancer, and colectomy is usually recommended.

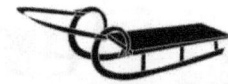

Please see (Feldman M., et al. Sleisenger and Fordtran's Gastrointestinal and Liver Disease. 9th Edition. Saunders/Elsevier, Philadelphia, 2010, Table 112.19, page 2007, "algorithm for the management of dysplasia-associated lesion or mass (DALM), flat dysplasia, indefinite dysplasia, or no dysplasia found on surveillance colonoscopy in patients with ulcerative colitis", and Figure 112.20, page 2008, "Recommended Algorithm for Management of Polypoid lesions [in chronic UC".Biopsies of the colon taken for dysplasia/CRC surveillance in a patient in the UC ideally should be taken when the UC is inactive (i.e., in remission).

➢ Diagnosis

SO YOU WANT TO BE A GASTROENTEROLOGIST!

It may be difficult to distinguish dysplastic from regenerative mucosa in IBD. For this purpose, several markers have been developed, such as Ki-67, p53, sucrase isomaltase and Sialyl-Tn antigen.

- Give the characteristics of AMACR (α-methylacyl-CoA racemase) which make it a promising diagnostic marker for dysplasia in IBD.

AMACR

  o Specificity > 99%

  o Sensitivity
    – LGD   96%
    – HGD   80%
    – Adenocarcinoma   71%

  o A combination of immunohistochemistry for AMACR and histopathological evaluation is useful.

➢ Endoscopy

- Give the endoscopic and pathological features of five types of dysplasia in patients with IBD.

Lesion	Endoscopic	Pathological Features	Approximate Risk for CRC
o Sporadic adenoma	– Circumscribed polypoid lesion, pedunculated or sessile	▪ Circumscribed lesion ▪ Tubular, tubulovillous or	5%

459

 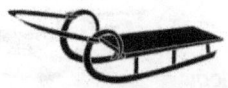

- Typically outside the actively or previously inflamed colonic mucosa
  - villous architecture
  - Crypts uniformly lined with adenomatous epithelium

Lesion	Endoscopic	Pathological Features	Approximate Risk for CRC
o DALM, adenoma like	– Circumscribed polypoid lesion – Mostly sessile – In (previously) inflamed areas of the colonic mucosa. – Often undistinguishable from sporadic adenomas	▪ Tubular, tubulovillous or villous architecture ▪ Dysplastic mucosa ▪ Generally lamina propria inflammation. ▪ Dysplastic crypts may be mixed with normal crypts	5%
o DALM, nonadenoma like	– Irregular – Diffuse – Masses or plaque like lesions in actively or previously inflamed areas of the colonic mucosa	▪ Dysplastic mucosa ▪ Crypts lined with dysplastic epithelium ▪ Occasionally admixed with non dysplastic crypts and inflamed lamina propria	60%
o LGD in flat mucosa	– No gross abnormality	▪ Crypts lined with dysplastic epithelium ▪ High ratio of nucleus to cytoplasm ▪ Nuclei remain confined to the basal half of the cell	18%
o HGD in flat mucosa	– No gross abnormality	▪ Nuclei extend into the luminal parts of the dysplastic epithelium	36%

*Risk may apply to HGD in both flat and raised mucosa.

Abbreviation: CRC, colorectal cancer; DALM, dysplasia associated lesions or masses; HGD, high grade dysplasia; LGD, low grade dysplasia

Adapted from: van Schaik FD, et al. *Nature Review Gastroenterology and Hepatology* 2009; 11:671-8, page 674

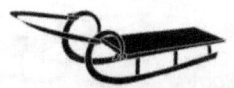

A patient with chronic distal UC for 30 years is found to have a polypoid lesion at the junction of the junction of the UC and non-UC mucosa.

- Give features which helps to distinguish a non-adenoma-like DALM (dysplasia-associated lesion or mass) from a sporatic adenoma (SPO-Ad).

Feature	DALM	SPO-Ad
o Age of patient	– Younger	▪ Older
o Duration of UC	– Longer	▪ Shorter
o Extensive	– More	▪ Less
o Size of lesion	– Larger (~ 18 mm)	▪ Smaller (~ 5 mm)
o Endoscopic appearance	– Large – Plaque – Ulcerated	▪ Pedunculated ▪ Sessile
o Molecular markers		
– Beta catenin	– 8%	▪ 40%
– P53	– 29%	▪ 5%
o Treatment		▪
– HGD	– Prompt colectomy	▪ Polypectomy, plus post polypectomy surveillance
– LGD	– Controversial *	

Abbreviation: HGD, high grade dysplasia

*It is controversial whether the patient with low grade dysplasia (LGD) should also have prompt colectomy, or continued intense surveillance with multiple biopsies.

- o When given the following statistics (M. A. Peppercorn and RD Odze, UpTodate May 2012), many patients will choose to have colectomy, rather than colonoscopy plus biopsy performed at least once per year with quadrant biopsies every 10 cm from cecum to rectum:

- o 70% of UC and 30% of CC (crohn colitis) already have dysplasia at portion of the colon.
  - – 19% to 33% already have CRC
  - – 34% will have CRC in 1 year

- o Progression
  - – 50% LGD → HGD/CRC
  - – 10% within 32 months LGD → HGD/CRC within 10 years
  - – 15% LGD → CRC in 10 years

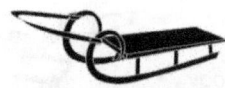

➤ Histopathology

• Give histopathological features which help to distinguish dysplasia from regenerative changes in the inflamed UC tissue.
  o Lack of surface maturation
  o ↑ mitoses (typical and atypical)
  o Back-to-back gland pattern
  o ↑ nuclear size
  o Variation in the size and shape of nuclei (pleomorphism)
  o ↑ nuclear/cytoplasmic ratio
  o Altered nuclear polarity
  o Stratification of nuclei
  o Hyperchromaticity

Features	Dysplasia	Regenerative Changes
o Changes in		
– Crypts	Yes	Yes
– Surface epithelium	Yes	No
o Positive tissue IHC for		
– AMACR	Yes	No
– Sialosyl-TN	Yes	No

Abbreviations: AMACR, alpha-methyl-acyl-CoA-racemase (a mitochondrial and peroxisomal enzyme with ↑ expression in dysplasia)

CRC (Colorectal Cancer) **Surveillance in Ulcerative Colitis (UC) and in Crohn Colitis** (CC)

➤ Risk factors
  o The risk of developing colorectal cancer (CRC-Ca) in a person with UC is related to
    - The extent and duration of the disease, as well as
    - Associated PSC, histological severity of UC, or possibly a family history of CRC-Ca, or a history of post-inflammatory pseudopolyposis
    - After 8 to 10 years of pancolitis, the cumulative risk of UC-CRC is about 0.5% to 1% per year

463

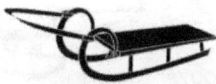

- o The longer duration of colitis (UC, ulcerative colitis; or CC, Crohn colitis), the higher the risk of developing CRC. For example, with 10 and 20 yr UC, the risk of CRC is 2% and 8%, rising to 18% at 30 yr (some authorities quote lower figures of ~ 3% and 8% at 20 and 30 yr, respectively). If the UC patient also has PSC, the 10, 20 and 25 years risks of CRC are 9%, 31% , 50%, respectively. In addition to the duration of the disease, and presence of PSC, other factors which may increase the absolute risk include disease onset before 15 yr, and presence of a stricture.

- Give three additional factors in addition to duration of UC and the presence of PSC which ↑ risk of CRC in IBD, and give the approximate value of the relative risks (RR).

Risk Factors	RR (95% CI)
o Extent of colonic involvement	
– Pancolitis	14.8 (11.4 – 18.9)
– Left-sided disease	2.8 (1.6 – 4.4)
– Proctitis	1.7 (0.8 – 3.2)
o First degree relative with sporatic CRC	
– < 50	9.2 (3.7 – 23.0)
– > 50	2.5 (1.4 – 4.4)
o Histopathology	
– Gross	
▪ Shortening of colon	28.4 (1.6 – 512.2)
▪ Stricture	5.7 (1.7 – 18.9)
▪ Pseudopolyps	21 (1.2 – 3.7)
– Inflammation	
▪ Colonoscopic	5.1 (2.7 – 11.1)
▪ Microscopic	3.0 (1.4 – 6.3)

Farraye FA et al., *Gastroenterology* 2010; 138: 746 – 774.

- Give the influence of male gender on the risk of UC-CRC after 10 years of pancolitis.

The risk of UC-CRC is higher in males than females, but this gender-effect is seen only in boys diagnosed before age 4 years.

	RR of UC-CRC
o Crohn disease (CD)	
– Any site	2.5
– Colon only	5.6
– Age at CD diagnosis < 3 years	30

- Give the effect of **CRC in IBD on family risk** of CRC.

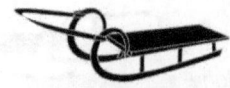

The effect of a patient with UC (ulcerative colitis) who develop CRC (colorectal cancer) on the risk to their family

- o UC plus CRC
  - Non-UC family member
    - ↑ CRC risk
- o UC plus non-UC family member with CRC
  - ↑ CRC risk n UC patient
- o In UC plus stricture or bypassed loop of colon
  - Watch out for CRC
- o UC + CRC in resected colon
  - 90% had dysplastic mucosa in other parts of colon
- o UC plus dysplasia
  - 30% also have CRC
- o The clinical problem: which UC is continuous, dysplasia is patchy, so multiple colonic biopsies taken at surveillance colonoscopy may miss the dysplasia that would raise the alarm that 30% could already have CRC.

➤ Pathology

SO YOU WANT TO BE A GASTROENTEROLOGIST!

The current guidelines suggest that for quadrant mucosal biopsies every 10 cm from cecum to rectum must be taken when colonoscopy is performed for CRC surveillance in UC or CC (Crohn colitis), as per standard guidelines such as those recommended by ACG, ASG, BSG, CDG. Areas of mucosal irregularity should also be biopsied.

- • Give the **number of colonic mucosal biopsies** which need to be taken at the time of colonoscopic surveillance for persons with chronic UC or CC, which detect dysplasia with 90% confidence.
  - o Thirty-three
  - o Now ask the patient if she/he is satisfied to wait 1 to 2 years for their next colonoscopy with biopsies with the chance that the dysplasia miss rate is at least 10% (and as high as 70%), and the risk of their already having a missed CRC is 19% to 33%.

Eyes on the Future

- o With the improvement in the detection of dysplastic lesions and using targeted colonic mucosal biopsies using chromocolonoscopy, this is likely to replace the current practice of blind non-targeted sampling.

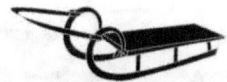

- Give the mucosal biopsy findings at screening or colonoscopic surveillance in persons with UC or Crohn colitis when indicated early colectomy.
  - HGD in flat mucosa → colectomy
  - HGD or LGD in polypoid lesion → colectomy if
    - Polyp is not completely removed
    - There is adjacent dysplasia
    - There is invasive cancer

Abbreviations: HGD, high grade dysplasia; LGD, low grade dysplasia

---

SO YOU WANT TO BE A GASTROENTEROLOGIST!

- A patient with colitis (Crohn colitis or Ulcerative colitis) has a polypoid mucosa on endoscopy, with the appearance of inflammatory pseudo-polyps.
- Mucosal biopsies are taken to confirm the histopathology of the suspected inflammatory polyps.
- As expected the biopsies show long crypts, and in the lamina propria there is a mixed inflammatory infiltrate.

- Give the additional histological findings you would search for which would diagnosis a second type of recurrent, inflammatory pseudopolyp.
  - Cap polyposis appears just like inflammatory pseudopolyposis, but is likely due to repeated mucosal prolapse, and has a surface cap of fibropurulent exudate.

➢ Differential

- Give features which help to distinguish UC-CRC from sporatic CRC (SPO-CRC).

Features	UC-CRC	SPO-CRC
o Age of diagnosis of CRC, years	~ 40	~ 60
o Location of dysplasia	May be distant from CRC UC CC 30%	Associated with polyp
o Location of CRC	R~ = LC CC 23% to 70%	LC > RC

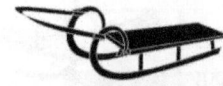

Mastering the Boards: Gastroenterology   A.B.R. Thomson

Features	UC-CRC	SPO-CRC
o Mutation		
– RAS protooncogene		
▪ %	~ 20%	50%
▪ Timing	Late	Early
– LOH for p53		
▪ Timing	Early	Late
▪ In non-dysplastic tissue	Yes	No
– Small SRC activation		
▪ Timing	Early	Late
▪ Correlate with degree of dysplasia	Yes	No
o Pathology		
– Anaplastic	Often	Less often
– Mucinous	Often	Less often
o Synchronous	More common in UC-CRC than in SPO-Ca	

Abbreviations: LOH, loss of heterogeneity; RC, right colon; LC, left colon; SPO-Ca, spontaneous CRC

Note:

- o The BSG (British Society of Gastroenterology) but not the AGA/ASG guidelines suggest that surveillance in Crohn colitis (CC) may be every 5 years rather than more frequently if their Crohn colitis involves < 50 cm of the colon.

- o It is possible that 5-ASA, folic acid, calcium, ASA, or NSAIDs may reduce the risk of sporadic CRC, as well as CRC associated with IBD.

- o There is no evidence yet that azathioprine, 6-MP or anti-TNF therapy reduces the rate of development of IBD-associated dysplasia/CRC.

"Ships in harbor are safe,
but that's not what ships are built for."

John Shedd

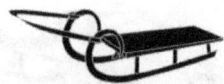

OTHER FORMS OF COLITIS

Radiation Colilis

➢ Pathophysiology

- Give the molecular mechanisms responsible for the acute and chronic damage to the GI tract causes by radiation.
    - o Acute
        - – ↑ expression of P53 (a tumour suppressor gene) → ↑ apoptosis
    - o Chronic
        - – Radiation increases the translation by the gene which codes for TGF-β (transforming growth factor-beta)
        - – ↑ TGF
            - → fibrogenic cytokine → ↑ initiates stromal injury & fibrosis
            - → Proinflammatory cytokine
                - - ↑ WBC migration to the wall of intestinal blood vessels
                - - ↓ normal degradation of extracellular matrix
            - → ↑ CTGF (connective tissue growth factor) – maintains the activation of fibrogenesis

➢ Clinical

- Give the symptoms associated with 4 types of lesions associated with chronic radiation enteritis.

Lesion (s)	Symptoms
o Stricture	– Obstruction
o Abscess	– Infection
o Fistula	– Fistulization
o Ulceration	– Bleeding
o Mucosal damage	– Malabsorption

Adapted from: *Sleisenger & Fordtran's gastrointestinal and liver disease: Pathophysiology/Diagnosis/Management* 10th Edition, 2016, Table 40-1, page 669.

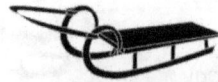

- Give the acute and chronic symptoms of radiation-associated damage to the colon.

  - Acute
    - Onset 6 weeks of radiation therapy
    - Usually stops after radiation treatment is completed
    - Symptoms may persist for 1 year after cessation of radiation therapy
    - In ~ 1/3 patients bleeding stops spontaneously within 6 months
    - Most often affects rectosigmoid portion of colon

  - Chronic
    - Symptoms begin 9 months to 30 years after radiation therapy
    - Should be could "proctopathy" (chronic radiation proctopathy), since there is not an inflammation infiltration (no proctitis)
    - Fistula changes
    - May be associated with late (> 30 years) malignant transformation and CRC

➢ Endoscopy

  - Mucosa
    - Pale
    - Friable
    - Telangiectasias

  - Small or large abnormal areas

➢ Histopathology

  - Biopsy posterior and lateral walls of rectosigmoid to avoid area of maximum radiation exposure (uncertain if this ↓ risk of fistula formation)

  - Changes may be continuous or patchy (i.e., skip lesions)

- Give the histopathological features seen on small bowel biopsy which accompany chronic radiation damage.

o Arterioles; (intima vasculopathy)	– Obliterative endarteritis – Foam cells – Loss of vessel wall → ischemia
o Mucosa	– Atrophy – May be continuous or patchy (i.e., skip lesions)
o Submucosa	– Thickening • Hyaline • Collagen • Fibrosis • Telangiectasias

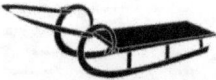

- o Lymphatics   – Constriction
  - $\downarrow$ flow $\rightarrow$ edema
  - $\uparrow$ inflammation

- o Ulceration, necrosis
  $\rightarrow$ perforation

- o Crypts   – Normal or decreased

- ➢ Treatment
  - o Medications
    - – Constipation
      - Infliximab 5 mg/kg on day 0, 14 and 42 (2 and 6 weeks)
      - Stool softers, and other symptomatic measures
    - – Obstruction (from strictures)
      - Endoscopic dilation for short and straight stricture
      - Try to avoid surgical resection ($\uparrow$ risk of dehiscence)
    - – Bleeding (from ectatic vessels)
      - Sucralfate enema, 2 g bid PR for 8 weeks (good response 4 weeks 77%; 8 weeks 92%)
      - Metronidazole 400 mg PO tid
    - – Hormonal therapy
      - Estrogen +/- progesterone (evidence from only 1 case series)
    - – Steroids, 5-ASA, SCFA enemas
      - No proven benefit
  - o Amifostine is an organic thiophosphate which acts as a scavenger of free radicals, and which is under study as a radioprotective agent of the GI tract and bladder.

  - o Endoscopic therapy
    - – Formalin 4% to 5%, soaked gauze through sigmoidoscope, at 2 to 4 week intervals, for as long as required to stop bleeding
    - – Cessation of bleeding
    - – 2/3 require only 1 session
      - 1 month   60%
      - 1 month   76% to 93%
    - – Bipolar (Bi) and Heater Probe (HP)
      - Reduction in severe bleeding over 1 year (vs control group [CG])

Bi	CG		HP	CG
75%	33%		67%	11%

TG therapeutic gain   Bi   42%

                              HP   56%

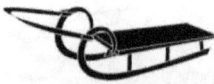

- o Hyperbaric O_2 (HO_2)

	HO_2	PL
Clinical response	89%	63%

- o Surgery
  - – Not recommended as first line therapy because of high risk of complications

Sleisenger and Fordtran's Gastrointestinal and Liver Disease. 10th Edition. Saunders/Elsevier, Philadelphia, 2016, Table 40.3, page 670)

Microscopic Colitis

➢ Definition

- o A chronic inflammatory condition causing chronic watery diarrhea, typically seen in middle-aged women, whose colonoscopy shows apparently normal mucosa but the mucosal biopsies are either lymphocytic or collagenous colitis.

➢ Types

- o Microscopic colitis (MC) is comprised of LC (lymphocytic colitis) and CC (Collagenous colitis).
- o MC is comprised of lymphocytes > 20/100 epithelial cells
- o MC occurs in a bowel which is endoscopically normal (implication; mucosal biopsies must be taken from endoscopically normal-appearing mucosa)

➢ Causes/associations

- • Give medications used for with microscopic colitis.
  - o Loperamide (or other antidiarrheals)
  - o Bismuth subsalicylate
  - o Mesalamine
  - o Cholestyramine
  - o Budesonide
  - o Prednisone
  - o Azathioprine/6-mercaptopurine
  - o Methotrexate

Source: Chande, N. *Can J Gastroenterol* 2008; 22: pg 687.

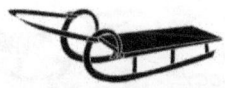

➢ Clinical

- Give features which help to distinguish between LC and CC.

Feature		LC	CC
o	Definition	Colitis, ↑ lymphocytes but no ↑ collagen layer or glycoprotein tenascin	Subepithelial collagen layer > 10 μm Type I, III, VI collagen plus ↑ glycoprotein tenascin
o	Incidence, persons per 10^5 per year	3	1
o	Distribution	-	80% cecum and TC
o	Association with celiac disease	9%	2%
o	Possible drug damage	– BBs – Bisphosphonates – PPIs – SSRIs – Statins	NSAIDs (~60%) SSRIs
o	Autoimmune markers		ANA (~50%) pANCA (~14%)

Abbreviations: ANA, antinuclear antibodies; BBs, beta-blockers; CC, collagenous colitis; LC, CD, Crohn colitis; lymphocytic colitis; pANCA, perinuclear antineutrophil cytoplasmic antibodies; SSRIs, selective serotonin reuptake inhibitors; TC, transverse colon

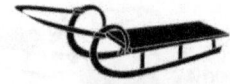

Mastering the Boards: Gastroenterology　　　　　　　　A.B.R. Thomson

➢ Endoscopy

Clinical Tip

The patient with IBS-like symptoms has a colonoscopy, which is normal. You are asked if this excludes IBD

    o No, it does not
- Very mild and early UC or CD may be seen only on mucosal biopsy of the colon
- CD may be in the small bowel, beyond the reach of the colonoscopy
- The patient may have MC (microscopic colitis, either collagenous colitis or lymphocytic colitis), where biopsies are positive and diagnostic, but colonic mucosa appears normal on colonoscopy.

➢ Treatment
    o Budesonide 9 mg po od

Diversion Colitis

➢ Definition
    o "….. an inflammatory process that occurs in the diverted segment of colon and rectum after surgical diversion of the fecal stream" (Sleisenger and Fordtran's Gastrointestinal and Liver Disease. 10th Edition. Saunders/Elsevier, Philadelphia, 2016, page 2301).

➢ Demography
    o 3x more frequent for surgery for IBD then for non-IBD colonic disorders (87% versus 28%)

    o "an inflammatory process that occurs in segments of the colorectum that are diverted from the fecal stream by surgery.

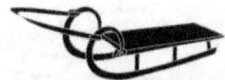

- ➢ Pathogenesis
  - o Diversion colitis (DC) may develop in the surgically diverted segment of colon. DC is speculated to be due to decrease in the diverted segment of obligate anaerobes and therefore in SCFAs (short-chain [length] fatty acids).
  - o If possible, the continuity of the colon may be restored, with resolution of the colitis. In the event that the continuity of the bowel cannot or should not be restored, the deficiency of SCFAs and the impaired metabolism of the colonocytes can be restored by giving enemas of SCFAs.
  - o Such SCFA enemas must be prepared by a pharmacist who is capable of compounding the preparation for the individual patient.
  - o ↓ obligate anaerobes in diverted colon loop
    - − ↓ SCFAs
    - − ↓ major energy source for colonocytes

- ➢ Clinical
  - o May occur in persons with no pre-existing IBD
  - o Few (6% to 30%) have symptoms, yet most have histopathological changes of colitis
  - o Onset of symptoms is months to years after diversion

- ➢ Endoscopy
  - o Severity of diversion colitis
    - − Mild   52%
    - − Moderate   44%
    - − Severe   4%
  - o Colitis in non-bypassed ("in continuity") colon 0%
    (Note: there are case reports of symptomatic UC developingin the "in continuity" colon in persons with established diversion colitis)

- ➢ Histopathology
  - o Inflammatory cells
    - − Neutrophils, diffuse infiltration
    - − Lymphocytes
    - − Mononuclear cells
  - o Aggregates
    - − Neutrophils
    - − Lymphoid follicular hyperplasia
  - o Crypts
    - − Cryptitis
    - − Abscesses
  - o Paneth cells
    - − Metaplasia

474

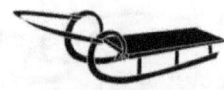

- Prominent lymphoid follicular hyperplasia in mucosa and submucosa
- Aphthous ulcers (erosions over lymphoid follicles)
- If the diversion was for Crohn disease, granulomas may occur in the bypassed bowel
- May be difficult to distinguish from acute UC

SO YOU WANT TO BE A GASTROENTEROLOGIST!

A patient with Crohn disease of the ileum undergoes a surgical diversion of the colon. Post-operatively, proctitis develops.

- Give features which favour the proctitis being recurrent Crohn disease (CD) versus diversion colitis (DC).

Features	CD	DC
o Linear ulcers	+++	+
o Transmural inflammation	+++	+
o Architectural changes in crypts	+++	+
o Epitheloid granulomas	+++	+
o Lymphoid follicular hyperplasia	+	+

➤ Treatment
- SCFA (short chain fatty acid) enemas
    - Prepared by "compounding" pharmacies, as sodium salts
        - Acetate   60 mmol   ⎤ Mix in 22mmol/L NaCl, with an enema
        - N-butyrate   40 mmol   ⎬ volumeof 60 mL, given bid per rectum
        - Proprionate   30 mmol   ⎦ (PR) or per mucous fistula.
        - Chloride (to achieve osmolality of 280 to 229 mOsm/L; 22 mmol
        - Hydroxide adjust pH to 7.0
- 5-ASA enemas (only case report evidence)
    - Switch from, or add to SCFA enemas
- Surgical reanastamosis
    - Especially early if patient has Crohn disease, to reduce likelihood of formation of stricture

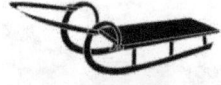

NSAID-Associated Colitis

- o A high local concentration of NSAIDs may cause inflammation in any part of the GI tract, especially in the stomach but also in the small intestine and in the colon.

- o The development of diaphragms across the small or large intestine are pathognomic for NSAIDs damage.

- o In the absence of "diaphragm disease", there are histopathological features which might help to distinguish NSAIDs damage from for example, in the stomach or duodenum, non-NSAIDs, non-H.pyloric peptic ulcer, or in the colon, non-specific colonic ulcers.

- Give features which help to distinguish NSAID-associated lesions from idiopathic ("non-specific") lesions in the colon.

Feature	Non-Specific Colonic Ulcers	NSAIDs Ulcers
o Peak, age and onset, years	- 40 to 50	▪ Any age
o Site in colon	- Right	▪ Right
o Number of ulcers	- Single	▪ Usually multiple
o Round	- Yes	▪ Not necessarily
o Demarcation of edge	- Yes	▪ Not necessarily
o Diaphragm	- No	▪ Yes

Infectious Colitis

- Give common causes of **pocto-sigmoiditis** in MSM (men who have sex with men).

  - o Chlamydia

  - o GC (gonorrhea)

  - o HSV

  - o Syphilis, T. palladium

- Give the most common infectious causes of **fulminant colitis and toxic megacolon** in **HIV/AIDs**.

  - o MAC

  - o CMV (cytomegatovirus)

  - o E.histolytica

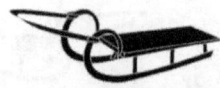

- Give the CD4 counts below which certain infectious causes of colitis become more common in HIV/AIDs.

Infection	CD4 counts
o CMV	≤ 100
o MAC	≤ 50

HSV (Herpes Simplex Virus)

➤ Pathology
- o May cause an "attack" of UC recurrence
- o "saddle" distribution of S2-S4 neuropathy (almost pathognomic)
- o Usually left-sided only
- o Multiple small round ulcers
- o Raised borders central exudates
- o Found at the edge ("rim") of the ulcers

➤ Treatment
- o Acyclovir
- o Famciclovir
- o Valacyclovir

Clinical gem – Take mucosal biopsy from rim ("high up") on the lesions suspected of being caused by HSV.

CMV colitis
- o May complicate UC and cause a recurrence of symptoms/inflammation
- o May cause severe colitis

- Give the features of CMV colitis which are suggestive of this diagnosis.

➤ Pathology
- o Ischemic changes
- o Intranuclear inclusion bodies ("owl's eye" appearance)

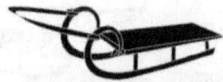

➤ Endoscopy

   o Redness

   o Friability

   o Ulcers
- Long
- Deep
- Serpiginous
- Discrete, clean-based

Entamoeba Histolytica-Associated colitis

➤ Clinical

   o Fulminant colitis/toxic megacolon

   o Perforation

   o Strictures (when E. histolytica infection is chronic)

478

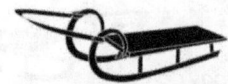

> Laboratory

  o Wet mount of stool samples
    - Motile trophozoites
    - Ingested erythrocytes

> Histopathology

  o May be indistinguishable from UC

  o Classically, "flask-shaped" mucosal ulcers

> Treatment

  o Metronidazole, followed with

  o Paromomycin or iodoquinol

Cryptosporidium

  o Cryptosporidium is the most common parasitic infection in HIV/AIDs, but it can be easily confused with isospora belli

  o Both cryptosporidium and isospora belli are acid fast, and are localized to the luminal membrane.

Acid fast staining

  o TB

  o MAC

  o Isospora belli

  o Cryptosporidium

Note: Tropheryma whippelii macrophages in Whipple disease are not acid fast.

- Give features which help to distinguish between Isospora belli versus cryptosporidial infection of the GI tract.

Feature	Isospora belli	Cryptosporidium
o Geographical location (recent travel)	Haiti, Africa	World-wide
o Acid-fast staining of stools	+	+
o Charcot-Leyden crystals in stool	+	-
o Localization of organism on mucosal biopsy		
- BBM	+	+
- ICV	+	-
o Sensitivity to TMP-SMX	+	+

Abbreviations: LM, luminal membrane; ICV, intracytoplasmic vacuoles; TMP-SMX, trimethoprim-sulfamethoxazole

479

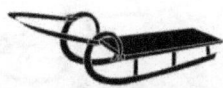

Typhlitis *(aka Necrotizing enteropenic enterocolitis)*

➢ Causes/associations

    o Organ transplantation

    o Infection
- HIV/AIDs

    o Cancer chemotherapy
- Cytosine arabinoside
- Solid tumour combination

    o Polymicrobial
- E.Coli, Staphylococcus, Streptococcus, Enterococcus, Klebsiella
- Aspergillus, Candida

➢ Pathology

    o Both MAC and T.whippeli are PAS-positive

    o Only T.whippeli is diastase resistant

    o Usually affects cecum, ileum, rarely sigmoid colon

    o May become transmural, with necrosis, gangrene (intramural air), and perforation

➢ Endoscopy

    o Avoid colonoscopy
- High risk of perforation because of colonic necrosis
- Surgical resection risk of mortality ~50%

➢ Treatment

    o Appropriate antibiotics for polymicrobial infection against organisms noted above

    o GMCSF (granulocyte-macrophage colony-stimulating factor)

    o Avoid surgical resection
- Risk of mortality ~ 50%

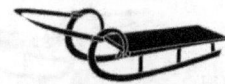

Clostridium Difficile Infection (CDI)

➢ Terminology

    o Antibiotic-Associated Diarrhea (AAD)

    o Pseudomembranous Enterocolitis (PMEC)

    o Clostridium difficile-Associated Diarrhea and Colitis (CDADC)

➢ Microbiology

    o PMEC (PMC and PME) is caused by non-invasive C. difficile, S. aureus, and non-infectious conditions such as the seriously ill ICU patient.

➢ Risk factors

    o The usual
        – Recent use of antibiotics
        – Dirty hospitals
        – Dirty hands

    o C.diffcile is a "big deal" organism these days, because of
        – Its widening disease scope, present in as well as out of hospital, with as well as without recent.
        – Some strains cause severe CDA
            • ↑ morbidity / ↑ mortality

    o Hand washing with the alcohol-containing dispensers which are now found throughout most hospitals!! (only soap and water destroys C.difficile)

    o HIV and IBD (even in the absence of use of antibiotics), antineoplastic chemotherapy

    o Newly recognized
        – Anybody-that means even healthy persons in the community
        – Recent use of PPIs
        – Post-partum women
        – Patients with UC and CD

Abbreviations: UC, ulcerative colitis; CD, Chronic disease; PPIs, proton pump inhibitors

---

Clinical Tip

Another watch out: A normal colonic mucosa on sigmoidoscopy does **not** exclude C. difficile infection beyond the reach of the scope, in the colon or small intestine

---

481

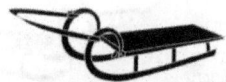

> Pathogenesis

- Give the way in which a Clostridium difficile infection (CDI) causes pseudomembranous colitis in a patient with a history recent of antibiotic use.

    o Antibiotics deplete regular gut microbiotica, which normally outnumber the C.*difficile* which is present.

    o C.*difficile* can resist antibiotics as a spore and then will outgrow normal microbiotica when antibiotics are discontinued.

    o Toxins A and B are produced by the greater numbers of C.*difficile*, causing diarrhea.

> Pathology

    o There is overlap between AAD, PMEC and CDADC

    o PMC (pseudomembraneous colitis) or PME (pseudomembraneous enteritis): the pseudomembrane is comprised of inflammatory and cellular debris, may be seen only on biopsy and not on colonoscopy, and may be associated with underlying ulceration.

> Diagnosis

    o Diagnostic tests include
        - Tissue culture cytotoxicity assay
        - EIA (enzyme-linked Immunoassays) for toxin A and B
        - Culture followed by testing for toxin A and B
        - PCR (polymerase chain reaction) to detect the genes for the toxins
        - Colonoscopy: AAD plus PMC = C. diffcile colitis (sigmoidoscopy is not adequate, since 20% of PMC involves only the right side of the colon)

> Treatment

❖ Initial therapy

    o Mild CDI
        - General management
        - Stop offending antibiotics
        - Contact precaution, especially hand hygiene
        - Supportive therapy

    o Antibiotics (bacteriostatic)
        - Metronidazole 500 mg po tid, or 250 mg po qid, for 10 to 14 days
        - If metronidazole ineffective and symptoms persist, vancomycin 125 mg po qid, for 10 to 14 days
        - If patient requires antibiotics for non- C. Difficile indication, continue metronidazole or vancomycin ("concomitant antibiotics") for 1 week after other antibiotics for non- C. difficile infection is stopped.

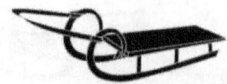

- Note: Risk of VRE (vancomycin-resistant enterococci) is similar with both metronidazole and vancomycin.

- o Repeat stool cultures
  - Not indicated if symptoms subsided (50% will have C. difficile spores for up to 6 weeks in persons who have become asymptomatic)
  - Not indicated to treat C. difficile spore; even if person is toxin-positive, they may be an asymptomatic carrier.

- o Treatment options for recurrent C. difficile infections include
  - Repeat causes of metronidazole or vancomycin
  - Pulsed dose of vancomycin
  - Prolonged doses of vancomycin
  - Rifaximin
  - Cholestyramine or colestipol binding resins
  - Probiotics
  - IV pooled human immunoglobulin
  - Fecal transplantation

❖ Recurrent CDI

- o ~20% of C. difficile diarrhea patients recur after initially successful treatment with metronidazole or vancomycin. Because post-infectious IBS (irritable bowel syndrome) may present with similar symptoms, repeat testing of stool for C. difficil toxin is appropriate.

- o Recurrence rates
  - Usual treatment 31%
  - Pulse 14%
  - Taper 45%
  - Recurrence usually within 3 weeks to 12 weeks
  - Of these with 1 recurrence, at least 25% will have a second recurrence
  - ½ due to relapse from original strain of C. difficile
  - ½ due to reinfection with a different strain

➢ Treatment

- o Repeat vancomycin or metronidazole (usual treatment)

- o Associations with metronidazole failures
  - Transfer from another hospital
  - CDI on hospital admission
  - Recent use of cephalosporin

- o Intermittent (pulse) therapy
  - Antibiotic-free interval allows C. difficile spores to germinate, and be susceptible to being destroyed by next interval dose of antibiotic

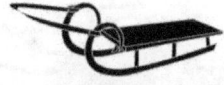

- o Tapered vancomycin
  - – Sequential therapy
    - ▪ Vancomycin, followed rifaximin for 14 days (88% response) previous exposure to rifaximin may cause rifaximin resistant C. difficile infection
  - – Fidaxomicin (bactericidal)
    - ▪ 200 mg po bid for 10 to 14 days
    - ▪ Response
- o Anion-binding resins
  - – Adjuvant therapy with tapered vancomycin
  - – Cholestyramine or colestipol
- o Probiotics inconclusive results
- o Immunotherapy
  - – Monoclonal antibodies (MAb)
    - ▪ Adjuvant to antibiotics (Ab), to reduce rate of recurrence

	Ab + MAb	Ab
Rate of recurrence	7%	25%

  - – IVIG (intravenous immunoglobulin) – no proven benefit

SO YOU WANT TO BE A GASTROENTEROLOGIST!

Because CDI is a common and serious complication of hospitalization and poor hand hygiene, including poor contact precaution by staff, alcohol-based hand sanitizers are being increasing placed in/outside patient rooms.

- • Give why this practice may be challenged.
  - o C. difficile spores are destroyed by soap and water
  - o Washing with alcohol allows spores to survive, germinate and potentially cause more CDI

Relapse or reinfection of difficile leading to recurrent symptoms occurs in about 25% of persons.

- • Give risk factors for recurrent CDI.
  - o Age > 65 years
  - o Need for concomitant antibiotics (antidote for medical condition, plus antibiotic for CDI)
  - o Co-morbidities
  - o ↓ host immune response (low anti-toxin antibody levels
  - o Exposure to asymptomatic carriers

Note: Answering development of antibiotic resistance is not correct recurrence of CDI after initial treatment with metronidazole does not signify metronidazole resistance.

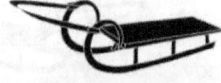

Severe CDI

➤ Defnition
- o No consensus definition

➤ Guidelines
- o Suggested guideline parameters
  - – WBC > 20,000 cells/µL
  - – Serum creatinine ≥ 1.5 x pre-infection level
  - – Scoring system (maximum 8 points)
    - ▪ One point each for
      - – Age. > 60 yr
      - – > 38.3 °C
      - – WBC > 15,000 WBC/µL within 48 hours of enrollment
      - – Serum albumin < 2.5 mg/dL
    - ▪ Two points each for
      - – PMC (pseudomembranous colitis) on endoscopy
      - – Admission to ICU
  - – Severe disease ≥ 2 points

➤ Complications
- o Patient
  - – Shock
  - – Death (within 30 days)
- o Colon
  - – Megacolon
  - – Perforation
  - – Need for colectomy
  - – Risk of complications for the hypervirlent stain of C. difficile, NAP (north American Pulsed Field type I), 11%

485

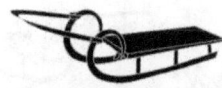

- ➢ Treatment
- • Pharmacological
  - ○ Vancomycin 125 mg po qid
  - ○ For severe disease, vancomycin (VAN) is superior to metronidazole (MET)

	VAN	MET
Cure rate for severe CDI	97%	76%

  - – If patient with severe CDI is NPO (such as with megacolon or ileus), consider use of
    - ▪ Vancomycin by enema, 500 mg in 100 mL normal saline q 8 hour
    - ▪ Adding metronidazole 500 mg IV q 8 hour
- • Surgery
  - ○ Indications
    - – Worsening of patient
      - ▪ age ≥ 65 years
      - ▪ SIRA (systemic inflammatory response syndrome)
      - ▪ Multiorgan failure
      - ▪ Peritoneal signs
    - – Colon
      - ▪ Megacolon
      - ▪ Severe ileus
      - ▪ Microperforation
      - ▪ Necrotizing colitis
    - – Laboratory
      - ▪ WBC ≥ 20,000 WBC/µL, and/or
      - ▪ Plasma lactate, between 2.2 and 4.9 mEq/L
  - ○ Procedures
    - – Subtotal colectomy and ileostomy, secondary closure of ileostomy with ileorectal anastomosis
    - – Diverting loop ileostomy, and colonic lavage (intraoperative PEG solution; post-operative autograge flushes of vancomycin into the ileostomy
- • Transplantation of stool (fecal bacteriotherapy, aka fecal microbiota transplantation [FMT])
  - ○ Increasing evidence that this is beneficial for recurrent CDI

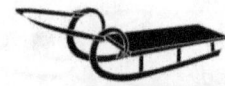

COLONIC POLYPS AND CANCER: NON-FAMILIAL FORMS

Colonic Polyps

➤ Definition: "A gastrointestinal polyp is a discrete mass of tissue that protrudes into the lumen of the bowel" (Feldman M., et al. Sleisenger and Fordtran's Gastrointestinal and Liver Disease. 9th Edition. Saunders/Elsevier, Philadelphia, 2010, page 2155).

Caution: An adenoma is neoplastic, because it shows cellular dysplasia.

➤ Demography: Some approximate percentages to remember
- Age 50, asymptomatic, average risk
  - Likelihood of finding
    - Adenomatous polyp, ~30% (5:3 M to F)
    - AAP (adenoma with advanced pathology, ~8%)
  - Greater risk of large or right-sided adenoma in African Americans > 60 yr
  - Adenoma recurrence, 19% per year
  - Incident
    - Adenomas, 5% per year
    - AAP, 0.4% per year

➤ Terminology

o Deminative polyp	– ≤ 5 mm
	– 1/3 to ½ have adenomatous changes
	– few have severe dysplasia/villous changes
	– 0.1% have carcinoma
o AAP (advanced adenomatous polyps, aka adenoma with advanced pathology)	– Villous architecture, or
	– HGD, or
	– Carcinoma
o Flat adenoma	– Flat, or slightly raised
	– May be multiple
	– D > 2x T (diameter is more than two times the thickness) of the lesion
	– Usually < 1 cm (T < 0.5 cm)
	– Represent ~10% of adenomas (% depends on techniques used for detection, e.g., chromoendoscopy shows that 7% to 36% of all adenomas are flat!)
	– More HGD/cancer risk
o Serrated adenomas	– Histopathological features for both adenomatous plus hyperplastic polyp

487

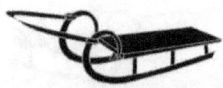

- o Aberrant crypts
  - – Small, raised foci of irregularly-shaped crypts when viewed from lumen by magnifying endoscopy
  - – Hyperplastic or adenomatous (when adenomatous, are preneoplastic)
- o "multiple". e.g., multiple polyps or multiple CRCs ≥ 2
- o Synchronous
  - – Two polyps or one identified at the same time e.g., the index polyps is seen in the descending polyps, and a second polyps seen in the cecum at the time of the same colonoscopy
  - – About 40% of colons with one polyp will have one or more synchronous polyps
- o Metachronous
  - – A polyp or CRC is identified at the index colonoscopy, and a polyp or CRC identified six months later is metachronous.
- o Malignant
  - – The term malignant polyp refers to an adenoma in which a focus of carcinoma has invaded beyond the muscularis mucosae into the submucosal
  - – Note that some non-adenomatous polyps (e.g., hamartoma, juvenile [when polyps are multiple]) may also become malignant (i.e., the above definition refers to "adenoma", but when non-adenomatous polyps develop CRC, they are still referred to as being "malignant".
  - – Colonic cancers which have a polypoid appearance may also be called a "malignant polyp".
  - – About 5% of adenomatous polyps
- o Mucosal
  - – Submucosa pushes mucosa to appear as a small bump
  - – Seen in ~10% of screening colonoscopies
  - – No clinical importance
- o Inflammatory
  - – Inflammation and granulation tissue resulting from regeneration of ulcerative tissue
- o Juvenile
  - – ↑ lamina propria, with edema
  - – Dilated cystic glands filled with mucus
  - – Inflammatory cells
  - – ↑ vascularity
- o Peutz-Jegher
  - – Hamartomatous lesion characterized by glandular epithelium supported by an arborizing framework of well-developed smooth muscle that is contiguous with the muscularis mucosae

488

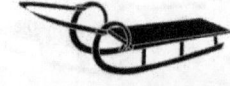

> Pathology

- Give a classification of colorectal polyps.

  o Neoplastic   – Adenoma
                                    – Carcinoma

  o Non-neoplastic   – Hyperplastic
                                      – Mucosal polyps
                                      – Juvenile
                                      – Inflammatory

  o Hamartomas   – Peutz-Jegher Syndrome
                                      – Juvenile

- Another useful classification of colorectal polyps

> Mucosal lesions

  o Adenoma
  - Tubular
  - Tubulovillous
  - Serrated villous

  o Pathological features
  - Immature goblet or columnar cell
  - ↑ cellularity of crypts
  - ↑ mucin
  - ↑ hyperchromatic (↑ basophilia)
  - Elongated nuclei
  - "picket fence" pattern of nuclei

  o Carcinoma
  - Carcinoma in situ
  - Intramucosal

  o Invasive

  o Hyperplastic

  o Inflammatory

  o Juvenile (retention)

  o Peutz-Jegher syndrome (hamartomas)

  o Normal mucosa in a polypoid configuration

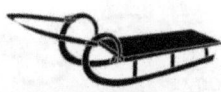

- ➢ Submucosal Lesions
  - o Colitis cystica profunda
  - o Pneumatosis cystoides intestinalis
  - o Lymphoid polyp (benign and malignant)
  - o Lipoma
  - o Carcinoid
  - o Metastic neoplasms

Adapted from: Sleisenger and Fordtran's Gastrointestinal and Liver Disease. 10th Edition. Saunders/Elsevier, Philadelphia, 2016, Box 126-1, page 2214.

- • And a futher alternate approach to a classification of colonic polyps, based on predominant glandular pattern (may be mixed, e.g., serrated adenoma)
  - o Epithelial cells
    - – Adenomatous, hyperplastic, serrated
    - – Mucosal
    - – Inflammatory
  - o Hamartomas
    - – Juvenile
    - – Peutz-Jegher syndrome
    - – Cowden disease
    - – BRR syndrome
    - – Neurofibromatous
  - o Submucosal
  - o Colitis cystica coli
  - o Pneumatosis cystoides coli

"The superior man is modest in his speech, but exceeds in his action."

Confucius

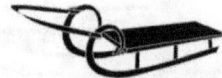

- Give the histopathological findings of mild, moderate and severe dysplasia.

Feature	Mild (70%)	Moderate (20%)	Severe (5%)
o Nuclei	– Basal position – Hyperchromatic – Elongated – Elongated – Uniform size	Stratified Pleomorphic	↑↑ ↑↑
o N/C ratio	– Ratio	Normal	↑
o Nucleoli	– Normal	Normal	↑↑
o Cribriform**	-	+/-	+
o Mucin	↓	↓↓	
o Distribution of changes in crypt	– Partial	Entire	Entire
o Architecture	– Branching – Budding – Crowding	↑	↑↑↑

*cribriform appearance, aka glands within glands

- o Note:
  - – Common practice
    - > LGD – Includes mild plus moderate dysplasia
    - > HGD – includes severe dysplasia plus carcinoma in situ
  - – Recall that if an adenomatous polyp has HGD, cancer, or a villus architecture, it is considered to meet the criteria for being called an AAP (**adenoma with advanced pathology**)

Abbreviations: HGD, high grade dysplasia; LGD, low grade dysplasia; N/C ratio, ratio of nucleus to cytoplasm

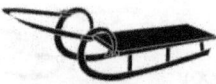

- Give the histopathological terms used to describe non-invasive and invasive colonic cancer.

Name	Through Basement Membrane	Into Lamina Propria	Through Muscularis Mucosae
o Non invasive			
– Carcinoma in situ	-	-	-
– Intramucosal cancer	+	+	-
o Invasive			
– Malignant polyp	+	+	+

×××

SO YOU WANT TO BE A GASTROENTEROLOGIST!

- Give the anatomical reason why carcinoma in situ and intramucosal carcinoma are considered to be non-invasive lesions, with no potential to metastasize.

  o Carcinoma in situ and intramucosal cancer of the colon are contained in the mucosa, which lacks lymphatics, and thus there is no potential to metastasize.

- Give the histopathological characteristics of an AAP (adenoma with advanced pathology):

  o AAP are adenomatous polyps which have one or more of the following:
    – Villous architecture
    – Presence of high grade dysplasia (HGD)
    – Carcinoma

➢ Size: For purposes of considering their malignant potential, colonic polyps are categorized as
  o Diminutive < 5 mm
  o Small > 0.5 < 1 cm
  o Medium 1 to 2 cm
  o Large > 2 cm

492

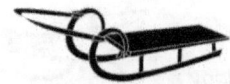

- Give the approximate malignant potential of colonic adenomas based on their size, histology and dysplasia.

			(%)
o	Size	< 1 cm	1
		1-2 cm	10
		>2 cm	45
o	Histology	Tubular	5
		Tubular Villous	25
		Villous	40
o	Dysplasia	Mild	5
		Moderate	20
		Severe	35
o	Site (colorectal cancer)	Cecum/Asc. Colon	25
		Transverse	15
		Descending	5
		Sigmoid	25
		Rectum	20

Clinical recommendation:

Rather than using an adjective to describe the size of a polyp in a colonoscopy dictation (e.g., small, medium, large), give their actual estimated size.

"Dedication, Determination, and Hard work will feed life into your dreams."

LaDonna M. Cook

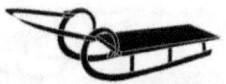

- Give the predictive value of a distal polyp for the approximate frequency of a proximal synchronous AAP (adenoma with advanced pathology).

  o ↑ with size of distal polyp

  o Varies with histopathology of distal polyp

Distal Colonic Lesion	AAP
– No polyp	3%
– Hyperplastic	3%
– Adenoma	1%
– Advanced adenoma (AA)	
▪ Tubular > 1 cm	9%
▪ Villous	12%
▪ HGD	12%
▪ Cancer (invasive)	25%

  o Note:
    – Only 30% of proximal CRCs have a distal colonic marker lesion, and
    – Only half of persons with proximal AAP have a distal marker

Adapted from: Feldman M., et al. Sleisenger and Fordtran's Gastrointestinal and Liver Disease. 9th Edition. Saunders/Elsevier, Philadelphia, 2010, Table 122.9, page 2169.

- Give the possible use of all of this information about the predictive value of a distal lesion.

  o If you do sigmoidoscopy for CRC screening, you have an idea when you see a distal lesion, you must follow up with a colonoscopy.

  o But, because many proximal lesions do not have a distal marker, you really should be arranging for your patient to have colonoscopy, regardless of what the distal colon shows.

➤ Postulated Progression of Colonic Mucosa to Sporatic Adenoma

  o Normal crypt   -   Proliferative compartment at the base of the crypt
       ↓
  o Aberrant crypt   -   Expansion of proliferative compartment to entire crypt
       ↓
  o Unicryptal adenoma   -   Monoclonal expansion
       ↓
  o Sporatic adenoma   -   Polyclonal expansion

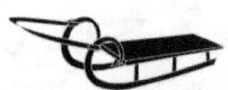

- Give the cumulative risk over time of a 1 cm colonic polyp developing into CRC.

Time Interval (years)	Cumulative Risk of Cancer at Polyp Site	Approximate Annual Rate
5	2.5%	0.5%
10	8%	0.8%
20	24%	1.2%

➢ Genetics

- Give the molecular pathways of tumour initiation and progression of CRC.

  - Tumour initiation
    - ↓ function of APC genes such as β-catenin, AXIN7 number, and of junction
    - Germline plus somatic mutation in FAP; 2 acquired somatic mutations in APC in sporatic adenomas from loss of function of both APC alleles

  - Tumour progression
    - ↑ K-Ras oncogene
      - The larger the adenoma, the greater the number of adenomas positive for K-Ras (small, 9%, large, 58%)
    - DCC
      - Small tubular/tubulovillous adenoma, 12% with foci of cancer, 73%

Abbreviation: DCC, deleted in colon cancer gene

  - Stability genes
    - MMR (DNA mismatch repair) gene
      - Germline mutations
        - hMLH1
        - hMSH2
        - hMSH6
    - BER (base-excision repairs) gene
      - MUTYII (mutated BER gene; aka MYN)
      - MMR gene mutations load to MSI (microsatellite instability)
      - MSI in 15% sporatic and 55% of HNPCC CRC (colorectal cancers)

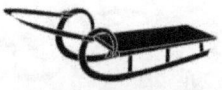

SO YOU WANT TO BE A GASTROENTEROLOGIST

- Give biochemical changes that occur during the development of CRC.

    - ↑ CEA (carcinoembryonic antigen)

    - ↑ matrix metalloproteinases
        - MMP-1
        - MT1 – MMP

    - ↑ EGF (vascular endothelial growth factors) increase angiogenesis and vasculization

    - ↑ selectins (on endothelium)

    - ↑ sialoglycoproteins (on tumour)

SO YOU WANT TO BE A GASTROENTEROLOGIST!

- Give the name of the gene in the APC gene family which increases the risk of colon cancer (CRC) in Ashkenazi Jewish persons, and the genes which may be altered and increase the risk of CRC from the metabolism of nutrients and environmental agents.

    - In Ashkenazi Jewish persons
        - I 1307 K

    - Environmental risk
        - Methylene tetrahydrofolate reductase
        - N-acetyltransferase-1 and -2

"Don't judge each day by the harvest you reap but by the seeds you plant."

Robert Louis Stevenson

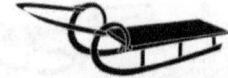

> Risk factors

- Give factors which alter the **risk for development** of colonic adenomas or CRC (colorectal cancer).

  - ↑ risk
    - Lifestyle
      - ↑ fat diet (especially red meat)
      - Obesity
      - Alcohol
      - Smoking (cigarettes)
      - Low calcium intake
    - Medical conditions
      - Ureterosigmoidostomy
        - Polyps (adenomas juvenile and hyperplastic) and CRC at stoma
        - Adenomas and CRC at stoma
      - Acromegaly: pooled odds ratio
        - Adenomas, 2.4
        - CRC, 4.3
      - Infection
        - Streptococcus bovis bacteremia,
        - JC virus

  - ↓ risk by increasing dietary intake
    - Carbohydrate
    - Fibre
    - Calcium
    - Folate
    - Fresh fruit and vegetables
    - Physical exercise
    - Chemopreventive compounds
      - NSAIDs, ASA, Coxibs
      - Calcium, 20% ↓ risk of adenomas
      - Selenium, 20% ↓ risk of CRC
      - HRT (hormone replacement therapy)
      - UDCA (ursodeoxycholic acid)

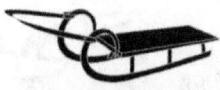

Screening and Surveillance for Non-polyposis Syndromes

➢ Terminology

- o **Primary prevention** "identifying genetic, biological, and environmental factors that are etiologic or pathogenetic and subsequently altering their effects on tumour development" (Sleisenger and Fordtran's Gastrointestinal and Liver Disease. 10th Edition. Saunders/Elsevier, Philadelphia, 2016, page 2276).

- o **Secondary prevention** "….. identify existing preneoplastic and lesion and to treat them thoroughly and expeditiously" (Sleisenger and Fordtran's Gastrointestinal and Liver Disease. 10th Edition. Saunders/Elsevier, Philadelphia, 2016, page 2276).

- o **Case finding**: the investigation of the patient with symptoms and/or signs suggestive of the diagnosis (such as CRC).

- o **Screening**: the investigation of an asymptomatic person to find an early pathological lesion or condition.

- o **Surveillance**: the investigation of a person at regular intervals after and index lesion has been discovered by screening or case finding.

➢ Colonoscopic screening and surveillance

- o Improvement in survival from CRC
    - 10 yr global benefit LC > RC
    - Split dosing of preparation for colonoscopy is best prep'
    - If you find a prox-polyp-look again, because of likely additional missed lesion
    - I serrated adenoma = risk of 3 adenomas
    - "ADR" – adenoma detection rate
    - ADR for second colonoscopy = 9.8% = pick – up for retroflexed view in cecum
    - ADR correlates well with RC serrated lesion detection

- o Watch out for
    - Three FOBT RCT's performed in 1993 to 1996 demonstrated a 13-21% reduction in CRC mortality (Winawer 09). The performance characteristics (sensitivity and specificity) of FIT (fecal immunochemical test) is comparable to FOBT1, without the need for dietary changes three days before FOBT.
    - CRC screening may be stopped at age 70 or 75, or at a time based on associated serious comorbidities.
    - Persons of African heritage have a risk of CRC shifted to an earlier age than do Caucasians, and their screening of African Canadians should begin at age 45.

498

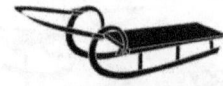

- The performance of screening colonoscopy done by skilled endoscopists or appropriately selected persons detects adenomas in approximately 15% of women and 25% of men, with 5-10% advanced adenomas (> 10 mm, villous, or with high grade dysplasia), < 1 % cancers, and a complication rate (perforation or bleeding) of about 1 per 1000 colonoscopies.
    - FDAs" (Flat & depressed adenomas)
        - Height < ½ of diameter
        - Aggressive biological behavior
            - ↓ K Ras and ADC mutations
            - Alternate neoplastic pathways
        - More advanced SX ↑ pathology
    - Lateral spreading tumour

  o Sessile or flat

  o Malignant potential is "significant"
    - LC   HP (Hyperplastic polyp)
                TSA (traditional serrated adenoma)
    - RC   SSA (Sessile serrated adenoma)
    - SSA/P   (without/with dysphasia/cancer)

  o The guidelines for CRC screening and surveillance are frequently being updated

  o Even following guidelines, CRC may develop in the interval between polypectomies. These "**interval cancers**" develop in about 0.6% of persons screened, having polypectomy, and then followed with an appropriate surveillance program.

  o While a single hyperplastic polyp normally does not have a malignant potential, followup is necessary if it is **serrated**, > 10 mm in size, or if these are **multiple hyperplastic polyps** above the rectosigmoid area

  o Colonoscopy screening provides its greatest benefit from the detection of left-sided lesions. In fact, the usefulness of colonoscopy to reduce the risk of right-sided CRC has been challenged.

  o Newer endoscopy equipment such as high-definition, narrow band imaging, or chromoendoscopy (including FICS [fujinon intelligent chromoendoscopy system], and the Pentax-scan) have yet to be shown to constantly improve polyp detection and CRC mortality

  o Persons with CRC associated with K-ras mutations do not respond as well to anti-EGFR therapy (Jiang Y, et al. *Cancer* 2009. In press.)

Abbreviations: EGFR, epidermal growth factor receptor; FICS, fujinon intelligent chromoendoscopy system; FIT, fecal immunochemical test

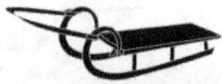

- Give factors which must be taken into account when stratifying risk and the need for screening for colorectal cancer (CRC).
  - Age >50 yrs
  - Personal history of colonic polyps or CRC
  - Family history - polyps, CBC, Lynch/FAP-associated tumours
  - High risk groups
    - IBD patients
    - African-Canadians
    - Smokers
    - Obesity (BMI>30, waist circumference>32-34")
    - Concurrent PSC (primary sclerosing cholangitis) in conjunction with UC
    - Dietary risk factors – low daily intake of fresh fruit, vegetables and fibre (possible); low intake of calcium and vitamin D; high intake of saturated fatty acids (especially red meat)

Fecal Testing for Occult Blood

A variety of stool and structure-based tests of the colon are included as options for screening for CRC. In the process of providing your patient with informed consent with regards to their making a choice about these tests, it is necessary for you to know the sensitivity of these investigations.

- Give tests for screening for CRC, and their approximate sensitivities for CRC and AA (advanced adenomas) in average risk persons presenting for colonoscopy.

Test	Sensitivity %	
	CRC	AA
❖ Stool-based		
○ Guaiac fecal occult		
– Standard	33-50	11
– "Sensitive"	50-75	20-25
○ FIT (fecal immunochemical test), 1-3 stool samples	60-85	20-50
○ DNA test, 1 stool sample		
– Old	51	18
– New	≥ 80	40
❖ Structure –based*		
○ CT colonography	Probably > 90	90
○ Colonoscopy (standard white light)	95	88-98**

* Flexible sigmoidoscopy is not reported here, because it demonstrates less than half of the colon, and its sensitivity will depend upon the distribution of CRC/AA.

** While sensitivities of 88% to 98% are reported, the work of Dr. L. Rabeneck (UofT) as well as others indicates that the miss rate is likely much higher, especially in the right colon.

500

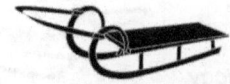

❖ Immunochemical FOBT (iFOBT)

Lesion	Sensitivity (%)
o Cancer	66
− Dukes' A	50
− Dukes' B	70
− Dukes' C/D	78
o HGD	33
o Adenoma ≥ 1 cm	20
o Advanced neoplasia	27
− Proximal	16
− Distal	31

o Test characteristics: Cancer

Fecal Hb Threshold	Sensitivity (%)	Specificity (%)
≥ 50 ng/ml	100	84
≥ 75 ng/ml	94	88
≥ 100 ng/ml	88	90

❖ Fecal DNA testing
- o Basis for Fecal DNA testing (fDNA)
  - Colorectal cancer is a disease of mutated genes
  - Mutations manifest through 3 pathways:
    - Chromosomal Instability
    - Microsomal Instability
    - Hypermethylation of promoter regions
- o Neoplasms shed cells that release DNA and have disordered apoptosis
- o Issues for Fecal DNA Testing
  - Performance is no better than iFOBTs or high-sensitivity guaiac-based tests
  - Testing interval not established
  - Management of positive fDNA test and negative colonoscopy is uncertain
  - Cost is greater than other non-invasive tests

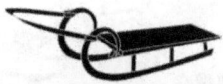

From the following table, calculate the absolute risk (AR) of CRC in a 55 year old patient whose father developed proven CRC at age 59, his 50 year old brother had an adenomatous colonic polyp, and a grandmother and an aunt of unknown age had CRC (baseline absolute risk for 50 year old, 6%).

Familial Setting	RR
o One first-degree relative with CRC	2.3
- < 45 yrs	3.9
- 45 – 59 yrs	2.3
- > 59 yrs	1.8
o Two first-degree relatives with CRC	3.8
o More than two first-degree relatives with CRC	4.3
o One second- or third-degree relative with CRC	1.5
o Two second-degree relatives with CRC	2.3
o One first-degree relative < 60 yrs with an adenoma	2.0

Abbreviation: AR, absolute risk; RR, relative risk

RR=(2.3 x 2.0 x 2.3)= 10.5; Absolute risk for average risk person over age 50, 6%; absolute risk for this person, (10.6 x 6%= RRxAR >60%)

Printed with permission: Winawer SJ. *Best Pract Res Clin Gastroenterol* 2007; 21(6): pg. 1035.

- Give the recommended age of onset (years) and interval (every "x" years) for CRC screening for each of the following groups.

Group	Age	Interval
o Average risk	50	10
o Family history:		
– One first-degree relative (parent, sibling or child) with a CRP or AP (adenomatous colonic polyp) at age < 60 or 10 yr younger than the earliest diagnosis in family	40	5
– One first-degree relative (parent, sibling or child) with a CRP or AP (adenomatous colonic polyp) at age > 60	40	10
– Two first-degree relatives with CRC at any age	40	5
– Two second-degree relatives (grandparents, aunt/uncle) with CRC at any age	40	10
– One second degree or third-degree relative (great-grandparent or cousin) with CRC at any age	40	10

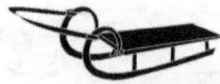

Group	Age	Interval
o Syndromic familial risk:		
familial adenomatous polyposis (FAP): genetic diagnosis, or clinical diagnosis from family history	10	1-2
o HNPCC: genetic diagnosis, or clinical diagnosis from family history	20, or 10 yr earlier than the youngest age of CRC in the family	1-2

Source: *World Gastroenterology Organization and International Digestive Cancer Alliance, chaired by Professor S. Winawek, USA.*

SO YOU WANT TO BE A GASTROENTEROLOGIST!

- Give the performance characteristics of FOBT and FIT for colonic adenomas and CRC.

❖ FOBT (fecal occult blood test, guaiac-based relying on the peroxidase reaction)
  - o Only adenomas > 1.5 cm bleed and thus FOBT sensitivity depends on the size of the lesions in the test group
  - o False negative for adenomas, 75%
  - o False positive (red meat, vegetables containing peroxidases [e.g., horseradish])
  - o PPV (positive predictive value): adenomas, ~30%; CRC, ~10%
  - o Annual FOBT (slide guaiac test for pseudoperoxidase activity of hemoglobin) results in 33% ↓ CRC mortality as compared with non-tested control group

❖ FIT (fecal immunochemical testing for human globin)
  - o Sensitivity (advanced adenomas), 25%
  - o Specificity (adenomas), 97% (93% for advanced adenomas)
  - o Fecal immunochemical tests (FIT) are preferred over guaiac-based fecal occult blood tests for CRC screening
  - o In a validation experiment performed at room temperature, conversion of test outcomes only occurred 10 days or longer after fecal sampling

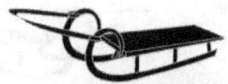

- Give the guidelines for screening and surveillance for the early detection of colorectal adenomas and cancer in individuals at increased risk or at high risk.

Risk Category	Age to Begin	Recommendation for Colonoscopy

- **Increased risk – patients with history of polyps at prior colonoscopy**
  - ○ Patients with small rectal hyperplastic polyps
    - -
    - ▪ Colonoscopy or other screening options at intervals recommended for average-risk individuals
    - ▪ An exception is patients with a hyperplastic polyposis syndrome.
    - ▪ They are at increased risk for adenomas and colorectal cancer and need to be identified for more intensive follow-up.
  - ○ Patients with 1 or 2 small tubular adenomas with low-grade dysplasia
    - – 5 to 10 years after the initial polypectomy
    - ▪ The precise timing within this interval should be based on other clinical factors (such as prior colonoscopy findings, family history, and the preferences of the patient and judgment of the physician)
  - ○ Patients with > 10 adenomas on a single examination
    - – < 3 years after the initial polypectomy
    - ▪ Consider the possibility of an underlying familial syndrome.
  - ○ Patients with sessile adenomas that are removed piecemeal
    - – 2 to 6 months to verify complete removal
    - ▪ Once complete removal has been established by colonoscopy subsequent surveillance needs to be individualized based on the endoscopist's judgment.
    - ▪ Completeness of removal should be based on both endoscopic and pathologic assessments.

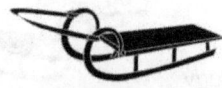

- **Increased risk – patients with colorectal cancer**
  - Patients with colon and rectal cancer should undergo high-quality perioperative colonoscopy to ensure there is no synchronous CRC.
    - 3 to 6 months after cancer resection, if no unresectable metastases are found during surgery: alternatively, colonoscopy.
    - 1 year after the resection or following the performance of the colonoscopy that was performed to clear the colon of synchronous disease.
    - In the case of nonobstructing tumours, this can be done by pre-operative colonoscopy.
    - In the case of obstructing colon cancers, CTC with intravenous contrast or DCBE can be used to detect synchronous neoplasms in the proximal colon.
  - Patient undergoing curative resection for colon or rectal cancer.
    - This colonoscopy at 1 year is in addition to the perioperative colonoscopy for synchronous tumours.
    - If the examination performed at 1 year is normal, then the interval before the next subsequent examination should be 3 years.
    - If that colonoscopy is normal, then the interval before the next subsequent examination should be 5 years.
    - Following the examination at 1 year, the intervals before subsequent examinations may be shortened if there is evidence of HNPCC or if adenoma findings warrant earlier colonoscopy.

Risk Category	Age to Begin	Recommendation for Colonoscopy

- **Increased risk- patients with a family history**

  o Either colorectal cancer or adenomatous polyps in a first-degree relative before age 60 years or in 2 or more first-degree relatives at any age.
  – Age 40 years, or 10 years before the youngest case in the immediate family.
  - Colonoscopy very 5 years.

  o Either colorectal cancer or adenomatous polyps in a first – degree relative age 60 or older or in 2 second – degree relatives with colorectal cancer.
  – Age 40 years.
  - Screening options at intervals recommended for average – risk individuals.
  - Screening should be at an earlier age, but individuals may choose to be screened with any recommended form of testing.

- **High risk**

  o Genetic diagnosis of FAP or suspected FAP without genetic testing evidence.
  – Age 10 to 12 years.
  - Annual FSIG to determine if the individual is expressing the genetic abnormality and counselling to consider genetic testing.
  - If the genetic test is positive, colectomy should be considered.

  o Genetic or clinical diagnosis of HNPCC or individual at increased risk of HNPCC.
  – Age 20 to 25 years, or 10 years before the youngest case in the immediate family.
  - Colonoscopy every 1 to 2 years and counselling to consider genetic testing.
  - Genetic testing for HNPCC should be offered to first-degree relatives of persons with a known inherited MMR gene mutation. It should also be offered when the family mutation is not already known, but 1 of the first 3 of the modified Bethesda criteria is present.

506

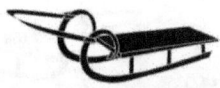

Mastering the Boards: Gastroenterology   A.B.R. Thomson

Risk Category	Age to Begin	Recommendation for Colonoscopy
o Inflammatory bowel disease, chronic ulcerative colitis and Crohn colitis	– Cancer risk begins to be significant 8 years after the onset of pancolitis or 12 to 15 years after the onset of left-sided colitis (UC or CC).	▪ Colonoscopy with biopsies for dysplasia. ▪ Every 1 to 2 years; these patients are best referred to a centre with experience in the surveillance and management of inflammatory bowel disease

Abbreviations: CC, Crohn colitis; CRC, colorectal cancer; CTC, computed tomographic colography; DCBE, double-contrast barium enema; FAP, familial adenomatous polyposis; FSIG, flexible sigmoidoscopy; HNPCC, hereditary nonpolyposis colon cancer (Lynch syndrome); MMR, mismatch repair; UC, ulcerative colitis

Printed with permission: Levin B, et al. *Gastroenterology* 2008;134(5): pg. 1588.

"Success must go hand-in-hand with effort and collaboration."

In Canadians, that means

"There's much more than just putting the puck in the net."

-- Actions Shape Character --

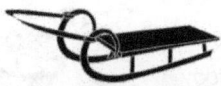

QUALITY ASSURANCE AND COLONOSCOPY

- o Quality assurance using a minimal set of indicators is essential to continuously improve the effectiveness of colonoscopy
- o Split-dose preparation is superior to single-dose preparation for both the quality of preparation and the tolerability
- o The use of variable stiffness colonoscopies is associated with a higher cecal intubation rate than are standard colonoscopies.
- o Of all advanced imaging techniques, panchromoendoscopy is the only one proven to improve the adenoma detection rate
- o Cold biopsy polypectomy seems to be associated with a high incomplete resection rate.

- • Give ways to ↑ polyp detection rate from colonoscopy.
  - o Access performance skills of endoscopist
    - − Identify the adequacy of
    - − Withdrawl time (> 7 min), and possibly retroflection of colonoscopy in rectum
    - − Polyp (or adenomatous polyp) detection rate
    - − Personal detection rate of adenomatous polyps on screening colonoscopy of average risk persons > 50 years of age (males, 25%; females, 15%)
    - − Rate of
      - ▪ Detection of CRC
      - ▪ Perforation
  - o Better bowel cleansing
  - o Better patient sedation
  - o Water instillation
  - o Insertion
    - − Cap-fit colonoscopy
    - − Overtubes
  - o Imaging
    - − Wide-angle colonoscopy
    - − Narrow-band imaging
      - ▪ Interference filters to illuminate the mucosa in narrow red, green and blue
      - ▪ Better visualization of the mucosal structure and vascular networks
      - ▪ Improve in the detection of dysplasia
      - ▪ Narrowing band imaging (NBI) was introduced to overcome the limitations of white light endoscopy (WLE) for adenoma detection.

508

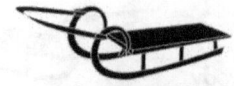

- There is no difference in detection of polyps or adenomas with NBI and WLE.
- There is no difference in miss rates of polyps or adenomas with NBI and WLE.
  - Chromoendoscopy
    - Dyes to stain the colonic mucosa
    - Sensitive and so can detect more dysplasia per (targeted) biopsy
    - Effective surveillance method
  - Electronic chromoendoscopy
    - Blue light for the excitation of tissue specific autofluorescence
    - Superior to conventional endoscopy for detecting dysplasia
  - Confocal laser microscopy
    - Imaging of the microarchitecture of the colonic mucosa and vasculature
    - Using a combination of chromoendoscopy and endomicroscopy, Kiesslich *et al*, reported a 4.75 fold increased detection rate of neoplastic lesions compared with conventional colonscopy alone.

Source: *Gastroenterology and Hepatology* 2009; 6:672

- Give causes of focal white patches on the mucosa seen on colonoscopy.
  - o Mucus
    - Cavity wasted away
  - o Leukoplakia
    - Biopsy diagnosis
  - o Pseudolipomatosis
    - Clear spaces in the mucosa and submucosal on biopsy
    - No individual cells seen in these spaces

Useful background: suggested excellent tables to review the following topics:
- o Endoscopic procedures for which antibiotic prophylaxis is recommended (Feldman M., et al. Sleisenger and Fordtran's Gastrointestinal and Liver Disease. 10th Edition. Saunders/Elsevier, Philadelphia, 2016, Table 40.1, page 654).
- o Side effects of medications used for sedation, analgesia, and reversal (Feldman M., et al. Sleisenger and Fordtran's Gastrointestinal and Liver Disease. 9th Edition. Saunders/Elsevier, Philadelphia, 2010, Table 41.2, page 684).
- o Risk factors for post-ERCP pancreatitis (Feldman M., et al. Sleisenger and Fordtran's Gastrointestinal and Liver Disease. 10th Edition. Saunders/Elsevier, Philadelphia, 2010, Box 41-1, page 684).

- Give the approximate risk of **serious complications** from endoscopic complications per 10^5 procedures.
  - EGD, 3-5
  - EGD removal of foreign bodies, 800
  - EUS, 20
  - EUS for malignant esophageal strictures, 2400
  - EUS-FNA   – Infection (of pancreatic cyst), 1400
                  – Pancreatitis, 100
  - PEG, 150-400
  - ERCP   – Pancreatitis (including injection of pseudocyst), 200-2500
                  – Bleeding (sphincterotomy), 100-200
                  – Ascending cholangitis, 100
                  – Acute cholangitis, 50
                  – Perforation, 50
  - DBE   – Diagnostic, 100
                  – Therapeutic, 400
  - Capsule endoscopy, 100-200
  - Sigmoidoscopy, 10
    - Balloon dilation of stricture, 1000
    - Placement of stents, 500
    - Decompression for acute pseudo-obstruction, 200
    - Therapeutic (polypectomy), 200
    - Diagnostic, 30

    > - Perforation/PPES, 1/1000
    > - Bleeding, 1/500
    > - Polypectomy, 1/1000

  - Colonoscopy
    - Perforation
      - Overall, 0.05 - 0.3%
      - Endoscopic ablation of angioectasias (R > L colon), 2.5%
      - Colonic decompression of Ogilvie syndrome (pseudo-obstruction), 20%
    - Bleeding
      - Overall, 0.1 - 0.6%
      - Polypectomy, 0.9%
    - Post-polypectomy electrocoagulation syndrome (PPES)
      - Abdominal pain, tenderness fever, WBC 1-5 d after polypectomy, 0.003% - 0.1%

Abbreviations: DBE, double balloon enteroscopy; EGD, esophagogastroduodenoscopy; ERCP, endoscopic retrograde cholangiopancreatography; EUS, endoscopic ultrasound; FNA, fine needle aspiration; PEG, percutaneous endoscopic gastroscopy

Source: Feldman M., et al. Sleisenger and Fordtran's Gastrointestinal and Liver Disease. 10th Edition. Saunders/Elsevier, Philadelphia, 2010, page 681-682.

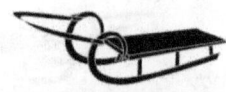

- In the context of the percutaneous endoscopic placement of a double balloon feeding tube, give the "buried bumper syndrome'.
  - If the two balloons of the PEG feeding tube are applied too tightly together, the intragastric balloon may migrate into the wall of the stomach.

- Give the recommendation regarding the need to continue the use of aspirin or clopidogrel with endoscopic procedures with low or high risk of bleeding

Endoscopic Procedure	Continue Aspirin	Continue Clopidogrel
Low risk of bleeding		
– EGD and colonoscopy ± biopsy	Yes	Yes
– EUS without FNA	Yes	Yes
– Digestive stenting	Yes	No
– ERCP stent placement of papillary balloon dilation without endoscopic sphincterotomy	Yes	Yes
– Argon plasma coagulation of angiodysplasia	Yes	Yes
– Colonic polypectomy < 1 cm	Yes	No
– Dilation of digestive stenosis	Yes	No
– EUS with FNA of solid mass	Yes	No
High risk of bleeding		
– Esophageal variceal band ligation	Yes	No
– EMR, ESD	No	No
– Percutaneous endoscopic gastrostomy	Yes	NA
– Endoscopic sphincterotomy	Yes	No
– Ampullary resection	No	No
– Endoscopic sphincterotomy + large balloon papillary dilation	No	No
– EUS with FNA of cystic lesions	No	No
– Colonic polypectomy > 1 cm	Yes	No

Note: Some authorities suggest that the risk of stopping aspirin (ASA) in a patient with an indication for ASA-prophylaxis is higher than the risk of bleeding, and that the ASA should always be continued.

Abbreviations: EGD, esophagogastroduodenoscopy; EMP, endoscopic mucosal resection; ERCP, endoscopic retrograde cholangiopancreatography; ESD, endoscopic submucosal dissection; EUS, endoscopic ultrasonography; FNA, fine-needle aspiration; NA not available

Printed with permission: Blero D, et al. Nat Rev Gastroenterol Hepatol. 2012;9(3):162-72

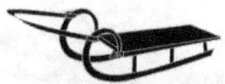

- Give the minimal set of quality indicators, auditable outcome measures and accepted standards in colonoscopy.

Quality Indicator	Outcome Measure	Standard
o Bowel preparation	– Quality of bowel preparation	▪ ≥ 90% described as "excellent" or "adequate" preferably assessed with a validated bowel preparation scale
o Cecal intubation	– Cecal intubation rate with photo-documentation of cecal landmarks	▪ ≥ 90% unadjusted (intention to scope) ▪ ≥ 90% in all colonoscopies and ≥ 95% in screening colonoscopies
o Adenoma detection	– Adenoma detection rate (number of patients with a least 1 adenoma/total number of patients)	▪ ≥ 25 in men and ≥ 15 % in women during screening colonoscopies ▪ ≥ 20% during screening colonoscopy
o Withdrawal time	– Time in minutes from cecal pole to anus	▪ ≥ 6 min inspection time in an intact colon
o Polyp retrieval	– Polyp retrieval rate	▪ ≥ 90% of polypectomy specimens
o Burden	– Gloucester comfort score	▪ Not established
o Complications	– Incidence of perforation	▪ ≤ 1:1,000 colonoscopies (diagnostic or therapeutic) ▪ ≤ 1:500 colonoscopies with polypectomy
	– Incidence of postpolypectomy bleeding	▪ ≤ 1:100 colonoscopies with polypectomy

Printed with permission: Hazewinkel C and Dekker E. Nat Rev Gastro Hep 2011; 8: 554-564, Table 1

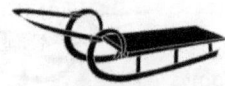

Recurrence Rates of Adenomatous Polyps

- Give the recommended follow-up interval for post-polypectomy colonoscopic surveillance.

Finding on Screening	Follow-up Interval
○ < 10 adenomas	
– 1-2 tubular adenomas < 1 cm	5-10 yrs
– 3-10 adenomas, or any adenoma with villous elements, high-grade dysplasia or $\geq$ 1 cm in size	3 yrs
– Patients with prior advanced adenomas after normal follow-up examination, or only 1-2 small tubular adenomas	< 3 yrs
○ >10 adenomas (possible familial syndrome)	
– Large sessile adenoma removed piecemeal	2-6 months to confirm complete removal
– Small distal hyperplastic polyps without adenomas	10 yrs
– Proximal colon hyperplastic polyps	Interval uncertain
– Sessile serrated adenomatous (SSA) polyp	Same as for adenoma

Adapted from: Rex DK. *2008 ACG Annual Postgraduate course book*: pg. 90; and Levin B, et al. *Gastroenterology* 2008;134(5):1588.

➢ Further information of rates of conversion of colonic adenoma to carcinoma

  ○ Overall, annual conversion rate of 0.25

  ○ Adenomas
- Annual rate of conversion, 3%
- > 1 cm, 3%
- Villous components, 17%
- Severe dysplasia, 37%

  ○ Mean doubling time of CRC, ~ 620 days

513

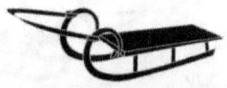

- o The index colonoscopy shows adenomatous polyp (s). The recurrence rates of adenomatous polyps or CRC are dependent on the number of index polyps, and the duration of follow up

# of Adenomas Removed at Index Colonoscopy	Types of Recurrent Lesion	Approximate Recurrence Rate at 10 yrs
1	Polyps	30%
> 1		70%
1	CRC	2%
> 1		10%

- o In addition to number of polyps and duration of follow-up after the index colonoscopy, other features which increase the cumulative risk of recurrence include:
  - – Patient
    - ▪ 60 years
    - ▪ CRC in a parent
  - – Polyp
    - ▪ Number
    - ▪ Size
    - ▪ Severe dysplasia
    - ▪ Villous
  - – Duration
- o The presence of one or more of the first three features (> 1 cm, severe dysplasia, villous architecture) allows an adenomatous polyps to be called AAP (advanced adenomatous polyp).
- o The risk of AAP recurrence depends on duration of follow up and the presence of three additional risk factors (ARF):
  - – ≥ 3 index adenomas
  - – > 60 years
  - – A parent with CRC
- o Timelines
  - – In order to determine when a respect colonoscopy needs to be performed after an initial procedure is free of polyps or shows polyp(s) which may recur, it is important to know the **natural history of polyps**, i.e., when polyps may occur after the index colonoscopy.
  - – For 1 cm polyps (history unknown), the cumulative risk of carcinoma (Ca) developing is approximately 1% per year:

Time Interval, Years	Risk of Ca Developing
5	2.5%
10	8%
20	24%

514

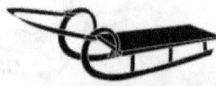

- For a polyp < 0.5 cm, it takes 2 to 3 years to become 1 cm in size (~0.25 cm per year)
- Thus, the rate of growth of adenoma is slow (~0.25 cm per year, before becoming the worrisome size of < 1 cm, and once 1 cm in size, the cumulative risk of the development of CRC is about 1% per year.

- Give the approximate polyp recurrence rates.

Time (years) After Index Polypectomy	Usual AAP	ARF
3	4%	10%
6	8%	20%

Abbreviations: AAP, adenoma with advanced pathology; ARF, additional risk factors

- Give the features of a malignant colonic polyp which suggest a favourable prognosis.

    o Differentiation margin   – Well or moderately clear, or > 2 mm margin

    o Invasion   – Submucosa   No
                         – Veins   No
                         – Lymphatics   No

Adapted from Sleisenger and Fordtran's Gastrointestinal and Liver Disease. 10th Edition. Saunders/Elsevier, Philadelphia, 2016, Table 126-8, page 2228.

SO YOU WANT TO BE A GASTROENTEROLOGIST!

- Give colonoscopic (gross) features which distinguish between an adenoma-like endoscopically resectable DALM and a non-adenoma-like endoscopically non-resectable DALM*.

Colonoscopic Features	Adenoma-Like	Non-Adenoma-Like
o Shape	Sessile/ Pedunculated	Sessile
o Borders		
– Circumscribed	Yes	No
– Clearly visible	Yes	No
o Surface	Smooth	Irregular
o Ulcer/necrosis	No	Yes
o Stricture	No	Yes
o Tethering of mucosa	No	Yes

* These may be referred to as areas of flat dysplasia

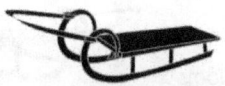

Mastering the Boards: Gastroenterology   A.B.R. Thomson

- Give the post-polypectomy recommendations for surveillance colonoscopy.

	Next Colonoscopy (yrs)	
❖ Non-serrated Lesions	10	No polyps
	5 – 10	1 – 2 TA (tubular adenoma) < 10 mm
	3	3 – 10 TA ≥ 1 TA > 10 mm ≥ 1 VA (villous adenoma)
	< 3	> 10 adenomas
	1	Adenoma plus HGD (high grade dysplasia)
❖ Serrated Lesions	10	Hyperplastic polyps (HPs) < 10 mm in rectosigmoid colon
	5	SSA < 10 mm (sessile serrated adenoma)
	3	SSA > 10 mm SSA plus dysplasia TSA (traditional serrated adenoma)
	1	SPS (serrated polyposis syndrome)

Adapted from: Sleisenger and Fordtran's Gastrointestinal and Liver Disease. 10th Edition. Saunders/Elsevier, Philadelphia, 2016, Table 129-9, page 2230.

From the "Acrin" trial of **CT colography** (NEJM 2008;359: pp 1207-1219), give the sensitivity (SENS), specificity (SPEC), positive predictive value (PPV) and negative predictive value (NPV) for detecting colonic polyps ranging from 5 to 10 mm.

➤ Efficacy and test performance characteristics

	>5mm	>6mm	>7mm	>8mm	>9mm	>1cm
SENS	65%	78%	84%	87%	90%	90%
>5mm	>6mm	>7mm	>8mm	>9mm	>1cm	>5mm
○ SPEC	89%	88%	87%	87%	86%	86%
○ PPV	45%	40%	35%	31%	25%	23%
○ NPV	95%	98%	99%	99%	99%	99%

Source: Johnson CD, Chen MH, Toledano AY, et al. *N Engl J Med.* 2008; 359(12):1207-17.

- Give the radiation risk from CTC (CT colography).
  - Average natural background radiation risk in USA is 3 mSv/year; average CTC effective dose, 2-5 mSv/year (Cash BD. *ACG Annual Scientific Meeting Symposia Session* 2009;97-100)
    - Primary tumours affected by radiation (thyroid, breast, lung) are shielded with CTC
    - Rates of case induction by radiation fall dramatically after 35 yr of age

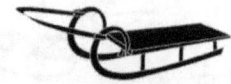

INTESTINAL POLYPOSIS SYNDROMES

Please see Feldman M., et al. Sleisenger and Fordtran's Gastrointestinal and Liver Disease. 10th Edition. Saunders/Elsevier, Philadelphia, 2016, Box 126-2, page 2235; Table 126-11, page 2236; Table 126-12, page 2239; Table 126-13, page 2240; and Table 126-14, page 2244.

➢ Classification

● Give the classification of multiple colonic polyps, based upon inheritance.

❖ Inherited
- o Adenomas
  - – FAP (familial adenomatosis)
  - – Variants of FAP
    - ▪ Gardner
    - ▪ Turcot
    - ▪ AFAP (attenuated FAP)
  - – MUTYH
  - – Bloom syndrome
  - – Familial tooth agenesis syndrome
- o Hamartomas
  - – PJS (Peutz-Jeghers Syndrome)
  - – JPS (Juvenile polyposis syndrome)
  - – PTEN hamartomas
    - ▪ Cowden disease
    - ▪ BRR (Bannayan-Ruvalcaba-Riley) syndrome
  - – Neurofibromatosis and ganglioneuromatosis
  - – Tuberous sclerosis

❖ Non-inherited
- o Inflammatory (pseudopolyps)
- o Cap polyposis
- o HPS (hyperplastic polyposis syndrome)
  - – ≥ 5 hyperplastic polyps proximal to sigmoid colon, 2 of which are 10 mm; or
- o Lymphomatous polyposis
  - – Hodgkin and NHL (non-Hodgkin lymphoma)
  - – MZL (mantle zone lymphoma)
- o NLH (nodular lymphoid hyperplasia)
  - – May be associated with Gardner syndrome
- o Cronkite-Canada syndrome

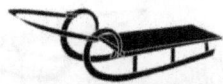

- Give the **polyposis syndromes**, based upon the adenomatous and hamartomatous subtypes.

Syndrome	Inheritance Pattern	Polyp Type	Commercial Gene Mutation Testing
o FAP	AD	Adenomatous	APC
o AFAP	AD	Adenomatous	APC
o MAP	AR (AD)	Adenomatous	MYH
o PJS	AD	Hamartomatous: Peutz-Jeghers polyps	STK11
o JPS	AD	Hamartomatous: Hamartomatous: juvenile	SMAD4 or BMPR1A
o CS	AD	Hamartomatous:juvenile, ganglioneuroma, lipoma, hyperplastic	PTEN

Abbreviations: AD, autosomal dominant; AR, autosomal recessive; AFAP, attenuated familial adenomatous polyposis; CS, Cowden syndrome; FAP, familial adenomatous polyposis; JPS, juvenile polyposis; MAP, modified adenomatous polyposis; PJS, Peutz-Jegher syndrome

➢ Genetics

CLINICAL GEM

- Most inherited GI conditions are autosomal dominant; only a few are autosomal recessive.

- So, learn the inherited GI conditions which are autosomal recessive, and all the others are dominant.

– Small intestine	▪ Abetalipoproteinemia
– Colon	▪ MUTYN
– Liver	▪ HH (hereditary hemochromatosis)
	▪ WD (Wilson disease)

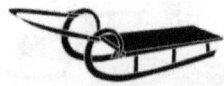

518

- Give inherited colon cancer syndromes, and for each give the affected gene(s), and the demonstrated mutation frequency (%) in the index case, and the likelihood (%) of finding a mutation in the index case.

Syndrome	Gene(s)	Demonstrated Mutation Frequency (%) Index Case
o FAP, AFAP	– APC, attenuated APC (dominant)	90
o MAP	– MYH (recessive)	100
o HNPCC	– MLH1, MSH2, MSH6	50-70
o Peutz-Jegher	– Germline mutation of serine/threonidine kinase gene (STK11) or chromosome 19	50
o Juvenile polyposis	– SMAD4 on chromosome 8; BMPR1A,on chromosome 10	50
o Cowden syndrome	– PTEN	90

Source: World Gastroenterology Organization and International Digestive Cancer Alliance, chaired by Professor S. Winawek, USA.

o FAP, AFAP, HNPCC and MAP are adenomatous polyp syndromes, PJS and JPS are hamartomatous and CS includes hamartomatous, juvenile, ganglioneuronia, lipoma or hyperplastic polyps

o Gene mutation testing includes: FAP and AFAP, APC gene; HNHCC, mismatch repair gene; MAP, MYN gene; PJS, STKII; JPS, SMAD4 or BMPRIA; CS, PTEN

Abbreviations: AFAP, attenuated familial adenomatous polyposis; CS, Cowden's syndrome; FAP, familial adenomatous polyposis; HNPCC, hereditary non-polyposis colon cancer (Lynch syndrome); JPS, juvenile polyposis syndrome ; MAP, MYH-associated polyposis; PJS, Peutz-Jegher's syndrome

Source: Burke, Carol A. Polyposis syndrome: making sense of genetic testing. *2009 ACG Annual Postgraduate Course*: 192-196.

"Always be true to yourself and follow your dreams!"

LaDonna M. Cook

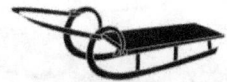

Mastering the Boards: Gastroenterology   A.B.R. Thomson

Familial Adenomatous Polyposis (FAP) Syndrome

➢ Demography

   o Prevalence and Penetrance
      - FAP $20/10^5$, 80% prevalence of CRC
      - Represents ~ 1% of all CRCs

• Give the median age of onset of CRC in the phenotypes of FAP.

Phenotype	Age, yrs
o Profuse	39
o Intermediate	39-50
o Attenuated (AFAP)	>50 (R colon)
o MYH (MAP)	>60 (recessive)

SO YOU WANT TO BE A GASTROENTEROLOGIST!

• Give the names, genetic mutations, and recommended frequency of surveillance colonoscopy in three **attenuated syndromes**.

   o AFAP (attenuated form of FAP)
      - < 100 adenomas, often in proximal colon
      - Some duodenal and gastric polyp associations as classic FAP
      - Loss of the 5' and 3' regions of FAP
      - CRC develops later than in FAP, ~5 years rather than 32 years
      - Surveillance colonoscopy of 2 year

   o APC gene pathway mutations
      - B-catenin
      - Axin

   o MUTYH (aka MYH) gene
      - 15-100 colonic adenomas
      - Defective MUTYH gene causes G:C → T:A translocation
      - Autosomal recessive
      - ↑ risk of CRC with biallelic MUTYH mutations
      - Colonoscopic screening age 18 to 20 with surveillance of 2 years
      - May be associated with outcomes and CHRPN (congenital hypertrophy of the retinal pigmental epithelium)

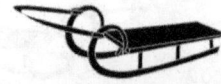

- ➢ Genetics
  - ○ Mutation of the tumour suppressor gene on the long arm of chromosome 5 q21 – q22 region
  - ○ MYH is a base-excision-repair gene on chromosome 1
  - ○ 70% of the germline defects in APC are inherited, while 30% occur spontaneously
  - ○ Mutations or deletions in the APC gene are present in 90% of FAP and 30% of AFAP
    - – Truncated germline mutation (stop codon) of first allele from affected parent causes APC mutation in all cells in the body
    - – Loss of normal phosphorylation of B-catenin, with loss of inactivation of B-catenin, leading to instability of chromosomes, and their segregation
    - – There may also be germline mutations of axin
    - – Unaffected parent passes on somatic mutations in the mutations in the mutation cluster region near the centre of all APC gene or lost second allele

- • Give the methods used for genetic testing in FAP to confirm the diagnosis of FAP in suspected cases, and to determine if a person from a family with FAP is a gene carrier.

  - ○ *In vitro* protein truncation in FAP
    - – Detects the presence of truncating mutations in vitro
    - – Detects a mutation in 80% to 90% of affected families known to have FAP
    - – Near 100% effective in family members once the presence of a mutation has been found in an affected person

  - ○ Gene sequencing
    - – Often preceded by single-strand conformational polymorphism (SSCP) or denaturing gradient gel electrophoresis (DGGE) to narrow the area of the gene where sequencing is to be performed
    - – Up to 95% effective in finding a disease-causing mutation if it is present
    - – Near 100% effective in family members once the presence of a mutation has been found in an affected person

  - ○ Linkage testing
    - – Used if other methods unsuccessful
    - – Two or more affected persons from two generations must be living for DNA to be obtained
    - – Effective in >95% of families, with >98% accuracy with present linkage markers

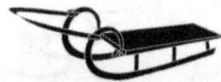

- Genotype-phenotype correlations:
  - These have not yet been found to be of precise use in the clinical setting
  - The following correlations have been made:
    - CHRPE (congenital hypertrophy of the retinal pigment epithelium): present in families with mutations distal to exon 9 of the APC gene
    - Dense polyposis: present with mutations in the mid portion of exon 15
    - AFAP/AAPC: found with mutation in the extreme proximal or distal end of the gene
    - Osteomas and desmoids (Gardner's syndrome): more commonly found with mutations in the distal portion of exon 15

Abbreviations: CHRPE, congenital hypertrophy of the retinal pigment epithelium; DGGE, denaturing gradient gel electrophoresis; SSCP, single-strand conformational polymorphism

Adapted from: Doxey BW, Kuwada SK, Burt RW. *Clin Gastroenterol Hepatol.* 2005;3(7):633-41; and Burt R, Neklason DW. *Gastroenterology* 2005;128(6):1696-716.

SO YOU WANT TO BE A GASTROENTEROLOGIST

- Give the role of APC gene function, nuclear β-catenin, the Wat signal pathway, the LEF (lymphoid enhancer factor) / TCF (T-cell factor) family in the development of CRC.

- Normal
  - APC (tumour suppressor) gene
    - Association with E-cadherin → cell-cell adhesion
    - Binds β-catenin → ↑ phosphorylation
    - ↓ β-catenin - ↓ stimulation of Wnt-Tcf signal pathway
      - ↓ proliferation
      - ↑ apoptosis

- APC gene mutation
  - ↓ cell-cell adhesion

  - ↓ β-catenin phosphorylation
    - ↑ unphosphorylated β catenin complex with LEF/TCF
    - ↑ Wnt-Tcf

  - Target genes
    - ↑ proliferation
    - ↓ apoptosis

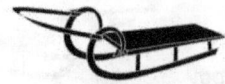

➤ Clinical

  o 100% will develop CRC by age 40 years

  o With AFAP, the adenomas develop later than with FAP, there are fewer polyps (< 100), the polyps tend to be on the right side of the colon, CRC develops at a later age, and 80% rather than 100% develop CRC

  o Screening must be done for gastric fundic gland polyps, periampullary polyps and for duodenal and cancer

  o Gardner's syndrome is FAP plus extraintestinal lesions: CHRPE (congenital hypertrophy of the retinal epithelium, thyroid cancer, sebaceous cysts, supernumerary teeth, osteomas, fibromas, lipomas

  o MAP was originally considered to be due to bi-allelic mutations in the base excursion repair gene (Y165C, G382D) MYN (recessive inheritance), but cases of mono-allelic mutations are being now described (autosomal dominant inheritances)

  o 10-500 adenomatous polyps, with a 50% risk of CRC

  o Classic FAP and its variants
    – Gardner syndrome
    – Turcot syndrome
    – Attenuated FAP (AFAP)

  o Synchronous CRCs occur in about half of FAP patients.

  o Even with recommended colonoscopic screening and surveillance, about a quarter already have CRC (perhaps time of recommended colectomy needs to be moved earlier).

Extracolonic Periampullary Adenomas in FAP

  o Stomach
    – A polyp in the fundic area of the stomach is a polyp in the fundus, and should not be called a fundic gland until the histopathology of the lesion proves this diagnosis of fundic gland polyps
    – In FAP, when polyps are seen in the fundic area of the stomach
      ▪ < 5% are adenomas
      ▪ 95% are fundic gland polyps (FGP) however at least a quarter of these FGPs already have epithelial dysplasia

  o Small bowel FAP polyps
    – Jejunum, 40%
    – Ileum, 20%
    – Distinguished from lymphoid hyperplasia
    – Low risk of malignancy

523

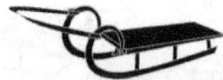

- o Duodenum
    - – Ampullary cancer
    - – Duodenal cancer
    - – ↑ risk of epithelial dysplasia is associated with
        - ▪ ↑ size
        - ▪ Site-associated duodenal polyposis
        - ▪ Association – Non-H.pylori antral gastritis
- o Duodenal FAP polyps
    - – Occur in 60% to 90% FAP patients
    - – Usually periampullary region, and > half involve the ampulla of Vater
    - – ~10% lifetime risk of duodenal cancer

- o About 60% to 90% of FAP patients have periampullary adenomatous polyps, and about 10% will develop duodenal cancer.

- o Clearly, FAP patients require surveillance with SV-EGD (side-viewing EGD, esophagogastroduodenoscopy).

- o Risk stratification for the development of duodenal cancer is based on the Spigelman classification.

- o This Spigelman classification provides guidance for EGD surveillance of these duodenal adenomas. Until EUS has refined our appreciation for any change in the currently recommended EGD surveillance guidelines, this remains the standard of care.

- o Screening with SV-EGD should begin at 2 years of age, and then be followed by regular SV-EGD surveillance.

- Give the recommended interval of duodenoscopic screening (visualization and biopsy) of duodenal polyps in FAP, using the Spigelman staging criteria.

Score	1	2	3
o Polyp count	1-4	5-20	>20
o Polyp size (mm)	1-4	5-10	>10
o Histologic type	Tubular	Tubulovillous	Villous
o Grade of intraepithelial neoplasia	Low-grade	Intermediate*	High-grade

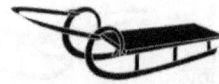

Grade	Surveillance Interval (years)
0	5
I, II	3
III	1
IV	3-6 months – pylorus preserving, pancreas sparing duodenectomy

Stage 0: 0 points, Stage I: 1-4 points, Stage II: 5-6 points, Stage III: 7-8 points, and stage IV: 9-12 points

*Intermediate grade is not existent in actualized classifications of intraepithelial neoplasia

Printed with permission: Schulmann K, et al. *Best Pract Res Clin Gastroenterol* 2007; 21(3): pg. 413.

Turcot Syndrome

> Definition: ".... a syndrome of familial colonic polyposis with primary tumours of the central nervous system" (Sleisenger and Fordtran's Gastrointestinal and Liver Disease. 9th Edition. Saunders/Elsevier, Philadelphia, 2010).

SO YOU WANT TO BE A GASTROENTEROLOGIST!

The Turcot syndrome is considered to be variant of FAP, and as such has a mutation in the APC gene.

- Give the reason why the Turcot syndrome may be misclassified, and should be considered either as a variant of HNPCC, or an overlap of both FAP and HNPCC.

  o In Turcot syndrome, the gene mutations are in FAP, or in DNA MMR, the same germline mutation seen in HNPCC.

- Give the difference in the CNS presentation of Turcot syndrome, depending upon which germline mutation is present.

  o Gene mutation in
    - APC
      - Medulloblastomas
    - DNA MMR
      - Glioblastoma multiforme tumours (familial tooth agenesis)
  o It may be surprising to learn, but there are actually at least two attenuated adenomatous polyposis syndromes.

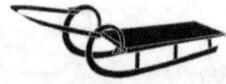

Garner Syndrome (GS)

- o A variant of FAP with numerous extraintestinal associations
- o Extraintestinal findings

- Give the extraintestinal associations of the Gardner syndrome (GS) variant of FAP.

  - o CNS — Medulloblastoma (Turcot syndrome)
  - o Eye — CHRPE (congenital hypertrophy of the retinal pigmented epithelium)
    - Multiple in 63%
    - Bilateral in 87%
  - o Teeth — Impacted teeth
    - Extra teeth
    - Supernumerary teeth
    - Familial tooth agenesis" is caused by mutation in APC pathway (AXIN2)
      - Both adenomatous and hyperplastic colonic polyps
  - o Bone — Osteomas
    - Jaw (in 90% of GS)
    - Cysts
    - Skull
    - Long bones
    - Exostoses
  - o Soft tissue tumours (benign) — Desmoid tumours (Diffuse mesenteric fibromatosis)
    - Fibromas
    - Lipomas
      - $300/10^5$ person-years
      - Treat with NSAIDs and tamoxifin chemotherapy, colectomy small bowel transplantation
      - May be a lethal association
  - o Mesentery — Mesenteric fibromatosis
  - o Endocrine tumours — Thyroid papillary tumour
    - Adrenal

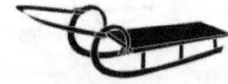

o Skin
- Desmoid tumours
- Fibromas
- Lipoma
- Sebaceous cysts
- Epidermoid (aka "inclusion") cysts

Abbreviations: CHRPE, congenital hypertrophy of retinal pigmented epithelium (pigmented spots on the fundus of the eye)

CHRPE

Cute Quotes

"The presence of multiple [CHRPE] lesions appears to be a reliable marker for gene carriage in FAP" (Feldman M., et al. Sleisenger and Fordtran's Gastrointestinal and Liver Disease. 9th Edition. Saunders/Elsevier, Philadelphia, 2010, page 2180; and page 2184; and 10th Edition, 2016, page 2242).

*Note: CHRPE is also seen in MUTYH.

Exam Alert

o The clinical examiner tells you that the patient has colonic polyps and hands you a fundoscope.

o She/he is expecting you to look for pigmented lesions in the ocular fundus, suggesting CHRPE in the Gardner variant of FAP.

MCQ Trick

o Remember: FAP in its classical form may be associated with dental abnormalities and osteomas of the jaw, without being considered to be a Gardner variant.

o Also remember, osteomas and CHRPH may occur in MUTYH.

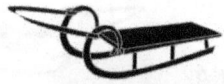

Desmoid Tumour

➢ Treatment

- Give the clinical management of FAP (familial adenomatous polyposis)

- Genetic testing

  - o Consider genetic testing between ages 10 to 12 years, as it will first be clinically useful.

  - o May need to begin in first decade of life to determine who should be screened for hepatoblastoma.

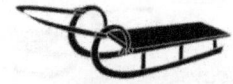

Mastering the Boards: Gastroenterology   A.B.R. Thomson

- GI tract screening

  - o Colon cancer risk > 90%

  - o Sigmoidoscopy in gene carriers every 1 to 2 years, beginning at age 10 years, or in all at-risk persons if genetic testing is not done or not informative.

  - o Colonoscopy every 2 years beginning at age 20 in families with AFAP/AAPC, or sometimes earlier, depending on the age of polyp emergence in other family members

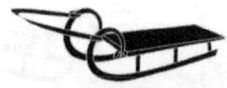

Mastering the Boards: Gastroenterology   A.B.R. Thomson

- Upper GI endoscopy
  - Upper GI tract (5-10% cancer risk for duodenal or peri-ampillary, 0.5% for gastric)
  - Begin when colon polyps emerge or by age 25 years
  - Repeat every 1 to 3 years, depending on the number of polyps, their size and histology
  - Side viewing should be performed as part of the examination to carefully identify and examine the duodenal papilla.
- Small bowel
  - Diagnostic imaging should be done before colectomy.
  - Should be done if numerous or large adenomas are present in the duodenum
  - Frequency determined by number and size of lesions found
- Pancreas (2% cancer risk) -periodic US (abdominal ultrasound) after age 20
- Hepatoblastoma (1.6 % of children <5 yrs) EUS (endoscopic ultrasound), AFP (alpha-fetoprotein) during first decade of life
- Non GI tract screening
  - Thyroid (2%) – annual thyroid exam starting age 20
  - Cerebellar meduloblastoma (<1%) – possible periodic head CT

Adapted from: Half EE, and Bresalier RS. *Curr Opin Gastroenterol* 2004;20(1):32-42.

- Give the recommended method, age to begin, interval of screening, and management of the person with FAP.

Screening Method	Age to Begin	Interval	Management
o Colonoscopy or flexible sigmoidoscopy –	10-12 years, or late teens if attenuated FAP	▪ If polyps are detected, screen annually until colectomy	- Colectomy is recommended when polyps become too numerous to monitor safely, or if polyps are ≥1 cm or exhibit advanced histology. - Removal of the rectum should be based on polyp burden and family history.

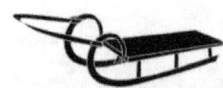

Mastering the Boards: Gastroenterology   A.B.R. Thomson

Screening Method	Age to Begin	Interval	Management
o Flexible sigmoidoscopy	– Within two years after colectomy	▪ Every 6 months to 3 years depending on polyp size and number	- Chemoprevention with NSAIDs may be considered
o EGD with end and side viewing instrument	– 20-25 years or at the onset of colonic polyps	▪ 3 yrs if stage[1] 0, II ▪ 2 yrs if stage[1] III ▪ 6-12 months if stage[1] 4	- Chemoprevention with NSAIDs is less effective for upper GI adenomas
o Physical examination	– 10 to 12 years	▪ Annually	
o Physical exam, hepatic ultrasound, and alphafetoprotein	– 6 months	▪ Every 6 months during first decade of life	
o Determined by location of suspected desmoids, often abdominal CT	– When palpable mass or relevant symptoms present		

[1]Spigelman staging criteria

Printed with permission: Burt RW. *2007 AGA Institute Postgraduate Course.* pg. 236.

Trick Question

┌──┐

SO YOU WANT TO BE A GASTROENTEROLOGIST!

- Give the relative risk (RR) for the ↑ risk of breast cancer with GI cancers associated with BRCA2 mutations.

Site	RR
o Cholangiocarcinoma	5.0
o Pancreatic cancer	3.5
o Gastric cancer	2.6

Note: breast cancer is **not** associated with ↑ risk with colonic polyps, except for PJS (Peutz-Jegher syndrome; 54%) and CS (cowden syndrome; 25 to 50%).

Source: The Cancer risks in BRCA2 mutation carriers. The Breast Cancer Linkage Consortium. *J Natl Cancer Inst.* 1999;91(15):1310.

└──┘

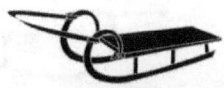

Mastering the Boards: Gastroenterology   A.B.R. Thomson

Hereditary Non-Polyposis Colon Cancer (HNPCC, aka Lynch Syndrome)

Definition Alert
- o HNPCC is a familial/inherited causes of colorectal cancer, but it does not cause colonic polyposis

➤ Genetics
- o Autosomal dominant, high penetrance
- o Germline mutation in DNR MMR (mismatch repair) genes in 80%
- o The 3 most common germline mutations in these DNA MMR genes are
  - – Chromosomes 2
    - ▪ hMSH2 (40% to 50%)
- o Chromosome 3
  - – hMLH1 (20% to 30%)

MCQ Alert
- o HNPCC/Lynch syndrome is a type of inherited CRC, but is not a polyposis syndrome.

- • Give the characteristics, associated cancers and genetic testing of Lynch syndrome.

Genes	Genetic Testing	Lifetime Cancer Risks		Other Features Reported in Some Case
o MLH1	– Full sequence of the coding	▪ Colon	50-80%	▪ Sebaceous adenomas, epitheliomas and Keratoxanthomas
o MSH2	– Regions of MLH1, MSH2, and MSH6	▪ Endometrium	20-60%	▪ Café-au-lait spots
o MSH6		▪ Stomach	11-19%	▪ Brain tumours
o PMS2	– Large deletion analysis with Southern blot or MLPA[1]	▪ Ovary	9-12%	▪ Hematological malignancies hav been reported in individuals with biallelic mismatch repair mutations
		▪ Hepatobiliary tract	2-7%	
	– MSI[2] and IHC[3] for the mismatch repair proteins	▪ Urinary tract infection	4-5%	
		▪ Small bowel	1-4%	
	– MLH1 methylation and BRAF testing to help differentiate sporadic MSI tumours from those due to Lynch syndrome	▪ Brain/CNS	1-3%	
		▪ Sebaceous carcinoma of the skin	1%	

[1]Microsatellite instability, [2]Immunohistochemistry, [3]Multiplex Ligation-dependent Probe Amplification

Printed with permission: Burt RW. *2007 AGA Institute Postgraduate Course.* 237.

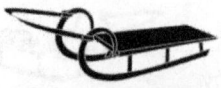

- The Amsterdam and the Bethesda Criteria were developed to justify the screening for MMR gene mutations.
  - Increasingly, screening for MMR genes is being performed in all persons diagnosed with colorectal cancer (CRC).

Amterdam Criteria (3-2-1)

- ≥ 3 first degree relatives with CRC
- 2 generations affect with CRC
- ≥ 1 < 50 yr old
- ≥ 1 first degree relative of the other family members

- Approaches

In families not meeting the Amsterdam criteria, three approaches have been suggested:

- The frequent presence of micro-satellite errors in tumour tissue is called micro-satellite instability (MSI)
  - MSI is present in >90% of colon cancers in HNPCC. MSI is present in only about 15% of sporadic colon cancers, and occurs usually by a different mechanism.
  - MSI is easily detected in tumour tissue and is often used as a marker that leads to the suspicion of HNPCC.
  - It has been suggested that MSI testing be done on tumours when one of the "Bethesda criteria" are met. They are as follows:
  - Individuals with cancer in families that meet the Amsterdam criteria
  - Individuals with two HNPCC-related cancers, including synchronous and metachronous colorectal cancers or associated extracolonic cancers*

- Apply MSI testing to the colon cancer tissue in the following situations and when positive, perform mutation findings in DNA from peripheral blood:
  - CRC diagnosis <50 yrs
  - CRC plus one first-degree relative with colon or endometrial cancer
  - CRC plus a previous colon or endometrial cancer
  - With this method, 24% of colon cancer cases will undergo MSI testing of the tumour, and 4% of colon cancer cases will have mutation finding in the MMR gene

- Use a specific logistic model applied to an extended family that includes kindred structure and known cancer cases
  - If the model predicts >20% chance of HNPCC, go directly to mutation finding.
  - If the model predicts <20% chance of HNPCC, first do MSI and if positive, go to mutation finding

533

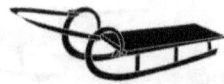

A.B.R. Thomson

- o The Amsterdam criteria for HNPCC do not include the extracolonic cancers (Lynch tumours) which may occur in these families
  - – The Bethesda guidelines contain reference to both the colonic and extracolonic cancers, and serve as guidelines as to who with CRC should be tested for microsatellite instability (MSD).
  - – The Bethesda criteria were developed to identify persons whose tumours should be tested for microsatellite instability, the tumour fingerprint, the DNA MMR gene mutation.
- o Go directly to MMR mutation finding if one of the first three Bethesda criteria for testing tumour tissue is positive, but use age <50 years, rather than 45 yrs. In one study this approach gave a sensitivity of 94%, and a specificity of 49%.
  - – Over 95% of families in whom mutations have been found have mutations of either the MSH2 or MSH1 genes, which are responsible for replication error repair.
  - – These types of errors usually occur during DNA replication.
  - – They are most often one or several base pairs in length.
  - – Mutation of the MMR genes leads to rapid accumulation of relocation error.
  - – Frequently are found in DNA repeats, singlets, doublets, or triplets, called microsatellites
  - – Individuals with CRC and a first-degree relative with CRC and/or diagnosed at age < 45 yrs, and an adenoma diagnosed at age <45 yrs.
  - – Individuals with CRC or endometrial cancer diagnosed at age <45 yrs.
  - – Individuals with right-sided colorectal cancer with an undifferentiated pattern (solid/ cribriform) on histopathology diagnosed at age <45 yrs.
  - – Individuals with signet-ring-cell-type colorectal cancer diagnosed at age <45 yrs.
  - – Individuals with adenomas diagnosed at age <40yrs.
  - – Endometrial, ovarian, gastric, hepatobiliary, or small bowel cancer or transitional cell carcinoma of the renal pelvis or ureter.
  - – Genetic errors that accumulate when the MMR genes are mutated and dysfunctional are quite specific and include genes such as TGF-beta and BAX.
  - – Mutations in any one of the MMR genes leads to HNPCC.

Adapted from: Sleisenger and Fordtran's Gastrointestinal and Liver Disease. 10th Edition. Saunders/Elsevier, Philadelphia, 2016, Box 127-2, page 2263; and Box 127-3, page 2264.

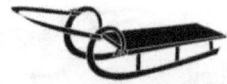

Bethesda Criteria (for testing tumour tissue)

- o Persons who have had 2 Lynch tumours

- o Persons with a Lynch tumour with a first degree relative under 50

- o Persons with a Lynch tumour in at least 2 first- or second-degree relatives at any age

- o CRC diagnosed before age 50

- o CRC with MSI-related histological features diagnosed before age 60

- ❖ The revised Bethesda guidelines

  - o Colorectal cancer under 50 years of age

  - o Synchronous or metachronous Lynch syndrome related cancers[1] regardless of the age at diagnosis

  - o Colorectal cancer that exhibits histological features associated with the MSI[2] prior to age 60 years

  - o Individuals with colorectal cancer and a first-degree relative with a Lynch syndrome-related tumour[1], and at least one of the two diagnosed under age 50 years

  - o Individuals with colorectal cancer who have two or more first- or second-degree relatives affected with Lynch syndrome related cancers[1], regardless of age

[1]Lynch syndrome related cancers for these guidelines include colorectal, endometrial, stomach, ovarian, pancreas, ureter and renal pelvis, biliary tract, brain (usually glioblastoma), sebaceous gland adenomas, and keratoacanthomas.

[2]MSI associated histologic features include tumour infiltrating lymphocytes, Crohn-like lymphocytic reaction, mucinous/signet-ring differentiation, or medullary growth pattern.

Printed with permission: Burt RW. *2007 AGA Institute Postgraduate Course:* pg. 237.

Please also see Sleisenger and Fordtran's Gastrointestinal and Liver Disease. 10th Edition. Saunders/Elsevier, Philadelphia, 2016, Box 127-3, page 2264.

- ➢ Sequence of testing for HNPCC

  - o Diagnosis of CRC

  - o Although multiple colonic tumours occur in HNPCC (~35%), only about 10% of persons with sporatic (non-HNPCC) CRC may have multiple polyps.

  - o Although the mean average of development of CRC is younger in HNPCC than in sporatic tumours (4 versus 67 years, respectively) in the individual patient it may be difficult to distinguish the two conditions.

535

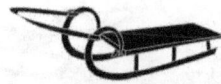

- Give the cancer risk and the **screening recommendations** for Lynch syndrome (HNPCC) tumours.

Cancer	Cancer Risk	Screening Recommendations
o Colon	80%	- Colonoscopy, q 1-2 yrs, beginning at age 20-25 yrs or 10 yrs younger than the earliest case in the family, whichever comes first
o Endometrial*	43-60%	- Pelvic exam, transvaginal ultrasound and/or endometrial aspirate q 1-2 yrs, starting at age 25-30 yrs
o Ovarian	9-12%	- Uncertain
o Gastric	13-19%	- Upper GI endoscopy q 1-2 yrs, start at 30-35 yrs
o Urinary tract	4-10%	- Ultrasound and urinalysis (urine cytology) q 1-2 yrs, starting at age 30-35 yrs
o Renal cell adenocarcinoma	3.3%	- Same as above
o Biliary tract and gallbladder	2.0-18%	- Uncertain, possible LFTs annually after age 30 yrs
o Central nervous system, usually glioblastoma (Turcot syndrome)	4%	- Uncertain, possibly annual exam and periodic head CT in affected families
o Small bowel	1-4%	- Uncertain, at least small bowel X-ray if symptoms occur

*Guidelines are empiric, except for colon

Adapted from: Burt RW. *2007 AGA Institute Postgraduate Course:*240.

- Give why HNPCC polyps might be missed.
    - o HNPCC polyps may occur sporatically
    - o The family may not have been carefully detailed (especially forgetting to use the Bethesda criteria and include high risk "Lynch" extraintestinal cancers).
    - o The clinical suspicion of HNPCC may not be properly recorded on the pathology requisition.
    - o Failure to diagnosis HNPCC has serious consequences for the patient and their family (not to mention the physician, who may be exposed to malpractice claims).
    - o Sometimes the pathologist may consider that an adenomatous polyp is truly an HNPCC polyp from the histopathology.

(Please see Sleisenger and Fordtran's Gastrointestinal and Liver Disease. 9th Edition. Saunders/Elsevier, Philadelphia, 2010, Table 123.6, page 2206).

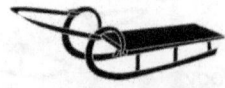

- ➤ Pathology
- • Give characteristic endoscopic and pathologic features of tumours that are highly suggestive of microsatellite instability (MSI) (Lynch syndrome).
  - ○ Endoscopic
    - Multiple
    - Synchronous
    - Metachronous
    - Right-sided
  - ○ Microscopic
    - Lymphocytes infiltrating the CRC tumour
    - Mucinous histology ("signet ring")
    - Poor differentiation
    - Lack of "dirty" necrosis

Please see Sleisenger and Fordtran's Gastrointestinal and Liver Disease. 10th Edition. Saunders/Elsevier, Philadelphia, 2010, Table 122.1, page 2172; and 10th Edition, 2016, page 2270.

Muir-Torre Syndrome
  - ○ Extracolonic cancer in HNPCC is known as the Muir-Torre variant
  - ○ A rare subset of HNPCC associated genetically with
    - MSI
    - Loss of expression
      - hMLH1
      - hMSH2
  - ○ Associated cancers
    - Skin
      - Keratoacanthomas
      - Sebaceous adenomas
    - Carcinomas
      - Basal call
      - Squamous
  - ○ GI tract
    - Stomach
    - Small intestine
    - Biliary tree
  - ○ GU
    - Ovary
    - Uterus
    - Ureter
  - ○ CNS
    - Brain

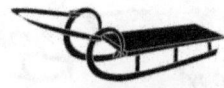

- Give the screening and management guidelines for Lynch syndrome (HNPCC).

Cancer	Screening	Age to Start	Treatment

- Annual screening

  - Endometrial /Ovarian | Endometrial biopsy (for pre-menopausal women) and transvaginal ultrasound (preferably day 1-10 of cycle) for premenopausal women CA125 | 30-35 yrs (or 5-10 yrs before the earliest diagnosis in the family) | Consider prophylactic TAH/BSO after childbearing Consider oral contraceptives for premeno-pausal women. |

  - Urinary tract | Pelvic and abdominal US | 30-35 yr | |
    | Urinalysis with cytology | 30-35 yrs | |

- Screening q 1-2 yr

  - Colon | Colonoscopy | 30-35 yrs | Consider colectomy if cancer or advanced adenoma is found. |
    | | 20-25 yrs (or 10 yrs before the earliest diagnosis in the family) | |

  - Stomach | EGD | 30-35 yrs | |

  - Small bowel | Small bowel enteroclysis (CTE, MRE) | 30-35 yr | |

  - CNS | MRI | CNS symptoms | |

  - Biliary tract, gallbladder | Liver function tests | 30-35 yr | |

Abbreviations: TAN/BSO, total abdominal hysterectomy, bilateral salpingo-oophorectomy; CNS, central nervous system; EGD, esophagogastroduodenoscopy

Printed with permission: Burt RW. *2007 AGA Institute Postgraduate Course.* pg. 240.

538

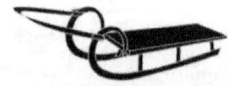

HYPERPLASTIC/SERRATED POLYPOSIS SYNDROMES

➤ Definition

- o 1 or more hyperplastic polyp proximal to the sigmoid, in a person with a first-degree relative with HPS or

- o Serrated polyposis syndrome = hyperplastic polyposis (serrated polyps proximal to sigmoid colon, of which ≥ 2= 10 mm)

- o > 30 hyperplastic polyps throughout the colon (not just proximal to the sigmoid colon)

Serrated = distortion of crypts "boot-/bell-shaped"

Abbreviation: LC, left colon; RC, right colon

➤ Demography

- o During screening colonoscopy, hyperplastic polyps occur in 10% of persons (please remember that in screening colonoscopies for average risk persons, 25% of males and 15% of females over age 50 years will have adenomatous polyps).

- o Smoking is a risk factor for both adenomatous and for hyperplastic polyps.

➤ Gene mutations

- o BRAF

- o DNA methylation

➤ Pathology

- o Both of adenomatous and hyperplastic polyps may occur in the same colon, especially if there is a family history of CRC or HNPCC.

- o If the patient has a hyperplastic polyp identified on sigmoidoscopy (usually small [< 5 mm], and biopsy shows long crypts and a papillary configuration of the colonocytes), they need to have a full colonoscopy, since a distal hyperplastic polyp is a marker for a proximal lesion (approximate risks):
  - Proximal neoplasia, 25%
  - Proximal advanced neoplasia, 5%

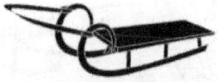

- Give the pathology/histopathology and genetic mutations of HP, SSA/P and TSA.

	HP	SSA/P	TSA
Gross/endoscopy			
o Site	DC	PC	DC
o Shape (sessile)	+	+	-
o Size	< 5 mm	> 5 mm	> 5 mm
o Appearance	Pale	Mucus cap	Lobular
Histopathology			
o Irregular bases of crypts	-	+	-
Genetic mutations			
o K-Ras	+/-	+	+/-
o BRAF	+/-	-	+/-

Abbreviation: DC, distal colon; HP, hyperplastic polyps; PC, proximal colon; SSA/P, sessile serrated adenoma/polyps; TSA, traditional serrated adenoma

Adapted from: Sleisenger and Fordtran's Gastrointestinal and Liver Disease. 10th Edition. Saunders/Elsevier, Philadelphia, 2016, Table 126-10, page 2231.

➤ Surveillance

- Give the surveillance recommendations after resection of serrated polyps.

Resected Polyp	Recommended Surveillance Interval
o Typical hyperplastic polyp	No surveillance recommended, unless multiple, large and proximally located
o Sessile serrated adenoma (non dysplastic)	5 years if < 3 lesions, all < 1 cm size; 3 years if ≥ 3 lesions, or any ≥ 1 cm size
o Sessile serrated adenoma with dysplasia (SSAD)	3 years after ensuring complete resection
o Traditional serrated adenoma (TSA)	
o Suspected type I hyperplastic polyposis (serrated adenomatous polyposis)	1-3 years, with resection of polyps > 5 mm

Printed with permission: Huang C.S. Am J Gastroenterol 2011;106:229-240,Table 3, page 237.

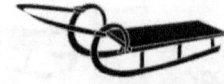

Hamartomatous Polyposis Syndromes (HPS)

➢ Classification

- Give a classification of hamartomatous polyposis syndromes.
  - ○ PJS (Peutz-Jegher syndrome)
  - ○ JPS (Juvenile polyposis syndrome, aka familial juvenile polyposis)
  - ○ PTEN tumour syndrome
    - – Cowden disease
    - – BRR (Bannayan-Ruvalcaba-Riley) syndrome
  - ○ Neurofibromatosis (mutation in NF1 gene), and ganglioneuromatosis ↓ with MEN 2B)
  - ○ Tuberous sclerosis
    - – Hamartomas plus
      - ▪ CNS
        - – Epilepsy
        - – Mental challenge
      - ▪ Skin
        - – Adenoma sebaceum

Note: JPS, when associated with multiple polyps, is a diagnosis of exclusion (e.g., exclude PJS, CS, BRR, NFTS)

Syndrome	Gene (% Chance of Finding a Mutation in Proband)	Lifetime Cancer Risk		Other Features
○ Peutz-Jegher syndrome (PJS)	- STK11 (30-70%)	Breast Colon/rectum Pancreas Stomach Ovarian[1] Small bowel Lung Uterine/cervix[2] Testicle	54% 39% 36% 29% 21% 13% 15% 9% Rare	- Mucocutaneous pigmentation - Histologically characteristic gastrointestinal hamartomas, mostly small bowel, but in all areas

541

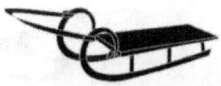

Syndrome	Gene (% Chance of Finding a Mutation in Proband)	Lifetime Cancer Risk		Other Features
○ Juvenile polyposis syndrome (JPS)	- SMAD4 (20%) - BMPR1A (20%) - ENG (rare)	Colon Upper GI cancers including stomach, pancreas, and small bowel	68% 21%	- GI juvenile polyps - Features of HHT[3] - Digital clubbing - Congenital defects
➤ Cowden syndrome (CS)	- PTEN (80-90%)	Breast Thyroid (especially follicular) Endometrium Kidney Colon and upper GI tract	25-50% 10% 5% ↑ CRC may be ↑	- Mucocutaneous papules - Macrocephaly - Hamartomas of the gastrointestinal tract, thyroid, and breast - Lhermitte-Duclos disease

[1]Sex cord tumours with annular tubules; [2]Adenoma malignum

Printed with permission: Burt RW. *2007 AGA Institute Postgraduate Course.* pg. 241.

"Abandon all hope, Ye who enter here

Lasciate ogne speranza voi ch'entrate."

Dante Alighieri

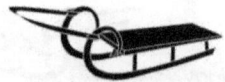

Peutz-Jeghers Syndrome (PJS)

- World Health Organization (WHO) diagnostic criteria for PJS: any one of the following:

➤ Diagnosis

   o ≥ 3 histologically characteristic PJS polyps

   o ≥ 1 PJS polyp in a person with a family history of PJS

   o Characteristic and prominent mucocutaneous pigment, in a person with a family history of PJS

   o ≥ 1 PJS, plus characteristic and prominent mucocutaneous pigmentation

   o Intestinal
      - Colon, 39%
      - Pancreas, 36%
      - Stomach, 29%
      - Small bowel, 13%
      - Esophagus, 0.5%

   o Extra-intestinal
      - Breast,, 54%
      - Ovary 21%
      - Lung, 15%
      - Uterus, 9%
      - Rarely cervix, ovary, testicle

Clinical Pearl

- Give the way to distinguish freckles from the brown pigmentation of PJS.

   o These are the common sites of pigmentation in PJS
      – Nose*
      – Lips
      – Mouth (buccal mucosa)*
      – Hands
      – Feet
      – Perianal and genital regions

   o In RJS, Freckles do not occur near the nostrils of the nose, or on the buccal mucosa of the mouth

---

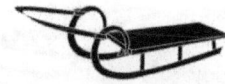

Mastering the Boards: Gastroenterology   A.B.R. Thomson

> Genetics

  o Autosomal dominantly inherited syndrome of histologically specific hamartomatous polyps together with characteristic mucocutaneous pigmentation

  o Occurrence estimated to be 1 on 150,000 live births

  o Arises from mutations of the STK II (serine threonine kinase II, also called LKB I) gene on chromosome 19p13.3

  o Autosomal dominant germline mutation in the STK II (LKB I) gene, with mutations seen in 90% of persons with PJS

  o 50% of mutations are inherited, and 50% are spontaneous, appearing de novo

- Give the gene mutation and lifetime cancer risk from affected organs in the Peutz-Jeghers syndrome (PJS, hamartomatous polyposis syndrome).

Gene (% Chance of Finding a Mutation in Proband)	Lifetime cancer risk		Other features
o STK11 (30-70%)	Breast	54%	- Mucocutaneous pigmentation
	Colon/rectum	39%	
	Pancreas	36%	- Histologically characteristic gastrointestinal hamartomas, mostly small bowel, but also in other areas
	Stomach	29%	
	Ovarian[1]	21%	
	Small bowel	13%	
	Lung	15%	
	Uterine/cervix[2]	9%	
	Testicle	Rare	

[1]Sex cord tumours with annular tubules; [2]Adenoma malignum

Printed with permission: Burt RW. *2007 AGA Institute Postgraduate Course.* pg. 241.

> Clinical

  o Mucocutaneous pigmented macules
    - May be present at birth on buccal mucosa, lips, peroral region, fingertips or toes, hands or feet, perianal or genital area
    - Occur in over 95% of cases
    - Most common in the perioral and buccal areas (94%), but also occurs:
      ▪ Around the eyes
      ▪ On palmar and plantar surfaces
      ▪ On an around the genetalia and anus

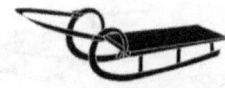

- o Pigmented
  - – Face
  - – Lips
  - – Buccal mucosa
- o Sex cord tumours
  - – Men
    - ▪ Sertoli cell testicular tumour
  - – Women
    - ▪ Ovary
- o Breast cancer
- o Appears in infancy and begins to fade at puberty, except on the buccal mucosa, which provides a clinical feature for diagnosis even in adult life
- o Polyps occur in small intestine (> 75%), colon (42%), stomach (38%), and rectum (28%) (colon plus rectum, 70%)
- o Histology and morphology:
  - – Distinctive histology of hamartomatous polyps
  - – May be sessile or pedunculated, ranging in size from mm to cm
- o Clinical presentation age 10-20 years from time of initial small bowel obstruction
- o Distribution
  - – Stomach, 38%
  - – Small bowel, 78%
  - – Colon, 42%
  - – Rectum, 28%
- o Clinical presentation
  - – Benign complications from the polyps (bleeding, obstruction and intussusceptions) predominate in the first three decades of life
  - – Cancer may arise in polyps even though they are hamartomas

➢ Overall malignancy risk:

- o GI and non-GI cancers are common in PJS, with a combined frequency of all cancers being 93% by age 65 yrs
- o Cancer risks and screening recommendations, which are all empiric, are given under management

545

 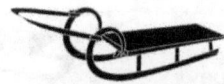

> Endoscopy

  o Cerebriform polyps on EGD

  o Smooth muscle arborization

  o Adenomatous changes occur in ~25% of PJS hamartomas, accounting for the development of adenocarcinomas

  o Cancer risk (hamartoma-carcinoma sequence) is 90% by age 65

- Give the **lifetime cancer risk** at GI and non-GI sites for FAP, HNPCC (Lynch syndrome) and Peutz-Jegher Syndrome (PJS).

		FAP (%)	HNPCC (%)	PJS (%)
o GI	– Stomach	<1	11-19	29
	– Duodenum	4-12	-	-
	– Small bowel	1	1-4	13
	– Pancreas	2	-	36
	– Hepatobiliary (hepatoblastoma)	<1	2-7	-
	– Colon	~100	~100	39
o Non-GI	– CNS	<1 (medulo-blastoma)	1-3 (glioblastoma)	-
	– Adrenal	2	-	-
	– Endometrium	<1	-	-
	– Ovary	-	20-60	9
	– Upper urinary tract	-	9-12	21
	– Skin	-	4-5	-
	– Breast	-		54
	– Lung	-	1	15
	– Testicle (Sertoli cell)	-		Rare

Adapted from: Burt RW. *AGA Institute Postgraduate Course book* 2007: pg. 235, 237 and 241.

"The future will bring personalized medicine based on genetics"

Grandad

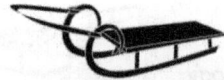

Juvenile Polyposis Syndrome (JPS)

➤ Demography

  ○ The incidence of inherited JP is ~$1/10^5$

  ○ 20-60% have a family history, and the remainder appear de novo

  ○ Juvenile polyps occur in 2% of children. The diagnosis of JP is made with the presence of 10 or more juvenile polyps in the GI tract.

➤ Genetics

  ○ At least a third of these will be found to have the autosomal dominantly inherited syndrome

  ○ Germline mutation in either the SMAD4 (MADH4) gene (in 35%) on chromosome 18q21.1 or in the BMPR1A (bone morphogenetic protein receptor 1A) gene (in 25%)

  ○ At least half of the affected families are found to have a disease from mutation of the SMAD4 gene

  ○ Half of the affected families have a disease causing mutation of the SMAD4 gene on chromosome 18

  ○ `Other genes may be involved (BMPRIA on chromosome 10)

  ○ Distinguish from PJS and CS

Syndrome	Gene	Chromosomes
– PJS	STK II	19p13.3
– JPS	SMAD4	18q21.1
– CS	BMPR1A	
	PTEN	10

Abbreviations: BMPR1A, bone morphogenetic protein receptor type 1A); CS, Cowden Syndrome; PTEN, phosphate and tensin homologue

➤ Clinical

  ○ Clinical management involves mainly screening for cancer prevention

  ○ Empiric guidelines have been developed for organs in which cancer develops

  ○ Cancer of colon (39%), esophagus (0.5%), stomach (29%), pancreas (36%), breast (54%), ovary (21%), lung (15%), uterus (9%)

  ○ Adenoma malignum of cervix

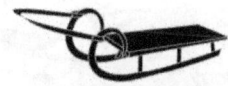

- o Ovarian sex cord tumours with annular tubules (SCTAT)
- o Testicular tumours
- o Symptoms: colonic bleeding and anemia usually occur in the first decade of life
- o The risk of colon cancer appears to be many-fold increased, and predominates the clinical presentations after the third decade of life
- o The average age of colon cancer diagnosis is approx 34 yrs
- o Gastric, duodenal and pancreatic cancers have been reported in JP, but their association is less certain
- o Congenital defects have been noted with the non-familial but not the familial form of JPS.
  - – Cardiac abnormalities
  - – Cranial abnormalities
  - – Cleft palate
  - – Polydactyly
  - – Bowel malrotations

Adapted from: Sleisenger and Fordtran's Gastrointestinal and Liver Disease. 10th Edition. Saunders/Elsevier, Philadelphia, 2016, page 2244.

- • Give the gene mutation and lifetime cancer risk from affected organs in the Juvenile Polyposis syndrome (JPS, hamartomatous polyposis syndrome).

Gene (% chance of Finding a Mutation in proband)	Lifetime Cancer Risk		Other Features
o SMAD4 (20%)	Colon	68%	- GI juvenile polyps
o BMPR1A (20%)	Upper GI cancers including stomach, pancreas, and small bowel	21%	- Features of HHT*
o ENG (rare)			- Digital clubbing
			- Congenital defects

* HHT, Hereditary hemorrhagic telangiectasia

Printed with permission: Burt RW. *2007 AGA Institute Postgraduate Course.* pg. 241.

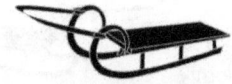

- ➢ Pathology
  - ○ The juvenile hamartomatous polyps demonstrate dilated cystic glands, columnar lining, abundant lamina propria which may contain an inflammatory infiltrate.
  - ○ These juvenile polyps may be seen in JPS, CS, and BRRS or Gorlin syndrome.
  - ○ The polyps are most commonly found in the colon, but may occur anywhere throughout the GI tract.
  - ○ Multiple juvenile polyps in colon (98%), stomach (14%), duodenum (2%), jejunum and ileum (7%).
  - ○ The full-blown syndrome may be characterized by hundreds of polyps.
  - ○ Polyps in JP differ from sporadic juvenile polyps in that new polyps almost always recur after polyps are removed and polyps always occur in adults.
  - ○ JP polyps have a smooth surface, are often covered by exudates, may be sessile or pedunculated and range in size from mm to cm's.
  - ○ Colorectal cancer (CRC) risk in JPS
    - – 20% by age 25 years
    - – 68% by age 60
  - ○ With the SMAD4 mutation, 23% have AVMs in brain, lung, and liver, consistent with HHT (hereditary hemorrhagic telangiectasia), and are more likely to have gastric polyps, massive gastric polyps, or gastric cancer.
  - ○ ↑ lamina propria
  - ○ Dilated cystic glands filled with mucus
    - – Cowden disease (aka multiple hamartoma syndrome)
      - ▪ Autosomal dominant
      - ▪ Facial trichilemmomas around eyes, nose, mouth
      - ▪ Polyps in
        - - Colon (hamartomas, ganglioneuromas)
        - - Esophagus (glycogenic acanthosis)
        - - Stomach
    - – Cancer
      - ▪ Breast
      - ▪ Uterus
      - ▪ Thyroid
      - ▪ **Not** in GI tract

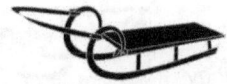

- BRR (Bannayan-Ruvalcaba-Riley) syndrome
  - Autosomal dominant
  - Macrocephaly
  - Delay in development
  - Pigment spots on penis
  - Thyroiditis
- Dilated cystic glands filled with mucus
  - GI
    - Meckel diverticulum
    - Malrotation of intestine
  - GU
    - Undescended testicle
    - Agenesis of one kidney
    - Bifid uterus and vagina
  - CNS
    - Macrocephaly
    - Hydrocephalus
    - Heart
    - ASD (atrial septal defect)
    - C of A (coarctation of aorta)
    - T of F (tetralogy of Fallot)

SO YOU WANT TO BE A GI PATHOLOGIST!

Juvenile polyps are hamartomas, and ordinarily should not be neoplastic. However, about 1/3 of JPS develop CRC, and a few even develop gastric cancer.

- Give a pathological explanation for this apparent contradiction.
  - JP and adenomatous polyps may occur in the same person
  - Hamartomatous plus adenomatous tissue may occur in the same polyp.

550

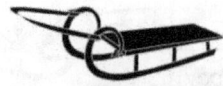

- ➢ Colon screening

  - o Multiple juvenile polyps in colon (98%), stomach (14%), duodenum (2%), jejunum and ileum (7%)

  - o This consists mainly of prevention of benign and malignant complications

  - o Only empiric guidelines are available

  - o CRC

  - o Colonoscopy, beginning with symptoms or in early teens, if no symptoms occur. Interval determined by number of polyps but at least every 3 years once begun.

Adapted from: Sleisenger and Fordtran's Gastrointestinal and Liver Disease. 10th Edition. Saunders/Elsevier, Philadelphia, 2016, page 2244.

Cowden Syndrome (CS)

- ➢ Genetics

  - o CS occurs in $< 1/10^5$

  - o Autosomal dominant

  - o Mutations of the PTEN gene on chromosome 10

  - o Germline mutations in PTEN gene seen in 85% of CS affected persons

  - o Skin lesions (99%)

  - o Colon cancer risk is estimated at 17%. Additionally, this condition must be distinguished from other hamartomatous diseases

- ➢ Pathology

  - o A juvenile-like polyp which contains neural components is characteristic for CS (Jass JR. *Pathol Res Pract* 2008:431-447).

Clinical Trick

- • Give the ↑ risk of colorectal cancer (CRC) in Cowden syndrome, and the recommended screening for CRC.

  - o Read on, read the fine print, and be surprised.

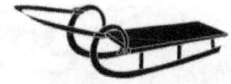

- ➢ Clinical (criteria for phenotypic diagnosis)
  - o 90% of affected persons have mucocutaneous papillomatous papiles (hamartomas), as well as hamartomas of the infundibulum of the hair follicles (trichilemmomas)
  - o Other important features of CS include hamartomas of GI tract, tumours of breast and thyroid, macrophaly, and mental impairment
  - o 40% have involvement of esophagus (glycogen acanthosis), stomach and colon (hamartomas)
  - o Any part of GI tract from stomach to rectum may have hamartomas, juvenile polyps, adenomas, lipomas, inflammatory polyps, ganglioneuromas, or lymphoid hyperplasia
  - o Multiple hamartomatous polyps occur in the colon and throughout the GI tract. A number of different types of hamartomas occur:
    - – Juvenile polyps (by far the most common)
    - – Lipomas
    - – Esophageal glycogenic acanthosis
    - – Inflammatory polyps
    - – Ganglioneuromas
    - – Lymphoid hyperplasia
  - o Cowden syndrome is the presence of multiple facial trichilemmomas (the hallmark sign, most commonly around the mouth, nose and eyes):
    - – Café-au-lait spots
    - – Vitiligo
    - – Papillomatous papules
    - – Acral keratoses
    - – Cysts, as well as squamous cell and basal cell carcinomas
  - o Oral mucosal lesions
    - – These are histologically similar to the trichilemmomas
    - – They develop a few years after the skin growths and are present in approximately 85% of patients
    - – They include pinpoint, red, flat-topped papules on the outer lips and small, flat, papillomatous or verrucous papules of the oral mucosa, gingiva and tongue
    - – Cobblestone-like pattern in mouth from coalesced trichilemmomas in 40%
  - o Thyroid abnormalities:
    - – Two-thirds of patients have multinodular goiter histologically arising from nodular hyperplasia or follicular adenomas
    - – There is an approximate 3-10% risk of thyroid papillary carcinoma

552

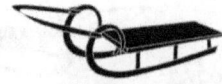

- o Breast lesions:
    - – 75% of affected females have breast lesions, including fibrocystic disease and fibroadenomas
    - – There is a 30-50% incidence of breast carcinoma, with frequent bilateral occurrence, and a median age at diagnosis of 41 yrs
    - – Genitourinary abnormalities (44% of affected women)
        - ▪ Multiple uterine leiomyomas (fibroids) and/or bicornuate uterus
- o ↑ risk of endometrial cancer
- o Additional benign soft tissue and visceral tumours have been observed:
    - – Hemangiomas
    - – Lipomas
    - – Lymphangiomas
    - – Neurofibromas
    - – Uterine Leiomyomas
    - – Meningiomas
- o Developmental or congenital abnormalities also occur:
    - – Hypoplastic mandible
    - – A prominent forehead
    - – A high-arched palate

- • Give the gene mutation and lifetime cancer risk from affected organs in the Cowden syndrome (CS, hamartomatous polyposis syndrome).

Gene (% Chance of Finding a Mutation in Proband)	Lifetime Cancer Risk		Other Features
o PTEN (80-90%)	- Breast	25-50%	- Mucocutaneous papules
	- Thyroid (especially follicular)	10%	- Macrocephaly
	- Endometrium	5%	- Hamartomas of the gastrointestinal tract, thyroid, and breast
	- Kidney	↑	
	- Colon and upper GI tract	CRC may be ↑	- Lhermitte-Duclos disease (LDD)*

* Lhermittee-Duclos disease – Cerebellar dysplastic gangliocytoma

Printed with permission: Burt RW. *2007 AGA Institute Postgraduate Course.* pg. 241.

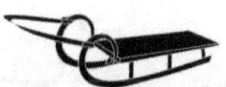

The Bannayan-Ruvalcaba-Riley (BRR) syndrome, is now believed to be related to Cowden syndrome (CS).

- o CS and BBR are referred together as the PTEN hamartoma tumour syndromes (PHTS)
- o BRR characteristics:
  - – Macrocephaly
  - – Lipomas
    - Pigmented macules on the glans penis
    - Other features of Cowden's syndrome
- o BRR also arises from mutations of the PTEN gene

➢ Diagnosis

- Specific clinical diagnostic criteria have been suggested by the *International Cowden Consortium* for the diagnosis of CS.

- Pathognomonic criteria
  - o Mucocutaneous lesions
    - – Trichilemmomas, facial
    - – Acral keratosis
    - – Papillomatous papules
    - – Mucosal lesions
  - o Major criteria
    - – Breast carcinoma
    - – Thyroid carcinoma (non-medullary), especially follicular thyroid carcinoma
    - – Macrocephaly (megalencephaly) (≥ 95th percentile)
    - – Lhermitte-Duclos disease (LDD, cerebellar dysplastic gangliocytoma)
    - – Endometrial carcinoma
  - o Minor criteria
    - – Other thyroid lesions (e.g., adenoma or multinodular goiter)
    - – Mental retardation (IQ ≤ 75)
    - – GI hamartomas
    - – Fibrocystic disease of the breast
    - – Lipomas
    - – Fibromas
    - – GU tumour (eg: renal cell carcinoma, uterine fibroids or malformation

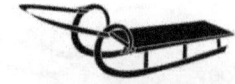

- Operational diagnosis in a person with mucocutaneous lesions alone if:
  - There are ≥ 6 facial papules, of which ≥ 3 must be trichilemmoma, or
  - Cutaneous facial papules and oral mucosal papillomatosis, or
  - Oral mucosal papillomatosis and acral keratoses, or
  - Palmoplantar keratosis ≥ 6
    - 2 major criteria but one must include macrocephaly or LDD
    - 1 major and 3 minor criteria
    - 4 minor criteria

- Operational diagnosis in a family where one person is diagnosed with CS
  - The pathognomonic criterion
  - Any one major criterion with or without minor criteria
  - Two minor criteria

➢ Screening

- Give the screening recommendations to detect early cancers associated with CS.

Cancer	Cancer Risk	Screening Recommendations
o Colon	– About 17%	▪ No recommendations
o Thyroid	– 3-10%	▪ Annual thyroid exam, starting in teens
o Breast	– 25-50%	▪ Annual breast exam, starting at age 25 yrs; annual mammography, starting at age 30 yrs
o Uterus/ovary	– Possible increase	▪ Uncertain

*Note: some authors suggest that there does not appear to be and ↑ risk of GI cancer.

Printed with permission: Zbuk KM, and Eng C. *Nat Clin Pract Gastroenterol Hepatol* 2007; 4(9): pg. 496.

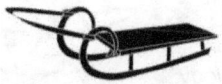

> Surveillance

- Give the surveillance recommendations for Cowden syndrome.

Women	Men
o Training and education in breast self-exam (BSE) and monthly BSE starting at age 18 years	– Annual comprehensive physical exam starting at age 18 years or 5 years younger than the youngest age of diagnosis of a CS cancer in the family (whichever is younger), with particular attention to breast and thyroid exam
o Semiannual clinical breast exam starting at age 25 years or 5-10 years earlier than earliest known breast cancer in the family	
	– Annual urinalysis; consider annual urine cytology and renal ultrasound, if family history of renal cancer
o Annual mammography and breast MRI screening starting at age 30-35 years or 5-10 years earliest known breast cancer in the family (whichever is earlier)	
	– Baseline thyroid ultrasound at age 18 years, and annual thereafter
o Blinded endometrial aspiration biopsies annually for premenopausal women starting at age 35-40 years, or 5 years before earliest diagnosis of endometrial cancer in the family; annual endometrial ultrasound in postmenopausal women	– Education regarding the signs and symptoms of cancer
	– Annual dermatologic exam
	– Advise about risk to relatives, and possibility of genetic testing for relatives
o Discuss options for risk-reducing mastectomy on case-by-case basis and counsel regarding degree of protection, extent of cancer risk, and reconstruction options	

Printed with permission: Zbuk KM, and Eng C. *Nat Clin Pract Gastroenterol Hepatol* 2007; 4(9): pg. 497.

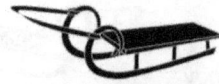

Mastering the Boards: Gastroenterology   A.B.R. Thomson

CROHKHITE – CANADA SYNDROME (CCS)

- Give the clinical features which might make you suspect Cronkhite-Canada Syndrome (CCS).

  o Skin and hair changes
    - Alopecia
    - Dystrophic nails

  o Protein-losing enteropathy

  o No family history of similar condition (CCS is not inherited)

  o GI hamartomatous polyps
    - Colon
    - Small intestine
    - Stomach

  o No ↑ risk of CRC (colorectal cancer)

SO YOU WANT TO BE A GASTROENTEROLOGIST!

For the Canadian GIs – CCS (Cronkhite-Canada Syndrome):
There are more than 5 inherited hamartomatous polyposis syndromes (e.g., PJS, JPS, Cowden disease, Bannayan-Ruvalcaba-Riley [BRR] syndrome, neurofibromatosis, ganglioneuromatosis, hereditary mixed [hamartomatous] polyposis syndrome, not to mention Devon family syndrome, and the **Cronkhite-Canada Syndrome** [CCS]).

- Give the typical clinical features of Cronkhite-Canada Syndrome (CCS), the histopathological differentiation from juvenile polyps, and the approximate risk of associated adenomatous changes and CRC.

  o Half of CCS patients have polyps from stomach to rectum. Their clinical characteristics are:

– Colon	▪ Multiple hamartomatous colonic polyps ▪ Associated adenomatous tissue in 40% risk of CRC, 9%
– Small bowel	▪ Diffuse mucosal damage ▪ SIBO (small intestinal bacterial overgrowth)
– Stomach	▪ ↑ risk of gastric cancer

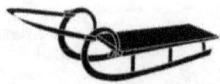

A.B.R. Thomson

- o There are numerous types of inherited adenomatous and hamartomatous polyposis syndromes, as well as non-inherited colonic polyposis comprised of hamartomatous, hyperplastic, lymphomatous or lymphoid tissue (NLH, nodular lymphoid hyperplasia).

- o One extremely rare inherited adenomatous polyposis syndrome associated with the risk of CRC is the **Bloom Syndrome**.

- • Give the features of the Bloom syndrome.

  - o Clinical inspection   – Short stature
      – Red face / telangiectasia
  - o Hematology   – Leukemia
      – Lymphoma
  - o Genitourinary   – Male sterility
  - o Gene mutation   – BLM

- • Give the extracolonic manifestations of **Tuberous sclerosis**.

  - o Skin
    - – Angiofibromas

  - o Brain
    - – Epilepsy
    - – Mental retardation

  - o Heart
    - – Cardiac rhabdomyomas

  - o Bone
    - – Bone cysts

  - o Kidney
    - – Renal cysts

  - o Colon
    - – Ganglioneuromas
    - – Hamartomas

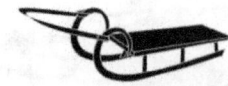

TUMOURS OF THE COLON

Colitis Cystica Profunda

➢ Definition: "….. dilated, mucus filled glands in the submucosal that can [protrude through the mucosa to] form solitary or multiple polyps" (Sleisenger and Fordtran's Gastrointestinal and Liver Disease. 9th Edition. Saunders/Elsevier, Philadelphia, 2010, page 2176).

➢ Speculated pathogenesis: "….. during the healing of a surgical wound or inflammation [colitis] …. the normal colonic glands… [are displaced] to beneath the epithelium" (Sleisenger and Fordtran's Gastrointestinal and Liver Disease. 9th Edition. Saunders/Elsevier, Philadelphia, 2010, page 2176; and 10th Edition, 2016, page 2309).

➢ Causes/associations
  o Colorectal cancer (CRC)
  o Inflammatory bowel disease (IBD)
    – Ulcerative colitis (UC)
    – Crohn disease (CD)
    – Infection
  o Polyps
    – Peutz-Jegher syndrome PJS)
  o Rectal prolapse
  o Solitary rectal ulcer syndrome SRUS)

  o Note:
    – Colitis cystica **superficialis**
      ▪ In mucosa of colon
      ▪ Associated with
        – Celiac disease
        – Pellagra

➢ Pathology
  o Mucus-filled cyst
    – Usually on anterior wall of rectum
    – Usually about 6 cm from anal verge

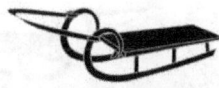

Pneumatosis Cystoides Intestinalis (PCI)

➢ Definition

  o "...... multiple gas-filled cysts located in the submucosal and subserosa of the intestine" (Sleisenger and Fordtran's Gastrointestinal and Liver Disease. 10th Edition. Saunders/Elsevier, Philadelphia, 2010, page 2306).

When PCI involves the colon, then aka **pneumatosis coli**

➢ Types

	Pneumatosis Cystoides Intestinalis (PCI)	Pneumatosis Linearis
o Age of patient	– Adult	▪ May be a child
o Predisposition	– COPD – Scleroderma	▪ Severe colitis (e.g., NEC)
o Pathogenesis	– Diffusion of gas in bowel lumen into cyst	▪ Complication of severe mucosal inflammation by gas forming bacteria

Abbreviations: COPD, chronic obstructive pulmonary disease; NEC, necrotizing enterocolitis

Pneumatosis Coli

➢ Definition

  o Only ~5% of PCI are in colon, and represent pneumatosis coli.

➢ Pathology

  o Thin wall cysts, unilocular, single or in clusters

  o Wall consists of endothelium and multinucleated giant cells

  o Do not communicate with lumen of bowel

  o Distinguish pneumatosis coli from pneumatosis linearis (gas in the wall of the bowel, often associated with AIDS, and usually associated with bowel wall necrosis)

➢ Treatment

  o O_2 therapy for at least 48 hours

  o Metronidazole
    – Resection for hemorrhage or obstruction of colon

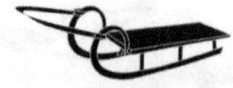

COLORECTAL CANCER (CRC)

➤ Demography

    ○ The age-standardized incidence of CRC (colorectal cancer) in Canada is approximately $25/10^5$ persons per year (26.9 for men, 21.3 in women) which means about 6% of the population will develop CRC in their lifetime.

    ○ Half CRCs are distal to the splenic flexure, but the proportion of right-sided tumours may be increasing.

    ○ Useful comparison: Approximate incidence of GI cancers (10^5/year)

Years of Age	<49	50-74	>75
Esophagus	<1	12	28
Stomach	<1	22	78
Colon	<1	150	400

Source: Canadian Cancer Surveillance, Health Canada

    ○ Lifetime risk of CRC 6%

    ○ Lifetime risk of dying form CRC 2.5%

    ○ Annual CRC mortality ↓ 33% for annual colonoscopy (2.5% → 1.6%, AR 0.8%↓)

    ○ Conversion rate (CR) to CRC
- Adenoma, 30%
- Synchronous risk 5%
- Metachronous risk 5%

➤ Molecular Genetics

    ○ There are 3-pathways in the adenoma-CRC pathway: chromosomal instability (CIS) pathway, microsatellite instability pathway (MIS), and the epigenetic pathway.

    ○ With the epigenetic pathway, DNA methylation in the promoter region of genes leads to gene silencing, which is essentially equivalent to inactivating metastasis. These epigenetic defects in methylation are replicated through cell division and a defective clone of cells is produced.

    ○ One of the methylation-induced inactivations is in MLH-1, one of the mismatch repair genes

    ○ Hyperplastic polyps (HP) are the earliest colonic lesion in the epigastric pathway

561

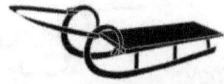

- o Large hyperplastic polyps (HP) (>10 mm) on the right side of the colon may develop into serrated adenomas, and have a malignant potential
- o 15% of all CRCs are thought to develop through this epigastric pathway of serrated adenomas
- o Because both Lynch Syndrome cancers and serrated adenoma cancers make a mismatch repair gene (MLH-1), the tumour morphology may be similar.
- o Quantitative Systematic Reviews have shown that guaiac-based fecal occult blood testing (FOBT) reduce CRC mortality by 13-16% on an intention-to-treat basis, and a 25% reduction when adjusted for screening attendance)

- Give examples of genetic changes associated with **sporatic** colorectal cancer (CRC).
  - o There are multiple genes which are altered in at least some patients with CRC, and these gene mutations may become important at different stages in the development of CRC.
  - o The gene mutations in CRC occur against a background of CIN
  - o Chromosomal instability (CIN) occurs in 80% of CRC
  - o Candidate genes for CIN include genes responsible for
    - Mitotic spindle checkpoint
    - DNA damage checkpoint
    - Control of number of centrosomes
  - o There are three important classes of these sporatic CRC-associated gene
    - Proto-oncogenes
    - Tumour suppressor genes
    - NMR genes
  - o Other important gene mutations include
    - RAS/RAF/MAPK pathway, with mutation in BRAF gene
    - Expression pattern of micro RNAs

- ❖ ↑ proto-oncogenes
  - o ↑ activation of proto-oncogenes
    - K-RAS
    - N-RAS
    - H-RAS

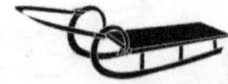

- o Role in sporatic CRC
    - – Activating point mutations (especially in K-RAS gene):
        - ▪ Adenomas   < 1 cm   10%
        -                > 1 cm   58%
        - ▪ Carcinoma   47%

❖ Loss of tumour suppressive genes

- o APC gene
    - – Allelic losses at chromosome locations
        - ▪ 5q
        - ▪ 17p
        - ▪ 18q
- o Truncation of the APC protein
- o Occur in 60% to 80% of sporatic adenomas/carcinomas
- o Loss of DCC (deleted in colon cancer)
- o Low of DPC4/SAMD4 (loss of activation of TGF-β receptors)
- o Loss of p53 tumour suppressor activity from deletion of chromosome 17p leads to loss of cells preventing damaged DNA from going from G1 to S phase of the cell cycle.
- o Loss of TP53 gene

❖ MMR (mismatch repair) genes

- o MSI (microsatellite instability)
- o Alterations in hMLH, hPMS1, hPMS2, hMSH2, hMSH3, hMSH6
- o ↓ repair of mismatches in base pairs → MSI → DNA replication errors → tandem repeat DNA sequences
- o Seen in only 15% of sporatic CRC

❖ Non-MMR gene changes

- o CIMP (CPG island methylator phenotype)
- o MSI may be caused by mutations in MMR genes, or by epigenetic silencing mechanism
- o Definition: Epigenetics is "…change in the genome that result in change expression or phenotype without a change in the sequence of DNA" (Sleisenger and Fordtran's Gastrointestinal and Liver Disease. 10th Edition. Saunders/Elsevier, Philadelphia, 2016, page 2212).
- o Hypermethylation of the hMLA, promotor, with inactivation of hMLH1.
- o Seen in 70% of sporatic MSI tumours.
- o Common pathway for the development of serrated adenomas.

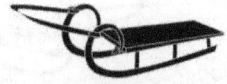

- Give examples of genetic changes associated with inherited CRC.
  - Familial Adenomatous Polyposis (FAP)
    - FAP – autosomal dominant inheritance of expression of gene changes
    - Only 80% penetrance of ARC gene – large protein, B-catenin pathway is important 2 hit hypothesis for FAP
    - Eye "CHRPE" congenital hypertrophy of the retinol pigment epithelium
  - Attenuated FAP (AFAP)
  - MUTYH-associated polyps (aka MYH-associated polyposis)
    - Suspect if patient has > 10 ad polys
    - Germline mutation in MYH base excision repair gene
    - Occurs in APC region
    - 25% of AFAP with > 15 adenomas have MUTYH mutations
    - May be associated with breast cancer
    - Parents, siblings rarely affected
    - Recessive inheritance
  - HNPCC
    - CRC in 50% - 80%
      - DNA mismatch
    - Younger age when CRC develops
    - Proximal colon
    - Glioblastoma (meduloblastomas in FAP)
    - Clinical criteria to suspect HNPCC
    - In family   - Amsterdam criteria I, II
    - In individual   - Bethesda

    - MSI-histology
      - Lymphocytes infiltrating tumour
      - Crohn-like lymphocytic reaction
      - Mucinous/signet ring appearance
      - Medullary growth pattern
    - MSI-Genetics
      - Test tumour for MSI (microsatellite instability) analysis, or IHC (immunohistochemistry) 90% of HNPCC tumours are positive
      - Test patient for same gene abnormality as for the index patient (proband)
      - Carrier with mutations need to be screened by colonoscopy

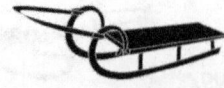

- Peutz-Jegher syndrome germline mutations of STK11/LKB1 (serine-threonine kinase gene) on chromosome 19q there may be genetic heterogeneity

- Juvenile polyposis
  - Autosomal dominant
    - Germline mutations in MADH4 (SMAD4), a tumour suppressor gene (in ~18%)
    - Germline mutations of BMPR1A (bone morphogenetic protein receptor 1A) (in ~ 21%)
  - Sporatic (in ~ 66%)

Note: Cowden syndrome (CS) is **not** associated with an ↑ risk CRC

SO YOU WANT TO BE A GASTROENTEROLOGIST!

We all know that the neurofibromas of the upper GI tract which occur in von Recklinghausen syndrome are caused by NF1 gene mutations.

- Give the gene that is mutated in sipple syndrome (aka MEN (multiple endocrine neoplasia) type 2B (bilateral medullary thyroid cancer and pleochromocytomas) associated with ganglioneuromatosis.

  - You need to take a break! The gene is RET.

➤ Environmental risk factors
  - Numerous environmental factors have been suggested to be associated with the development of adenomas, or their progression of CRC.
  - Despite contrary popular views, dietary fibre supplementation, or the intake of antioxidants have failed to be beneficial when studied in properly designed prospective studies.

- Give factors for which there is adequate and appropriate human data to suggest a beneficial effect on reducing adenomas or CRC.

  - Calcium   – 5% ↓ recurrence of adenomas over 3 years, with the small protective effect lasting for up to 5 years after the calcium was stopped.

565

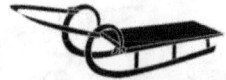

- o NSAIDs/ASA/Coxibs
  - ASA
    - Relative risk among users, 0.68
    - ↓ adenoma, 19% to 37%
    - ↓ advanced adenoma, 37% to 41%
  - Sulindac
    - FAP
      - Number 44% at 9 months, ↓ number by 76% at 1 year
      - ↓ diameter 35%
  - Coxibs
    - FAP
      - ↓ number 28%
      - ↓ number in 3 yr of
        - New adenomas ~40%
        - Advanced adenomas ~60%
  - DFMD (ornithrine decarboxylate inhibitor difluomethyornithine) plus sulindac
    - 70% ↓ new adenomas at 3 years
      - Statin use
    47% ↓ relative risk for CRC

- o Streptococcus Bovis
  - Strep. Bovis bacteremia - gram positive cocci, Biotype I
  - Found in blood in 10% - 15% of normal persons, especially older males
  - When endocarditis occurs with S.bovis, there is usually no typical pre-existing conditions (e.g., artificial valves, IV drug use)
  - S.bovis – in fecal cultures
    - Control 10%
    - CRC 56%
  - Scientific plausibility
    - CRC epithelial cells have receptors for S.bovis
  - S.bovis upregulates COX-2
    - Carcinogenic in rats
  - Recommendation and suggestion (R&S)
    - Colonoscopy for person with S.bovis in the blood (not if S.bovis is in stool)
    - Think of this issue as finding a source of the S.bovis bacteremia

566

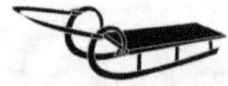

- Give the **pharmacological** or nutritional agents which have been shown possibly to be effective chemoprevention to reduce the risk of development or redevelopment of colorectal adenomas/CRCs.

  - o Drugs
    - – ASA
    - – Coxibs
    - – 5-ASA in IBD
    - – Hormone replacement therapy (HRT) in post menopausal women

  - o Nutrients
    - – Selenium
    - – Calcium (+ vitamin D)
    - – Non-western diet (low intake of saturated fats in red meat)
    - – High intake of green leafy vegetables
    - – Possibly folate, vitamins C, E, B-carotene
    - – Probably not dietary fibre

  - o Exercise

Adapted from: Arber N, and Levin B. *Gastroenterology* 2008;134(4): 1224-1237; and Meyerhardt JA, et al. *JAMA* 2007;298(7): 754-764.

➢ Pathology

Useful background: The TNM staging system for colorectal cancer and published survival rates for different stages.

T – Primary tumour (T)	
TX	Primary tumour cannot be assessed
T0	No evidence of primary tumour
Tis	Carcinoma in situ: intraepithelial or invasion of lamina propria
T1	Tumour invades submucosa
T2	Tumour invades muscularis propria
T3	Tumour invades through the muscularis propria into subserosa o into non-peritonealised pericolic or perirectal tissues
T4	Tumour directly invades other organs or structures and/or perforates visceral peritoneum

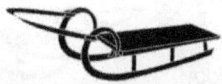

N – regional lymph nodes (N)

NX	Regional lymph nodes cannot be assessed
N0	No regional lymph node metastasis
N1	Metastasis in 1 to 3 regional lymph nodes
N2	Metastasis in 4 or more regional lymph nodes

M- Distant metastasis (M)

MX	Distant metastasis cannot be assessed
M0	No distant metastasis
M1	Distant metastasis

Stage	T N	M	5-year overall survival
Stage I	T1, T2 N0	M0	80-95%
Stage IIA	T3 N0	M0	72-75%
Stage IIB	T4 N0	M0	65-66%
Stage IIIA	T1, T2 NI	M0	55-60%
Stage IIIB	T3, T4 NI	M0	35-42%
Stage IIIC	Any T N2	M0	25-27%
Stage IV	Any T Any N	MI	0-7%

Printed with permission: Tejpar S. *Best Pract Res Clin Gastroenterol* 2007; 21(6): pg. 1074.

➤ Treatment

• Adjuvant or Neoadjuvant Chemotherapy and/or Radiotherapy

  ○ Benefit
    – Stage III   MR 33%
    – Colon Ca   recurrence 42% ↓

  ○ Use
    – T3/4 rectal cancer (locally advanced)
    – After resection of liver/lung metastases

  ○ Before curative surgery – Neoadjuvant

  ○ After curative surgery – Adjuvant

  ○ There are studies in progress assessing pre-operative (neoadjuvant) chemoradiotherapy, curative surgery, followed by 4 months of post-surgery (adjuvant) chemotherapy.

568

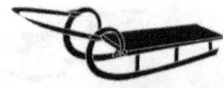

- The limitation to radiotherapy is its toxicity, but enhances of radiation therapy (e.g., capecitabine) may ↑ benefit without an ↑ toxicity
- Studies also examining possible benefit of infusion of 5-FU, leucovorin plus oxaliplatin (combination called FOLFOX).
- Adjuvant therapy within 8 weeks of resection for CRC
  - ↓ recurrence
  - ↑ survival
- 5-FU (5-fluorouracil) plus levamisole (levamisole increases tumour response rates from 12% for 5-FU to 23% for 5-FU + levamisole

Relative	Risk Reduction
– CRC	Overall
– Recurrence	Mortality

- **Dukes C / Stage III**   42%   33%
  - 5-FU plus leucovorin > 5-FU plus levamisole in efficacy after curative surgery for CRC
  - 5-FU plus leucovorin plus oxaliplatin in Stage III
    - ↑ 3 year disease-free survival
    - May also be small benefit in Stage II
  - For rectal CRC Duke B2 / Stage II (transmural extension) or Duke C / Stage III (positive lymph nodes)

5-year Rates	Radiation	Radiation plus Chemotherapy
No recurrence	35	60
Survival	40	50

Adjuvant or neoadjuvant chemotherapy for Stage II or III resected CRC is often given as 5-FU plus leucovorin.

- Give the mechanism of action of 5-FU and leucovorin.
  - 5-FU   – Binds to thymidylate synthetase → ↓ methylation of deoxyuridylic acid to thymidylic acid → ↓ DNA synthesis
  - Leucovorin   – ↑ binding of 5-FU to thymidylate synthetase, thereby ↓ DNA synthesis (please see above)

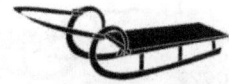

- Surgery
  - Recommended: Total mesenteric excision (TME) for CRC
  - Surgical resection for liver metastases
    - 10% to 25% at presentation
    - Resection
      - < 5 metastases in liver
      - No extrahepatic metastases
      - No extensive liver involvement (< 70%)
  - Non-operable, metastatic CRC
    - Chemotherapy
    - Photoabalation
    - Stents, colorectal

- Give complications for colorectal self-expandable metal stents. The mean % incidence is shown for your interest.

Complication	Mean Incidence (%)
o Re-obstruction	10
o Migration	10
o Perforation	4
o Bleeding	5
o Pain	5
o Death (from placement of stent)	1

Printed with permission: Baron, Todd H., et al. *Best Pract Res Clin Gastroenterol* 2004: pg. 220.

- Post-polypectomy colonoscopic surveillance

- Screening and surveillance
  - Please see previous section on Screening and Suveillance of Colonic Polyps
  - Miss rate of CRC on colonoscopy, 10%
  - While the lifetime risk of CRC in pancolitis LS ↑ 10x, (pseudopolyps not an ↑ risk of CRC in UC)

- Use of EUS of rectum in CRC
  - Sessile polyp
  - Determine resectability of rectal CRC (surgeon needs 5 mm tumour-free margin)

- Post-surgical colonoscopic follow-up
  - Colonoscopy 0→1→3→5 yr
  - CT yearly for 3 yr follow-up 0→1→3→5 yr

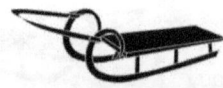

- CEA q 3 months for 3 yr
- Adjuvant chemotherapy with 5-FU can ↑ serum CEA (false elevation of CEA)
- Prior to resection for CRC, perform staging diagnostic imaging so that IOUS (intraoperative ultrasonography) does not need to be performed.
- "in patients whose tumour [CRC] recurs after hepatic resection, the liver is the initial site of recurrence in about 35% (Sleisenger and Fordtran's Gastrointestinal and Liver Disease. 9th Edition. Saunders/Elsevier, Philadelphia, 2010, page 2232; and about 75% of hepatic metastases appear within 2 yr after primary resection, 10th Edition, 2016, 2289).
- Risk of postoperative relapse of CRC
  - Stage II, 20% to 30%
  - Stage III, 50% to 80%
- Surveillance must be continued.
- Patients with small rectal hyperplastic polyps should be considered to have normal colonoscopies, and therefore the interval before the subsequent colonoscopy should be 10 years.
  - An exception is patients with a hyperplastic polyposis syndrome.
  - They are at increased risk for adenomas and colorectal cancer and need to be identified for more intensive follow up.
- Persons with one or two small tubular adenomas (<1cm) , and with only low grade dysplasia should have their next follow up colonoscopy in 5 to 10 years.
  - The precise timing within this interval should be based on other clinical factors (such as prior colonoscopy findings, family history, and the preferences of the patient and judgment of the physician).
- Patients with 3 to 10 adenomas, or any adenoma 1 cm, or any adenoma with villous features, or high grade dysplasia should have their next follow up colonoscopy in 3 years
- If the follow up colonoscopy is normal or shows only one or two small tubular adenomas with low-grade dysplasia, then the interval for the subsequent examination should be 5 years.
- Persons who have more than 10 adenomas at one examination should be examined at a shorter (<3 years) interval established by clinical judgment, and the clinician should consider the possibility of an underlying familial syndrome.
- Persons with sessile adenomas that are removed piecemeal should be considered for follow up at short intervals (2 to 6 months) to verify complete removal.
- Once complete removal has been established, subsequent surveillance needs to be individualized based on the endoscopist's judgment.
- More intensive surveillance is indicated when the family history may indicate hereditary nonpolyposis colorectal cancer.

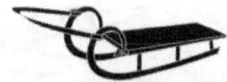

- o Every 5-10 years, except every 3 years for multiple, large, villous and proximal initial lesions.
- o Number- for each additional adenoma, OR=1.32
- o Size- for each additional 10 mm adenoma size, OR=1.56
- o Villous – OR =1.40
- o Proximal – OR =1.68

Note: Sessile serrated adenomas and serrated sessile hyperplastic polyps may have malignant potential, and surveillance should be performed for these. This is discussed in a later section.

Source: Winawer, Sidney J. Screening and surveillance for colorectal cancer: review and rationale. *2009 ACG Annual Postgraduate Course:*21- 25.

➤ Prognosis

The original Dukes staging system for CRC has been modified at least 6 times over the past 80 years (Sleisenger and Fordtran's Gastrointestinal and Liver Disease. 9th Edition. Saunders/Elsevier, Philadelphia, 2010, Table 123.9, page 2214), and has been largely replaced by the AJCC (American Joint Committee on Cancer), TNM (tumour-node-metastasis) staging of colorectal cancer (Sleisenger and Fordtran's Gastrointestinal and Liver Disease. 10th Edition. Saunders/Elsevier, Philadelphia, 2016, Table 127-6, page 2272).

- o Generally speaking, CRC of the left (distal) colon have a better prognosis than these of the right (proximal) colon, and CRC of the colon has a better prognosis than the rectum.

- • Give the appropriate 5 year survival rates for CRC base on the Duke Stage.

Dukes Stage		Approximate 5 Year Survival Rate
A	Limited to mucosa	
B1	Into muscularis propria (MP)	80
B2	Through MP	60
C	Regional node metastasis	40
C1	B1 plus regional node metastasis	
C2	B2 plus regional node metastasis	
C	1 to 3 nodes (N1)	50
	≥ 4 nodes (N2)	25
D	Distant metastases	0

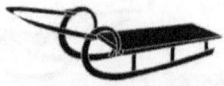

OSTOMIES

➢ Definition: an ostomy is a hernia, a "protrusion of abdominal contents through a muscular defect"

➢ To fix ostomy hernia
  o Move site of ostomy (recurrence rate of hernia is high, so move site)
  o Repeated obstruction – big bulge

➢ Types

	Ileostomy	Colostomy
o Protrusion	Yes	No
o Size	Smaller	Larger
o Smell	-	+++
o Hernia	+	+++

Stroma, 2 openings – loop ostomy

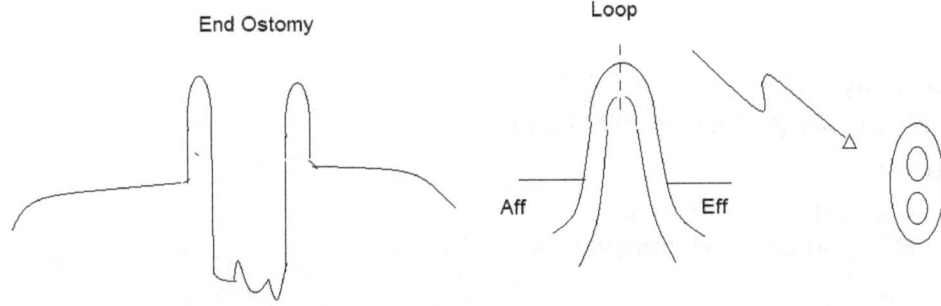

  o Ileoscopy protrudes – why?
    - Appliance comprised of 2 parts: face plate to protect skin
    - Ileum – damages skin – need face plate for protection
    - Colonscopy – Do not need to protect skin from stool
  o Placement site
    - Away from scars, umbilicus
    - Obesity
      ▪ Away from "trough" of skin folds, and can be seen by patients to clean/change (mark prop)

➢ Indications for ostomy
  o Acute inflammation, not safe for anastomosis
  o Protect an anastomosis downstream (prevent dehiscence; temporary diversion of fecal stream, giving distal anastomosis a chance to heal)

573

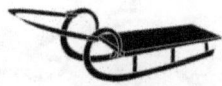

- Give how to determine which is the affected limb.
    - Ask the patient
    - Stool comes out of afferent limb
    - Protrudes a little
    - Check the operative report

    - DRE of ostomy
        1. Tip
        2. Skin
        3. Rectus abdominus

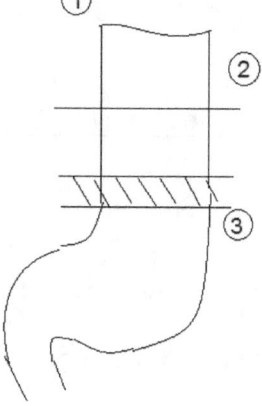

- Stomal output
    - Ileostomy
        - 1-2 L/day (decreases over time)
    - Colonostomy
        - Sigmoid, 200-250 mL/day
        - R. (right) colon, R. transverse- 0.5-1 L/day

➢ Types of ostomies

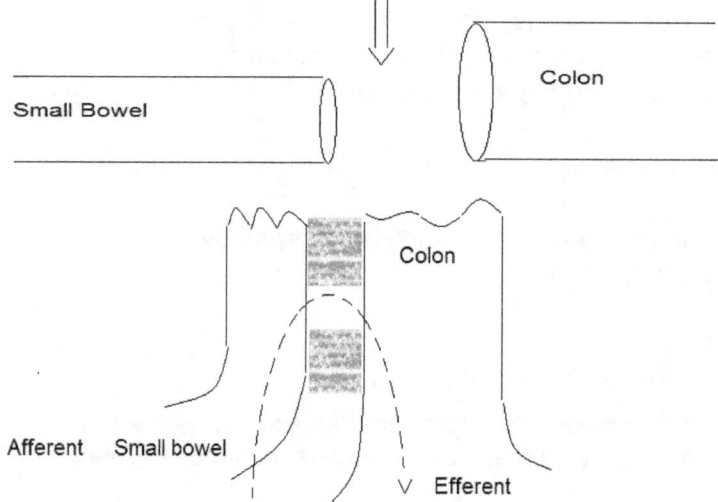

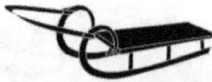

Side-to-side, but is functionally end-to-end

OR

- o End-to-end

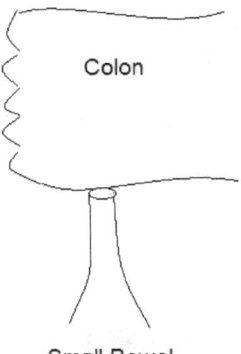

Colon

Small Bowel

- o Rectum vs anus
  - – Ileorectal anastamosis – above the pelvic floor
  - – Ileoanal anastamosis – below the pelvic floor

- o Digital rectal examination (DRE) findings
  - – Skin tag
  - – Squamous cell tumour
  - – Condyloma
  - – Pseudopolyp (in lower rectum)

"To save your world you asked this man to die,

Would this man, could he see you now, ask why?"

W. H. Anden

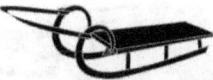

ENDOMETRIOSIS

➤ Definition: "... the presence of endometrial tissue outside the uterine cavity and musculature (Feldman M., et al. Sleisenger and Fordtran's Gastrointestinal and Liver Disease. 10th Edition. Saunders/Elsevier, Philadelphia, 2016, page 2311).

➤ Demography (occurrence in women)

  o Menstruating, 15%

  o Infertile, 30%

➤ Clinical

  o "symptoms are not always cyclical and might not fluctuate with hormonal levels" (Feldman M., et al. Sleisenger and Fordtran's Gastrointestinal and Liver Disease. 10th Edition. Saunders/Elsevier, Philadelphia, 2016, page 2311).

  o PV (per vaginal pelvic examination)

    – Before and after menstruation

    – Tender nodules in cul-de-sac

➤ Endoscopy

  o Site

    – Rectosigmoid (96%)

    – Appendix (10%)

    – Ileum (5%)

  o Colonoscopy

    – Compression by endometrial mass

    – Strictures (submucosal mass or partial narrowing, with intact mucosa)

    – Mucosa rarely abnormal → hematochezia

"You cannot solve a problem with the same mind that created it."

Albert Einstein

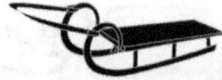

COLONIC OBSTRUCTION

Large Bowel Obstruction (LBO)

➢ Cause
- o CRC, 50%
- o Volvulus 10% - 15% (sigmoid, 75%; cecum, ~25%)
- o Diverticular disease, benign strictures 10%

• Give the effect of a competent ileocecal valve on the potential severity of LBO.
- o Yes, more severe because the colon cannot decompress into the small bowel

Acute Colonic Pseudo-Obstruction (ACPO, aka Ogilvie Syndrome)

➢ Definition
- o "…acute massive, colonic dilation that induces primarily the right side of the colon and is unexplained by mechanical cause."

➢ Pathophysiology

Please see above, Sleisenger and Fordtran's Gastrointestinal and Liver Disease. 9th Edition. Saunders/Elsevier, Philadelphia, 2010, page 2178.

➢ Pathology
- o Prederentially affects cecum > AC > TC
- o Presence of pain may herald ischemia/perforation
- o Risk of perforation   < 12 cm, 2%
                                     12-14 cm, 7%
                                       > 14 cm, 23%

Abbreviations: AC, ascending colon; TC, transverse colon

➢ Causes/associations
- o Causes seen by gastroenterologists are mostly secondary
- o Severe underlying medical or surgical illness (secondary causes)
- o ↑ age
- o ↑BMI
- o Use of patient-controlled analgesia (PCA)
- o Disease associations (secondary pseudo-obstruction)

Please see Sleisenger and Fordtran's Gastrointestinal and Liver Disease. 10th Edition. Saunders/Elsevier, Philadelphia, 2016, Table 124-2, page 2179; Box 124-5, page 2182.

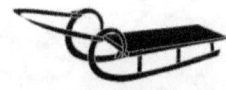

- Give causes of secondary pseudo-obstruction.

  o MSK
    - Amyloidosis
    - Scleroderma, dermatomyositis/polymyositis, SLE (systemic lupus erythematosus)

  o Muscle
    - Myotonic dystrophy
    - Duchenne muscular dystrophy

  o Metabolic
    - Diabetes
    - Thyroid disease
    - Hypoparathyroidism

  o Neurological
    - Parkinson disease
    - Spinal cord injury
      ▪ Spinal cord injury → "spinal shock" → paralytic ileus → 40% have persistent constipation
      ▪ Constipation is due to
        - ↓ postprandial response in descending colon
        - ↓ resting anal pressure

  o Psychiatric
    - Bulimia
    - Anorexia neurosa

  o Idiopathic
    - Neurofibromatosis
    - Myenteric ganglionitis

  o Cancer
    - Paraneoplastic visceral neuropathies

  o Infection
    - Chaga disease

  o Gastrointestinal
    - Celiac disease
    - Jejunal diverticulosis
    - Radiation damage
    - Enteric
    - Neuropathies
    - Myopathies
    - Menenchy myopathies

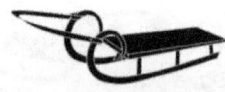

- ➢ Diagnostic imaging
  - ○ Plain abdominal films
    - – Sensitivity of plain abdominal films for SBO is poor only about 75% (this means that you miss the diagnosis of SBO in 25%!)
    - – It may be difficult to distinguish small bowel obstruction (SBO) from colonic obstruction (CO).

	SBO	CO
○ Air in the rectum	Yes	No
○ Dilation of both small and large intestinal		Yes (if ileocecal valve is incompetent)

- ➢ Treatment
  - ○ Acute: Neostigmine 2mg IV over 3-5 min with ECG monitoring to detect bradycardia. If no response in 4 minutes, repeat once (response rate>80%); if no response, perform decompression colonoscopy.
    - – Contraindications to neostigmine: signs of colonic ischemia or perforation, bronchospasm, bradycardia, creatinine >3mg/dL, pregnancy.
  - ○ Recurrence: Reduce the 35% risk of recurrence of megacolon by using 30g/day of PEG electrolyte solutions.
  - ○ Chronic: PEG electrolyte solution is useful; neostigmine, fibre and lactulose solution are ineffective.
    - – Note: There is no proven benefit of placement of decompression tube.

- ➢ Prognosis
  - ○ Fatality, 15%
  - ○ Recurrence, 50% (after rectal tube)
  - ○ ~15% develop colonic ischemia or perforation (when diameter of cecum > 12 cm)
  - ○ Mortality rate from perforation, ~40%
  - ○ Mortality from surgical decompression, ~30%
  - ○ Endoscopic decompression, perforation rate, 3%
  - ○ Neostigmine, initial benefit in > 60%

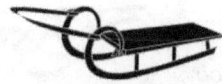

Volvulus of the Colon

➤ Causes
- o Occurs rarely in hospitalized patients with neurological disorders, diseases of intestinal smooth muscle, or may be idiopathic.
- o May be associated with disintegration of enteric nerves, or atrophy of the collagenous connective tissue membrane of the myenteric plexus and muscularis propria

➤ Sites
- o Sigmoid colon
  - – On diagnostic imaging
    - ▪ Distention of sigmoid colon
    - ▪ No haustra
    - ▪ Apex points to right shoulder
- o Cecal volvulus
  - – Less common (22%, vs sigmoid volvulus 75%)
  - – More frequently is complicated by ischemia (large diameter [large radius, R], high wall tension [T] [Laplace law, T= PR], so the bowel becomes ischemic because of ↓ capillary perfusion.
  - – On diagnostic imaging
    - ▪ Distention of cecum into the epigastric area or left upper quadrant
    - ▪ "bean-shaped"
    - ▪ Collapse of colon distal to cecum
    - ▪ Small bowel obstruction, single air-fluid level
- o Cecum in LUQ
- o Coffee-bean appearance
- o Dilated small bowel

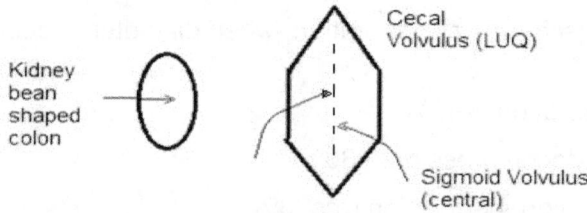

- o Tortion 180° to 360° clockwise or counter-clockwise orientation (50:50)
- o Dilated colon (megacolon)
  - – Rectum   > 6.5 cm
  - – AC   > 8 cm
  - – Cecum   > 10 (if > 13 cm, imminent perforation)

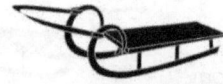

VASCULAR DISORDERS

Colonic Ischemia (CI)

➤ Demography

- o Incidence of
  - – CI in general population $7/10^5$ person-years
  - – IBS ~ $24/10^5$ person-years

➤ Causes/associations

- Give the lesions, syndromes or diseases associated with four types of vascular malformations, based on the most affected vascular structure.

Most Affected Vascular Structure	Lesions, Syndrome, Disease
o Venous	– Varices – Hemorrhoids
o Capillary	– Gastric antral vascular ectasia – Portal gastropathy
o Arteriovenous	– Angiodysplasia – Teleangiectasia
o Arterial	– Dieulafoy's lesion – Ehlers-Danlos syndrome – Pseudoxanthoma elasticum

Printed with permission: Regula, Jaroslaw. et al.*Best Pract Res Clin Gastroenterol* 2008;22(2): pg 314.

Please see Feldman M., et al. Sleisenger and Fordtran's Gastrointestinal and Liver Disease. 10th Edition. Saunders/Elsevier, Philadelphia, 2010, Box 118-2, page 2090.

- Give causes of acute and chronic mesenteric ischemia.
  - o Superior mesenteric artery (SMA)
    - – Embolism 50%
      - ▪ Atrial fibrillation
      - ▪ Left ventricle thrombosis
      - ▪ Ulcerated aortic plaque
    - – Thrombosis 15%

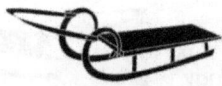

- Non-occlusive 25%
  - Vasospasm
  - Shock
  - Heart failure
  - Cardiac dysrhythmias
- Medications
  - 5-HT3 antagonist
  - 5-HT4 agonist
  - Cocaine
  - Digitalis
  - Dopamine
  - Oral contraceptive (OCA)
- Venous thrombus 10%
- Hypercoagulable conditions
  - Primary
  - Secondary
    - Cirrhosis, diabetes, hyperlipidemia, IBD, inflammation , intra-abdominal sepsis, paraneoplastic, perforation, postoperative, smoking, trauma
- Portal hypertension
- Oral contraceptive agent (OCA)
- Perforated viscous
- Pancreatitis
- Trauma
- Inflammatory bowel disease (IBD)

○ Focal segmental ischemia (5%)
- Mechanical
  - Trauma
  - Radiation
- Localized small vessel occlusion
  - Cholesterol emboli
  - Strangulated hernias
  - Vasculitis
  - Volvulus
  - Sickle cell disease

○ Irritable bowel syndrome (IBS), and its treatment (5-HT3 antagonists 5-HT4 agonists)

Trick MCQ

○ Chronic mesenteric ischemia (CMI)
- Not associated with smoking!

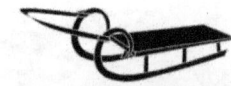

- o Chronic mesenteric ischemia
  - – Vessel lumen
    - ▪ Atherosclerosis and atheroma
    - ▪ Diabetes, hyperlipidemia, smoking
  - – Vessel wall
    - ▪ Celiac artery compression syndrome
    - ▪ Fibrovascular dysplasia
    - ▪ Mesenteric venous thrombosis
    - ▪ Takayasu's arteritis
    - ▪ Thromboangiitis obliterans

Abbreviations: IBS, irritable bowel syndrome; OCA, oral contraceptive agent; SMA, superior mesenteric artery

Adapted from: Sleisenger and Fordtran's Gastrointestinal and Liver Disease. 10th Edition. Saunders/Elsevier, Philadelphia, 2016, Box 118-2, page 2090.

- Give the names of classes of medications which are associated with the development of colonic ischemia (CI).
  - o AAHC (antibiotic-associated hemorrhagic colitis)
  - o Chemotherapy
  - o Cocaine
  - o Drugs
    - – 5-HT3 antagonists
    - – Decongestants (α1-adrenergics)
    - – HRT (hormone replacement therapy), OCP (oral contraceptive pill)
    - – NSAIDs

➢ Clinical

- Give clinical presentations of acute and chronic mesenteric ischemia.
- Acute
  - o Background clinical picture of underlying disease
  - o Acute onset of pain out of proportion to benign abdominal examination
  - o Rectal bleeding
  - o Urge to defecate/diarrhea
  - o Abdominal tenderness
  - o Confusion, sepsis, hypertension, fever, post prandial pain
  - o Rebound guarding

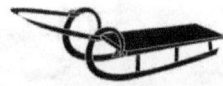

- o Consider risk factors (DM, AF, etc.), including drugs e.g., alosetron, tegaserod, cocaine, digitalis
- o Association with IBS (irritable bowel syndrome)

- Chronic
  - o Symptoms
    - – Post-prandial intestinal angina
    - – Fear of eating (sitophobia)
    - – Weight loss
    - – Nausea and vomiting
  - o Signs
    - – Abdominal tenderness out of proportion to benign abdominal examination
    - – Epigastric bruit (non-specific)
    - – Gastric ulceration
    - – Gastroparesis
    - – Gallbladder dyskinesia

Adapted from: Brandt L. *Sleisenger & Fordtran's gastrointestinal and liver disease: Pathophysiology/Diagnosis/Management* 2006: pg. 2566.

➢ Laboratory
  - o Lactic acidosis
  - o Ion gap metabolic acidosis
  - o Hypercoagulopathy
  - o Anemia
  - o Leucocytosis

➢ Diagnostic imaging

- Give the diagnostic imaging tests used to diagnose acute mesenteric ischemia (AMI).
  - o Abdominal film
  - o Colonoscopy or flexible sigmoidoscopy, with mucosal biopsy
  - o Doppler ultrasound (shows only proximal vessels)
  - o CT angiography
  - o MRI
  - o Angiography

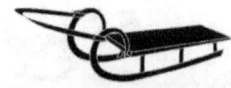

- o CTA/MRA (CT/MR angiography)

- o The splanchnic blood flow may be reduced without ischemia, so Doppler ultrasound must show > 70% stenosis and ↑ peak systolic velocity in SMA of 275 cm/sec, and 200 cm/sec in CA before the diagnosis of CMI is entertained.

- o Tests of provocation testing may be useful, such as GET (gastric tonometric exercise testing), looking for ↑ gastric-arterial PCO_2 gradient in patient on PPI and PCO_2 measured before, during and often exercise

- Give the diagnostic imaging findings suggestive of intestinal ischemia.

  - o Bowel lumen
    - – Calibre
    - – Content
    - – Transition point if associated obstruction
    - – Inraluminal hemorrhage
    - – Small bowel feces sign

  - o Bowel wall
    - – Thickness
    - – Homogeneity
    - – Enhancement pattern
    - – Length of involvement
    - – Pneumatosis

  - o Mesentery
    - – Edema
    - – Hemorrhage
    - – Patency of mesenteric vessels
    - – Mesenteric vascular engorgement
    - – Ascites
    - – Volvulus
    - – Intussusception

Printed with permission: Gore, et al. *Clin Gastroenterol Hepatol* 2008; 6: 849-59.

➢ Endoscopy

- o Segmental disease

- o Rectal sparing

- o All parts of the colon may be affected by CI (~23% sigmoid colon, 23% right side of the colon [IRC]), both pancolitis and right-sided colitis are common in persons with sepsis.

585

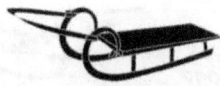

- o IRC has
  - – 2x ↑ risk of needing surgery
  - – 5x ↑ mortality rate
- o The presence of a circumferential ulcer has a worse prognosis than an ulcer in the longitudinal axis ("single-stripe" sign)
- o Superficial half of colonic mucosa preferentially affected
- o Hemorrhagic streaking (mucosal and submucosal hemorrhage)
- o Superficial ulceration
- o Deep ulcers
- o UC-like colitis
- o Liquefaction necrosis perforation
- o Stricture (reversible, irreversible, saccular stricture)
- o Pneumatosis linearis (colonic gangrene, HIV disease)
- o Carcinoma (pressure of CRC produces local ischemia)
- o Diverticulosis-associated ischemia
- o Isolated R-colon ischemia (IRCI) may herald a SMA occlusion

- ➢ Histopathology
  - o Fibrin plugs in capillaries
  - o Partial necrosis and ulceration
  - o Crypt abscesses
  - o Iron-laden macrophages in submucosa
  - o In IRC (but not other forms of CI), evaluation of vasculature is important
  - o CI is associated with vascular surgery
    - – Urgent surgery for ruptural AAA (~60%)
    - – Elective surgery on aortic valve (~7%)

Abbreviation: IRCI, isolated R-colon ischemia

Adapted from: Sleisenger and Fordtran's Gastrointestinal and Liver Disease. 10th Edition. Saunders/Elsevier, Philadelphia, 2016, page 2092.

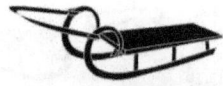

> Treatment

  o Supportive

  o Treat associated, underlying conditions

  o PTMA (percutaneous transmural mesenteric angioplasty), +/- stenting (PTMAS, percutaneous transluminal mesenteric angioplasty with stenting)

  o Early surgery with resection for infarction/gangrene/perforation

  o Embolectomy

  o Papaverine infusion

  o Revasculization surgery

  o Thrombolectomy

  o Broad spectrum antibiotics if micro-perforation is suspected

  o Laproscopy
    – If high index of clinical suspicion of infarction

Adapted from: *Sleisenger & Fordtran's gastrointestinal and liver disease: Pathophysiology/Diagnosis/Management* 2016, 10th edition, Figure 118-7, page 2082.

Hemangiomas

> Definition: Hemangiomas are well circumscribed, non-encapsulated hamartomas, single or multiple, involving just the colon or diffuse along the GI tract (GIT), with or without non-GIT tissues.

> Diagnostic imaging

  o Hemangiomas may be cavernous, capillary or mixed

  o Plain film
    – Multiple foci of calcification (phleboliths) in abnormal vascular channels
    – Soft tissue mass distorting/displacing rectal air column

  o Barium enema
    – The vascular lesion distorts/ displaces external surface of colon
    – Wall of rectum is thickened, causing a widened presarcral space
    – Lumen of colon
      ▪ Narrow
      ▪ Rigid
      ▪ Scalloped

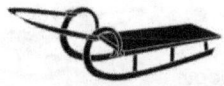

Congenital Arteriovenous Malformations (AVMs)

➤ Definition: "...congenital communications between arteries/veins, located primarily in the submucosa" (Sleisenger and Fordtran's Gastrointestinal and Liver Disease. 9th Edition. Saunders/Elsevier, Philadelphia, 2010, page 606).

➤ Pathology

- o Veins
  - – Dilated
  - – Tortuous
  - – Thick walls
  - – Hypertrophy of smooth muscle
  - – Intima thick/ scleroses

- o Arteries
  - – Dilated
  - – Wall atrophic
  - – Sclerotic degeneration

Abdominal Aortic Aneurysm (AAA)

➤ Demography

- o 85% occur in men
- o 95% are associated with atherosclerosis
- o 20% familial clustering (e.g.,association with Ehlers-Danlos syndrome type IV)

➤ Treatment (surgical resection)

- o Good risk patients with aneurysms which are
  - – Symptomatic
  - – Enlarging
  - – > 5 cm

➤ Surveillance

- o Management of asymptomatic aneurysms, ≥ 4 cm size: abdominal ultrasound every 3 to 6 mon (growth rate of AAA is about 0.35 cm per yr).

SO YOU WANT TO BE A GASTROENTEROLOGIST!

Most abdominal bruits increase in intensity with inspiration.

- • Give the clinical significance of an abdominal bruit which becomes louder on expiration.
  - o An abdominal bruit which becomes more intense on expiration suggests the Celiac axis compression syndrome (CACS).
  - o CACS is the presence of epigastric pain coming after meals, diarrhea, weight loss and an expiration intensifying abdominal bruit due to compression of the celiac axis by the median arcuate ligament of the diaphragm.

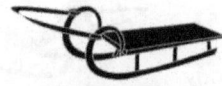

SO YOU WANT TO BE A GASTROENTEROLOGIST!

- Give why angiography is not as sensitive as abdominal ultrasound to determine the size of an AAA (abdominal aortic aneurysm).

    o If there is a laminated thrombus in the lumen of the aneurysm, the entire lumen cannot be visualized, and so the extent of the AAA cannot be correctly assessed by angiography.

- Give factors which increase the **risk of rupture** of an AAA.
    o Hypertension (systemic)
    o COPD (chronic obstructive lung disease)
    o Size

cm	5-year Risk
5.0	0
5.5 – 5.9	20% - 25%
6.0	35% - 40%
>7.0	75%

    o Morbidity, aortic graft enteric fistula, 2% (usually D3 or D4)
    o Mortality rate of elective repair in good risk patient, 1% - 4%

Abbreviation: D3; third part of duodenum; D4, fourth part of duodenum

Sleisenger and Fordtran's Gastrointestinal and Liver Disease. 10th Edition. *Saunders/Elsevier*, Philadelphia, 2016, page 633

- Give clinical features which suggest that an upper or lower GI bleed might be arising from on **aortoenteric fistula**.
    o Fever (from infection in the graft
    o History of AAA surgery
    o "herald bleed"

- In the context of an AAA, what is the significance of a loud abdominal bruit.
    o A loud abdominal bruit in a patient with an AAA suggests the development of a rupture of the AAA into the IVC (inferior vena cava).

589

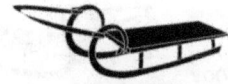

DIVERTICULAR DISEASE (DDC)

➢ Definition

- ○ 90% of colonic diverticulae are in the sigmoid

- ○ ~15% of DDC are in the right-side of the colon, with or without co-existing left-sided DDC (Right sided DDC is more frequent in Asian countries

- ○ 2x ↑ elastin deposits in muscle cells in taenia as well as ↑ type III collagen and ↑ tissue inhibitor of metalloproteinases, but no muscle hypertrophy

- ○ ↑ ICC (interstitial cells of Cajal)

➢ Demography

- ○ Diverticular disease is a significant contributor to the morbidity and health-care expenditures.

- ○ Affects ~ 25% of persons in "Westernized" countries

- ○ DDC ↑ prevalence with age

- ○ May be more common with ↑ intake of red meat and ↓ fibre

- ○ Associated with connective tissue disease, e.g., scleroderma, Ehlers-Danlos and marfan syndrome

- ○ Overweight, obesity, and physical inactivity among women increase
  - – Diverticular disease requiring hospital admission
  - – The risk for serious complications are even more pronounced.

Source: Hjern F, et al. Am J Gastroenterol 2012; 107: 296-302.

➢ Pathophysiology

- • Give the pathophysiology of diverticular disease.

  - ○ Motility
    - – ↑ ICC
    - – ↑ segmentation → ↑ high amplitude of contractions → ↑ pressure
    - – ↑ motility indices
    - – ↑ abnormal motility → ↑ retropropagation of some contraction waves
    - – Nerve activity
      - ▪ ↑ excitatory cholinergic
      - ▪ ↓ inhibitory non-adrenergic, non-cholinergic

590

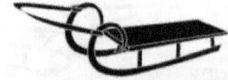

- – ↓ nerve responsiveness to
  - ▪ Antagonist of
    - – Acetylcholine
    - – Tachykinin
  - ▪ Substance P
- o Diet
  - – Dietary fibre
    - ▪ Role in pathogenesis and treatment remains controversial; recommend ↑ fibre intake on a person-by-person basis
- o NSAIDs
  - – NSAIDs and Diverticular complications
    - ▪ NSAID and aspirin use were associated with similar and ↑ risks (hazard ratios, HR) for diverticular bleeding compared with non-use of either drug (HR, 1.74 and 1.70).
    - ▪ Use of aspirin for 4 to 6 days per week was associated with higher risk of diverticular bleeding compared with higher and lower frequencies of aspirin use (HR, 3.13).
    - ▪ Longer duration of aspirin or NSAID use (≥ 10 years) was associated with greater risk for diverticulitis and diverticular bleeding.
    - ▪ Use of low-dose aspirin (81 mg daily) without concomitant NSAID use was associated with a great risk for diverticulitis.
    - ▪ NSAID use was associated with higher risk for diverticulitis than aspirin use when each was compared with non-use of either drug (hazard ratio 1.72 vs 1.25)
    - ▪ NSAID use was more strongly associated with complicated diverticulitis than with uncomplicated diverticulitis (HR, 2.55 vs 1.65)

Printed with permission: Strate LL, et al. Use of aspirin or non-steroidal anti-inflammatory drugs increases risk for diverticulitis and diverticular bleeding. Gastroenterology 2011;140(5):1427-33.

"All life is an experiment. The more experiments you make, the better."

Ralph Waldo Emerson

591

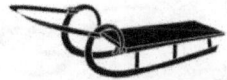

➤ Clinical

• Give symptoms and signs of diverticular disease.

Complication	Symptoms	Signs
o Diverticulitis	– Pain, fever & constipation or diarrhea (or both)	▪ Palpable tender colon, leukocytosis
o Pericolic abscess	– Pain, fever (with or without tenderness) or pus in stool	▪ Tender mass, guarding, leukocytosis, soft tissue mass on abdominal films or ultrasonograms
o Fistula	– Depends on site; dysuria, pneumaturia, fecal discharge on skin or vagina	▪ Depends on site; fistulogram, methylene blue
o Perforation	– Sudden severe pain, fever	▪ Sepsis, leukocytosis, free air
o Liver abscess	– Right upper quadrant pain, fever, weight loss	▪ Tender liver, tender bowel or mass, leukocytosis, increased serum alkaline phosphatase, lumbosacral scan (filling defect)
o Bleeding	– Bright red or maroon blood or clots	▪ Blood on rectal examination, sigmoidoscopy, colonoscopy, angiography

➤ Clinical classification
  o Stages of diverticular disease.
    – Stage 0   ▪ Development of diverticular disease
    – Stage I   ▪ Asymptomatic disease
    – Stage II   ▪ Symptomatic disease
                         – Single episode
                         – Recurrent
                         – Chronic (pain, diarrhea, IBD overlap/SCAD)

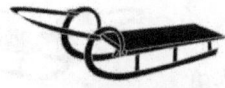

- Stage III
  - Complicated
    - Abscess
    - Phlegmon
    - Obstruction
    - Fistulization
    - Bleeding
    - Sepsis
    - Stricture

Abbreviation: SCAD, segmented colitis associated with diverticulum

Printed with permission: Sheth AA et al. *Am J Gastroenterol* 2008;103:1551.

o   EAES clinical classification

Grade	Clinical Description	Recommended Diagnostic Testing
o Grade I – Symptomatic, uncomplicated disease	-Fever, crampy abdominal pain	Colonoscopy *vs* barium enema to rule out malignancy, colitis
o Grade II – Recurrent, symptomatic disease	-Recurrence of above	CT scan *vs* barium enema
o Grade III – Complicated disease	-Abscess -Hemorrhage -Stricture -Fistula -Phlegmon -Purulent and fecal peritonitis -Perforation -Obstruction	CT scan

Abbreviation: EAES, European Association for Endoscopic Surgeons

Printed with permission: Sheth AA, Longo W, and Floch MH. *AJG* 2008;103: pp 1551-2.

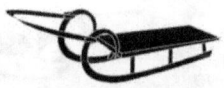

Mastering the Boards: Gastroenterology   A.B.R. Thomson

Clinical classification of complicated diverticulosis (diverticulitis; extramural disease)

- o Caused by obstruction by fecalith and perforation of diverticulum
  - Pericolic abscess (I) (microperforation)
  - Distant abscess (II)
  - Peritonitis (III)
  - Fecal peritonitis (IV)

- ➢ Pathology
  - o Pseudodiverticula colonic where vasa recta perforate the colonic wall between the mesenteric taenia and the two anti-mesenteric taeniae (but not between the two anti-mesenteric taeniae
  - o Non-specific inflammation
  - o Lymphocytes, PMN
  - o Granulomas
  - o Rectal sparing

- ➢ Complications

- • Give the complications of diverticulitis in immune-suppressed (IS) and non-IS patient.

Complication	IS	Non-IS
o Perforation	43	14
o Need for surgery	58	33
o Post-op mortality	39	2

Note: that the post-operative mortality rate in persons with a solid organ transplantation who develops diverticulitis is very high (25% to 100%).

- ➢ Diagnostic imaging

- • Give the diagnostic Imaging (DI) changes of acute diverticulitis.

  - o Plain film
    - Dilation
    - Abscess (soft tissue density)
    - Pneumoperitoneum (~10%)

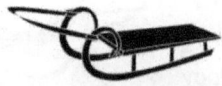

- o Ultrasonography
  - – Typical findings
    - ▪ Diverticular
    - ▪ Colonic wall, hyperechogenic
    - ▪ Abscess(es)
  - – Performance characteristics (equivalent to CT)
    - ▪ Sensitivity, 84% to 98%
    - ▪ Specificity, 80% to 93%

- o Gastrografin enema
  - – Diverticulosis
  - – Extravasation (Extraluminal mass)
  - – Sinus tract
  - – Fistula
  - – Performance characteristics
    - ▪ Sensitivity, ~75%
    - ▪ False-negative, ~30%

- o CT scanning with contrast
  - – Gold standard
  - – Typical findings
    - ▪ Diverticula
    - ▪ Periodic infiltration of fatty tissue (fat stranding)
    - ▪ Colonic wall thickened (> 4 mm)
    - ▪ Abscess(es)
  - – Performance characteristics
    - ▪ Sensitivity, 75% to 100%
    - ▪ Specificity, 93% to 98%

- ➤ Endoscopy
  - o Diverticulae Associated Colitis (DAC; aka SCAD [segmental colitis associated with diverticula])
    - – Note: not typical of IBD

  - o Multiple openings into diverticulae
    - – Sparing of orifices of diverticula
    - – Erythema on crest of fold
    - – Sparing of rectum (diverticula are usually in sigmoid colon)
    - – Usually mild disease

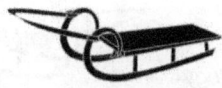

SO YOU WANT TO BE A GASTROENTEROLOGIST!

- Give the earliest signs of inflammation in colonic diverticula.

    - o Hyperplasia of the lymphoid tissue at the apex of the obstructed diverticulum.

A colonic biopsy is shown to you blindly, without any clinical information. The biopsy shows

- o Cryptitis
- o Chronic lymphocytic infiltration
- o Crypt abscesses
- o Granulomas

- Give the piece of information needed about the site of the biopsy before making the diagnosis of IBD.

    - o SCAD (segmental colitis associated with diverticulosis) may be histologically indistinguishable from IBD, so determine if the biopsy was taken from a colonic diverticulum!

- Give CT classifications of diverticulitis (e.g., Buckley, Hinchey).

    - o Buckley classification

	CT Findings
– Mild	▪ Bowel wall thickening, fat stranding
– Moderate	▪ Bowel wall thickening >3 mm, phlegmon or small abscess
– Severe	▪ Bowel wall thickening > 5 mm, frank perforation with subdiaphragmatic free air, abscess > 5 cm

596

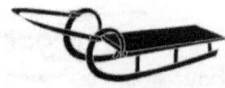

o Hinchey classification (perforated diverticulitis)

Grade		Finding		
I	–	Inflammation of pericolonic fat		
II	–	Pericolic abscess		
III	–	Abscess	▪	Pelvic
			▪	Distant
IV	–	Generalized peritonitis	▪	Purulent
			▪	Fecal

Printed with permission: Sheth AA, et al. *AJG* 2008;103: pp 1551. Please also see Sleisenger and Fordtran's Gastrointestinal and Liver Disease. 10th Edition. Saunders/Elsevier, Philadelphia, 2010, Table 121-1, page 2129).

➢ Treatment

- Treatment at age extremes
  - o Younger
    - – More frequent need for surgery because of more severe and more recurrent disease
  - o Older
    - – ↓ need for surgery, ↓ recurrent disease, but ↓ surgical morbidity is because of more frequent comorbidities in elderly,

- Acute
  - o Antibiotics
    - – Organisms
      - ▪ E. coli
      - ▪ Streptococcus
      - ▪ Bacteroids fragilis
    - – Metronidazole/clindamycin plus aminoglycoside/cephalosporin
  - o CT-guided percutaneous drainage of abdominal abscess(es)
  - o Endoscopic dilation +/- stent for stricture
  - o Surgery
    - – Required in ~25%
    - – Uncomplicated bowel preparation
      - ▪ Single-stage resection
    - – Complicated
      - ▪ Two stage resection, end colostomy, oversewing distal stump (Hartmann procedure); reanastomosis
    - – Fistula (colovesical, colovaginal)
      - ▪ Single stage resection

597

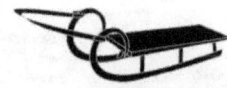

- Maintenance of SUDD (symptomatic uncomplicated diverticular disease; aka painful diverticular disease)
  - Patient-by-patient trial of
    - ↑ fibre intake
    - Anticholinergics
    - 5-ASA (aminosalicylic acid)
    - Locally acting antibiotics (e.g., rifaximin)
    - Sigmoid colectomy

- Recurrent diverticulitis
  - ~30% have second episode of diverticulitis, ½ within one year
  - "multiple recurrences don't appear less-favourable outcomes" (Feldman M., et al. Sleisenger and Fordtran's Gastrointestinal and Liver Disease. 9th Edition. Saunders/Elsevier, Philadelphia, 2010, page 2083).
  - "a recent decision analysis predict that performing colectomy after the fourth attack of diverticulitis rather than after the second attack would result in fewer deaths and colostomies while having a superior cost-effectiveness" (Feldman M., et al. Sleisenger and Fordtran's Gastrointestinal and Liver Disease. 9th Edition. Saunders/Elsevier, Philadelphia, 2010, page 2083).
  - Unfortunately, patients who have had a surgical resection
    - Recurrent diverticulitis, 10%
    - Further surgery, 2% to 3%

Diverticulosis and Hemorrhage

➤ Demography
  - ~5% of persons with colonic diverticula will have an arterial bleed
  - Just because a person with known diverticulosis has a LGIB does not prove that the LGIB is a diverticular bleed (may just as well be bleeding from angiodysplasia).

➤ Cause/associations
  - Precipitant NSAIDs may cause diverticular bleed, and more severe diverticular bleeding
  - Relative risk of LGIB (lower GI bleeding) from Coxib vs NSAIDs, 0.46%

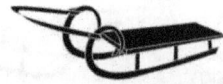

> Diagnosis

- o To make the diagnosis of a diverticular bleed, you need to show bleeding from the diverticulum
  - – Colonoscopy
    - ▪ Visible vessel
    - ▪ Adherent clot
  - – RBC scan
    - ▪ Sensitive to bleedy at 0.1 mL/ min
  - – Angiography
    - ▪ Sensitive to bleeding at 0.5 mL/min
    - ▪ Resection for LGIB
    - ▪ With site of resection determined by angiography, stops bleeding in 88% to 94% (i.e., 6% to 12% rebleed, presumably because correct bleeding site not identified by angiography)
  - – Enhanced CT

> Treatment

- o Superselective embolization of bleeding vessel stops LGIB in 67% to 100%, with risk of ischemia of only 20%
- o Endoscopic hemostatic therapy
- o Hemicolectomy

> Prognosis

- o Bleeding stops spontaneously, ~75%
- o Rebleeding, ~25%
- o Re-rebleeding, ~50%

"Change will not come if we wait for some other person, or if we wait for some other time. We are the ones we've been waiting for. We are the change that we seek."

Barack Obama

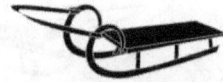

Intra-Abdominal Abscesses

➢ Causes/associations

• Give common causes of intra-abdominal abscesses.
  o Perforated
      – Stomach/ duodenum - peptic ulcer)
      – Small bowel - Crohn disease
      – Colon – diverticulitis
      – Appendix – appendicitis
      – Gallbladder – cholecystectomy
  o Trauma
  o Tumour

Adapted from: Minei, Joseph P. and Champine, Julie G. *Sleisenger & Fordtran's gastrointestinal and liver disease: Pathophysiology/ Diagnosis/Management* 2006; pg. 526; and 10th Edition, 2016, Box 28-2, page 440.

➢ Risk factors

• Give clinical risk factors for intra-abdominal abscess formation.
  o Systemic factors
      – Increasing age
      – Preexisting organ dysfunction
      – Transfusion
      – Malnutrition
      – Chronic Glucocorticoid use
      – Underlying malignancy
  o Local factors
      – Severity of illness/infection
      – Delay to surgery for underlying disease
      – Severity of trauma
      – Formation of an ostomy
      – Nonappendiceal source of infection

Adapted from: Sleisenger and Fordtran's Gastrointestinal and Liver Disease. 10th Edition. Saunders/Elsevier, Philadelphia, 2016, page Box 28-2, page 440.

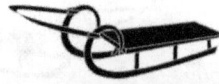

LOWER GI BLEEDING (LGIB)

➤ Causes/associations

• Give the common causes of hematochezia in adults.

Causes	Approximate Frequency (%)	Comments
o Diverticular disease	30	– Stops spontaneously in 80% of patients – In one series, the need for surgery may be unlikely if <4U red cell transfusion given in 24 h, but is required in 60% of patients receiving >4U in 24h
o Colonic vascular ectasia (AV malformation, angiodysplasia)	25	– Frequency of these lesions vary widely in clinical series – Acute bleeding appears to be more frequently due to lesion in proximal colon
o Colitis	10	– Ischemic colitis often presents with pain and self-limited haemotochezia. Colitis is segmental, most often affecting splenic flexure – Bleeding may also occur from other types of colitis, such as Crohn disease or ulcerative colitis (see Small Bowel question 40) – Bloody diarrhea is most frequent symptom of infectious colitis and inflammatory bowel disease of the colon
o Colonic neoplasia/post-polypectomy	10	– Post-polypectomy bleeding is frequency self- limited, and may occur ≤14 days after polypectomy
o Anorectal causes (including hemorrhoids, varices)	5	– Anoscopy/proctoscopy should be included in the rectal initial evaluation of these patients
o Brisk upper GI bleeding	5	– A negative nasogastric aspirate does not exclude this possibility
o Small bowel causes	10	– Frequency diagnosed by diagnostic imaging or enteroscopy after the acute bleeding episode has resolved.

Adapted from: Zuccaro G. *Best Pract Res Clin Gastroenterol* 2008; 22(2): pg. 227; Jensen DM. Lower GI. *2009 ACG Annual Postgraduate Course*:123-129.

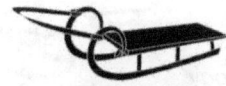

- Give the differential diagnosis of the causes of upper and lower gastrointestinal bleeding in persons with **HIV/AIDS** (excluding non-AIDS specific diagnoses).

  - o Esophagus
    - – Infection
      - • *Candida**
      - • Cytomegalovirus*
      - • Herpes simplex
      - • Idiopathic ulcer
  - o Stomach
    - – Infection
      - • Cytomegalovirus*
      - • Cryptosporidiosis
    - – Infiltration
      - • Kaposi's sarcoma*
      - • Lymphoma
  - o Small intestine
    - – Infection
      - • Cytomegalovirus*
      - • *Salmonella* sp.
      - • *Cryptosporidium*
    - – Infiltration
      - • Kaposi sarcoma*
      - • Lymphoma
  - o Colon
    - – Infection
      - • Cytomegalovirus*
      - • *Entamoeba histolytica*
      - • *Campylobacter*
      - • *Clostridium difficile*
      - • *Shigella* sp.
      - • Idiopathic ulcerations
    - – Infiltration
      - • Kaposi sarcoma*
      - • Lymphoma

  - o Infections
    - – C. difficile
    - – Campylobacter
    - – CMV
    - – Entameoba histolytica
    - – Histoplasmosis
    - – HPV
    - – HSV
    - – LGV
    - – Shigella sp.
    - – Tuberculosis
  - o Infiltration (cancer)
    - – CRC
      - • Lymphoma
      - • Squamous cell carcinoma
      - • Kaposi sarcoma
  - o Infections
  - o Perianal
    - – Abscess
    - – Fissure
    - – Trauma
    - – Fistula
  - o Idiopathic ulcers

*More frequent causes

Abbreviation: CRC, colorectal cancer

Adapted from: Wilcox, C. Mel. *Sleisenger & Fordtran's gastrointestinal and liver disease: Pathophysiology/Diagnosis/Management* 2006: pg 676.

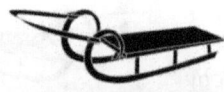

Non-HIV/AIDs Related Bowel Diseases

- Endoscopy
  - Hematochezia
    - Colonoscopy
  - Suspected rectal bleeding
    - Anoscopy and sigmoidoscopy with mucosal biopsy and with evaluation of anorectal pus for PMNs
    - Gram stain for gonococci
    - Tzanck prep, and culture for HSV, VDRL and PCR for C. trachomatis. Biopsy should be performed even if visual inspection of the anal canal is normal, since a normal appearance does not exclude high grade dysplasia.

Printed with permission: Yachimski, and Friedman. *Nat Clin Pract Gastroenterol Hepatol* 2008; 5 (2): 81.

Some words are surrogate markers ("**buzzwords**) which are often used to signal a clue to the diagnosis. For 4 of the following give the likely diagnosis from the "buzzword".

Buzzword	Implied Diagnosis
o Vimenton-positive	– Glomus tumour
o Actin-positive	– Leiomyoma
o S-100-positive	– Schwanoma
o Central umblication	– Pancreatic rest
o Dysphagia plus – Heliotrope rash – Shawl sign – Gottron knuckles – Proximal muscle wasting	– Dermatomyositis
o Wide-mouthed right-sided colonic diverticula	– Scleoderma (systemic sclerosis)
o Colitis plus Retinitis – "owl's eye" intranuclear inclusion bodies	– CMV
o Serpiginous ulcers	– CD (Crohn disease)
o Flask-shaped ulcers	– Entamaeba histolytica
o S2-S4 saddle distribution	– HSV neuropathy

603

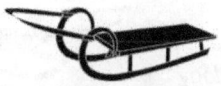

ABBREVIATIONS

AAA	Abdominal aortic aneurysm
AAD	Antibiotic-associated diarrhea
AAHC	Antibiotic-associated hemorrhagic colitis
AAP	Advanced adenomatous polyp
AC	Acute self-limiting colitis
AC	Ascending colon
ACC	Anterior cingulate cortex
ACPO	Acute colonic pseudo-obstruction
AD	Autosomal dominant
ADAL	Adalimumab
AFAP	Attenuated familial adenomatous polyposis
AIDS	Acquired immunodeficiency syndrome
AMACR	α-methylacyl-CoA racemase
ANA	Antinuclear antibodies
AR	Absolute risk
AR	Autosomal recessive
ARA	Anorectal angle
ARF	Additional risk factors
ASD	Atrial septal defect
ATP	Adenosine triphosphate
AVMs	Arteriovenous Malformations
AZA	Azathioprine
BBs	Beta-blockers
BER	Base-excision repairs
BMPR1A	Bone morphogenetic protein receptor 1A
BRR	Bannayan-Ruvalcaba-Riley
CBC	Complete blood count
CC	Collagenous colitis
CC	Crohn colitis
CCBs	Calcium channel blockers

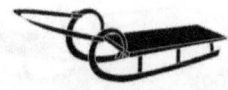

CCS	Cronkhite-Canada Syndrome
CD	Crohn disease
CDADC	Clostridium difficile-Associated Diarrhea and Colitis
CDI	Clostridium difficile infection
CEA	Carcinoembryonic antigen
Cg	Chromogranins
CGRP	Calcitonin gene-related peptide
CHRPE	Congenital hypertrophy of the retinal pigment epithelium
CIC	Chronic idiopathic constipation
CIMP	CPG island methylator phenotype
CIN	Chromosomal instability
CIS	Chromosomal instability
CMI	Chronic mesenteric ischemia
CMV	Cytomegalovirus
CNS	Central nervous system
CO	Colonic obstruction
COPD	Chronic obstructive pulmonary disease
CRC	Colorectal cancer
CRF	Corticotropin releasing factor
CS	Cowden syndrome
CTC	Computed tomographic colonography
DAC	Diverticulae associated colitis
DALM	Dysplasia-associated lesion or mass
DBE	Double balloon enteroscopy
DBP	Dibutyl phthalate
DCBE	Double-contrast barium enema
DGGE	Denaturing gradient gel electrophoresis
DRE	Digital rectal exam
EAES	European Association for Endoscopic Surgeons
EAS	External anal sphincter
EGD	Esophagogastroduodenoscopy

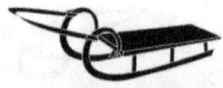

EGF	Endothelial growth factors
EGFR	Epidermal growth factor receptors
EIA	Enzyme-linked immunoassays
EMP	Endoscopic mucosal resection
ENS	Enteric neuron system
ERCP	Endoscopic retrograde cholangiopancreatography
ESD	Endoscopic submucosal dissection
EUS	Endoscopic ultrasound
FAP	Familial adenomatous polyposis
FAPS	Functional abdominal pain syndrome
FDA	Food and Drug Administration
FI	Fecal incontinence
FICS	Fujinon intelligent chromoendoscopy system
FIT	Fecal immunochemical test
FMT	Fecal microbiota transplantation
FNA	Fine needle aspiration
FOBT	Fecal occult blood test
FSI	Focal segmental ischemia
FSIG	Flexible sigmoidoscopy
GCS	Glucocorticosteroids
GERD	Gastroesophageal reflux disease
GMCSF	Granulocyte-macrophage colony-stimulating factor
GS	Gardner syndrome
HAPCs	High-amplitude propagated contractions
HGD	High grade dysplasia
HH	Hereditary hemochromatosis
HHT	Hereditary hemorrhagic telangiectasia
HNPCC	Hereditary non-polyposis colorectal cancer
HP	Hyperplastic polyps
HPS	Hyperplastic polyposis syndrome
HPV	Human papillomia virus

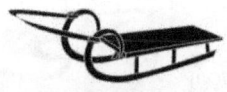

HRT	Hormone replacement therapy
HSV	Herpes simplex virus
IAS	Internal anal sphincter
IBS	Irritable bowel syndrome
IBS-D	Diarrhea-predominant IBS
IBC-C	Constipation-predominant IBS
IBS-M	Mixed: alternating diarrhea and constipation-predominant IBS
IC	Ileocecal
ICC	Interstitial cells of Cajal
ICC-IM	Interstitial cells of Cajal Intramuscular
ICC-MP	Interstitial cells of Cajal myenteric plexus
ICC-SM	Interstitial cells of Cajal submucosal
IL-10	Interleukin-10
IPAA	Ileal pouch-anal anastomosis
IPANS	Intrinsic primary afferent neurons
IRCI	Isolated R-colon ischemia
JPS	Juvenile polyposis syndrome
LBO	Large bowel obstruction
LC	Left colon
LC	Lymphocytic colitis
LCM	Laser confocal endomicroscopy
LEF	Lymphoid enhancer factor
LGD	Low grade dysplasia
LGIB	Lower GI bleed
LGV	Lymphogranuloma venereum
LM	Luminal membrane
LOH	Loss of heterogeneity
LP	Lamina propria
MAP	Modified adenomatous polyposis
MC	Microscopic colitis
MCP	Meta carpophalangeal joint

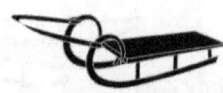

MET	Metronidazole
MIS	Microsatellite instability
MMR	Mismatch repair
MPOs	Myenteric potential oscillations
MSM	Men who have sex with men
MZL	Mantle zone lymphoma
NA	Not available
NAAT	Nucleic acid amplification testing
NBI	Narrowing band imaging
N/C	Ratio of nucleus to cytoplasm
NEC	Necrotizing enterocolitis
NK	Neurokinin
NLH	Nodular lymphoid hyperplasia
NMDA	N-methyl-D-aspartate
NNTs	Number needed to treat
NO	Nitric oxide
NPV	Negative predictive value
NSAIDs	Nonsteroidal anti-inflammatory drugs
OCA	Oral contraceptive agent
OCP	Oral contraceptive pill
OCT	Optical coherence tomography
Od	Once per day
PACAP	Pituitary adenyl cyclase-activating peptide
pANCA	Perinuclear antineutrophil cytoplasmic antibodies
PARs	Proteinase-activated and serine proteases receptors
PCA	Patient-controlled analgesia
PCI	Pneumatosis cystoides intestinalis
PCP	Pneumocystitis carini pneumonia
PCR	Polymerase chain reaction
PEG	Percutaneous endoscopic gastroscopy
PG	Pyoderma gangrenosum

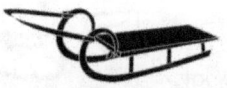

PHTS	PTEN hamartoma tumour syndromes
PI-IBS	Post-infectious irritable bowel syndrome
PIP	Proximal interphalangeal joint
PJS	Peutz-Jeghers Syndrome
PMC	Pseudomembraneous colitis
PME	Pseudomembraneous enteritis
PMEC	Pseudomembranous Enterocolitis
PML	Polymorphonuclear leucocytes
Po	By mouth
PPAR	Peroxisome proliferator-activated receptors
PPIs	Proton pump inhibitors
PPV	Positive predictive value
PRMA	Periodic rectal motor activity
PSC	Primary sclerosing cholangitis
PTMA	Percutaneous transmural mesenteric angioplasty
PTMAS	Percutaneous transluminal mesenteric angioplasty with stenting
RC	Right colon
RLQ	Right paracolic gutter
RMC	Rectal motor complex
RPR	Rapid plasma regain test
RR	Relative risk
SBO	Small bowel obstruction
SCAD	Segmented colitis associated with diverticulum
SCFA	Short chain fatty acid
SENS	Sensitivity
SIBO	Small bacterial overgrowth
SIRA	Systemic inflammatory response syndrome
SMA	Superior mesenteric artery
SPEC	Specificity
SPO-Ca	Spontaneous CRC
SRUS	Solitary rectal ulcer syndrome

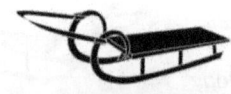

SSA	Sessile serrated adenoma
SSC	Secondary sclerosing cholangitis
SSCP	Single-strand conformational polymorphism
SSRIs	Selective serotonin reuptake inhibitors
STI	Sexually transmitted infections
STK II	Serine threonine kinase II
SUDD	Symptomatic uncomplicated diverticular disease
TAN/BSO	Total abdominal hysterectomy, bilateral salpingo-oophorectomy
TC	Transverse colon
TCF	T-cell factor
TID	Three times per day
TJs	Tight junctions
TME	Total mesenteric excision
TMP-SMX	Trimethoprim-sulfamethoxazole
TPHA	Treponema pallidum hemagglutination assay
TPPA	Treponema pallidum particle agglutination
TRPV1	Transient receptor potential vailloid -1
TSA	Traditional serrated adenoma
TSH	Thyroid stimulating hormone
UC	Ulcerative colitis
UDCA	Ursodeoxycholic acid
UP	Ulcerative proctitis
VAN	Vancomycin
VIP	Vasoactive intestinal polypeptide
VRE	Vancomycin-resistant enterococci
WD	Wilson disease
WLE	White light endoscopy

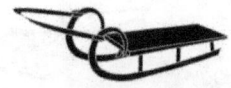

INDEX

Note: Page number followed by f and t indicates figure and table respectively.

A

AA. See Amino acids
AAA. See Abdominal aortic aneurysm
AAD. See Antibiotic-associated diarrhea
Abbreviations
    colon, 605–611
    esophagus, 131–135
    small bowel, 377–383
    stomach, 245–250
Abdominal aortic aneurysm (AAA)
    demography, 588
    loud abdominal bruit and, 589
    risk of rupture, 589t
    surveillance, 588
    treatment (surgical resection), 588
Aberrant pancreas. See Pancreatic rest
AC. See Acute self-limiting colitis
Achalasia
    causes, 62–64
    definition, 61
    diagnostic imaging, 64
    treatment, 64–67, 64t–67t
    types, 61, 62t
Acid rebound, 148
Acid-related disorder target intragastric pHs, 36, 36t
ACPO. See Acute colonic pseudo-obstruction
Acute colonic pseudo-obstruction (ACPO)
    causes/associations, 577–578
    definition, 577
    diagnostic imaging, 579, 579t
    pathology, 577
    pathophysiology, 577
    prognosis, 579
    treatment, 579
Acute erosive gastritis. See Reactive gastropathies
Acute mesenteric ischemia (AMI)
    causes/associations, 363
    clinical, 362
    diagnostic imaging, 363–364
    laboratory, 363
    pathophysiology, 362

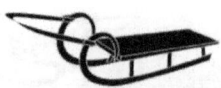

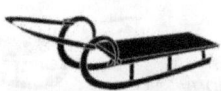

Mastering the Boards: Gastroenterology   A.B.R. Thomson

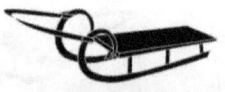

Mastering the Boards: Gastroenterology   A.B.R. Thomson

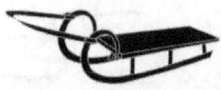

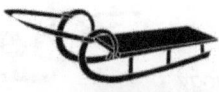

Mastering the Boards: Gastroenterology   A.B.R. Thomson

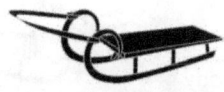

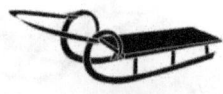

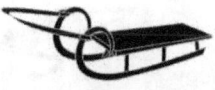

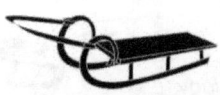

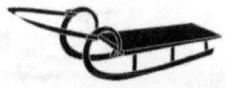

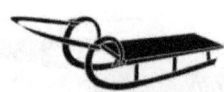

623

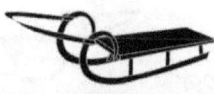

Mastering the Boards: Gastroenterology

A.B.R. Thomson

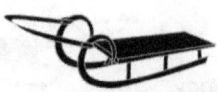

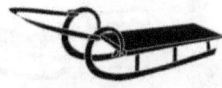

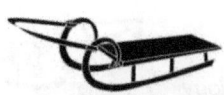

Mastering the Boards: Gastroenterology   A.B.R. Thomson

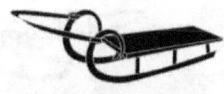

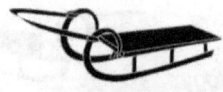

Helicobactor pylori (HP) infection
  demography, 149
  dyspepsia and pregnancy, 157
  negative PUD disease, 156–157, 156t
  pathophysiology, 149–151
  positive PUD
    pathophysiology, 154
    treatment, 155–156
  transmission
    diseases, 152–153
    epidemiology, 151–152
    modes, 151
Helicobactor pylori-negative peptic ulcer disease, 156–157, 156t
Helicobactor pylori-positive peptic ulcer disease
  pathophysiology, 154
  treatment, 155–156
Hemangiomas, 587
Hemorrhage
  cause/associations, 598
  demography, 598
  diagnosis, 599
  prognosis, 599
  treatment, 599
Hemorrhoids
  definition, 410
  endoscopy, 410
  treatment, 410–411
Hemospray®, 210
Hepatic venous pressure gradient (HVPG), 103–104
Hereditary hemorrhage telangiectasia (HHT), 376
Hereditary non-polyposis colon cancer (HNPCC)
  Amterdam criteria (3-2-1), 533–534
  Bethesda criteria (for testing tumour tissue), 535
  definition, 532
  genetics, 532–533, 532t
  lifetime cancer risk at GI and non-GI sites for, 546t
  Muir-Torre syndrome and, 537, 538t
  pathology, 537
  sequence of testing for, 535–536, 536t
Herpes simplex virus (HSV), 408t, 477
Heterotopic pancreas. See Pancreatic rest
Heterotropic gastric mucosa (HGM), 85
HGM. See Heterotropic gastric mucosa
HHG. See Hyperplastic, hypersecretory gastropathy
HHT. See Hereditary hemorrhage telangiectasia
High resolution esophageal manometry (HREM), 57
High resolution esophageal pressure topography (HREPT), 57

629

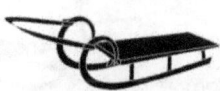

Mastering the Boards: Gastroenterology   A.B.R. Thomson

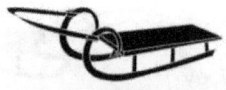

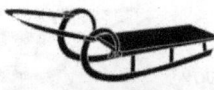

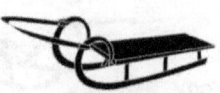

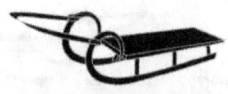

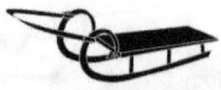

Mastering the Boards: Gastroenterology   A.B.R. Thomson

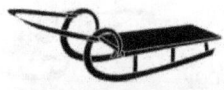

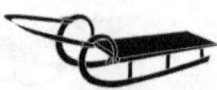

Normal esophagus reflux disease. See Non-erosive reflux disease (NERD)
NRCD. See Non-responsive celiac disease
NSAID-associated colitis, 476, 476t
NSAIDs. See Non-steroidal anti-inflammatory drugs
NSBB. See Non-selective beta blockers
Nuclear meducine scans, 370
Nucleotide-binding oligomerization domain 2 (NOD2), 293
Nutcracker esophagus, 58–59, 68
NVUGIB. See Non-variceal upper GI bleeding

O

Obscure GI bleeding (OGIB)
  diagnostic imaging/endoscopy, 368–371
    angiography, 370
    capsule endoscopy, 369
    CT enterography, 370
    double balloon enteroscopy, 369–370
    EGD, 369
    nuclear meducine scans, 370
  differential diagnosis, 371t–372t
  management, 372
  pathology, 368
  PHG vs. GAVE, 372t
  prognosis, 372
  from small bowel, 368
  treatment, 372
OCIF. See Osteoclastogenesis inhibitory factor
OGIB. See Obscure GI bleeding
Ogilvie syndrome. See Acute colonic pseudo-obstruction (ACPO)
Omeprazole, 39
OPG. See Osteoprotegerin
Oropharyngeal candidiasis, 81–82
Oropharyngeal dysphagia
  causes of, 11
  symptoms of, 12
Oropharynx, 3
Osler-Weber-Rendu syndrome. See Hereditary hemorrhage telangiectasia
    (HHT)
Osteoclastogenesis inhibitory factor (OCIF), 319
Osteopenia/osteoporosis, in IBD, 317–318
Osteoprotegerin (OPG), 319
Ostomies
  definition, 573
  indications for, 573–575, 574f, 575f
  ostomy hernia, 573
  types, 573, 573f, 573t, 574–575, 574f–575f

637

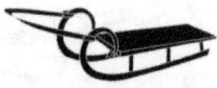

Mastering the Boards: Gastroenterology   A.B.R. Thomson

P

Pacemaker cells. See Interstitial cells of Cajal (ICC)
Pancreatic rest, 351, 351t
Pantoprazole, 39
Paraneoplastic visceral neuropathies (PVN), 374, 375
Parasympathetic nervous system (PNS), 180
Parietal cell, 144
PCI. See Pneumatosis cystoides intestinalis
Pepsin, gastric secretion of, 148
Peptic strictures, 31
Peptic ulceration, 178
Peptic ulcer disease (PUD)
  Helicobactor pylori-negative, 156–157, 156t
  Helicobactor pylori-positive, 154–156
Perianal fistulae (PF), 324
Periodic acid-Schill (PAS)-positive, 287–288
Peristalsis, 5–6
Peristaltic reflex, 183–184
Peutz-Jegher syndrome (PJS), 541t
  clinical, 544–545
  diagnosis, 543
  endoscopy, 546, 546t
  genetics, 544, 544t
  lifetime cancer risk at GI and non-GI sites for, 546t
  malignancy risk, 545
PF. See Perianal fistulae
PG. See Phlegmonous gastritis; Pyoderma gangrenosum
Pharyngeal swallow, 3
PHG. See Portal hypertensive gastropathy
Phlegmonous gastritis (PG), 219
PJS. See Peutz-Jegher syndrome
PMEC. See Pseudomembranous enterocolitis
Pneumatosis coli, 560
Pneumatosis cystoides intestinalis (PCI), 560, 560t
PNS. See Parasympathetic nervous system
Pocto-sigmoiditis in MSM, 476
Polymyositis, 374
PONV. See Post-operative nausea and vomiting
Portal hypertensive gastropathy (PHG), 117t
  GAVE vs., 372t
Postoperative ileus, 356
Post-operative nausea and vomiting (PONV), 197
Potassium (K$^+$), 335
Pouchitis, 456–458, 457t
  causes/associations, 453–454, 453t

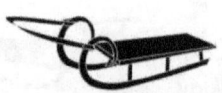

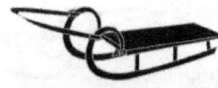

Mastering the Boards: Gastroenterology   A.B.R. Thomson

pharmacological, 450
surgical, 450–451

Q

Quality assurance, colonoscopy and, 508
  adenomatous polyps, recurrence rates of, 513–515, 513t, 514t, 515t
  buried bumper syndrome, 511
  efficacy and test performance characteristics, 516t
  endoscopic complications, 510
  endoscopic procedure, 511t
  focal white patches on mucosa, causes of, 509
  polyp detection rate, 508–509
  post-polypectomy recommendations, 516t
  quality indicators, outcome measures and standards, 512t
  radiation risk from CTC, 516

R

Rabeprazole, 39
Radiation colilis
  clinical, 468t, 469
  endoscopy, 469
  histopathological features, 469–470
  pathophysiology, 468
  treatment, 470–471, 471t
RCD. See Refractory celiac disease
Reactive gastropathies, 220
Reactive metabolite syndrome (RMS), 452
Rebound acid secretion, 35
Rectal pain "proctalgia," 405
Refractory celiac disease (RCD)
  definition, 282
  immunopathogenesis, 283–284
  treatment, 284
  types, 282–283
Refractory gastroesophageal reflux disease, 33
Refractory nausea/vomiting, 198
RMS. See Reactive metabolite syndrome
Rockall Risk Score Scheme, for assessing prognosis in NVUGIB, 203t
ROME III criteria
  for functional constipation, 422
  for functional defecation disorders, 422
ROME IV criteria, for IBS, 396
Roux-en-Y stasis syndrome, 200
Rumination syndrome, 84

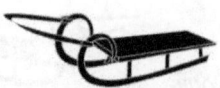

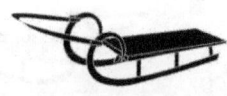

secretory IgA, functions of, 256
   treatment, 258
Small intestinal motility, 327
  clinical tests of, 330
  vs. colonic motility, 327–328
  intestinal cells of Cajal and, 328–329
  neurons with, 329
  regulation of, 330
Small intestine, malignant tumours of, 347
Smooth muscle, 6–7
Smooth muscle cells, 179, 180t
SNS. See Sympathetic nervous system
Sodium (Na^+)/H_2O absorption, 331–332
Solitary rectal ulcer syndrome (SRUS), 411
Somatostatin, 146
Sporatic gland polyposis, 226t
SRUS. See Solitary rectal ulcer syndrome
Standing-gradient hypothesis, 331
Steady-state phenomenon, 40
Stevens-Johnson syndrome, 452
STI. See Sexually transmitted infections
Stromal (mesenchymal) tumours, 226–229
  endoscopic diagnosis, 227
  genetic mutations, 227
  markers for, 227
  pathology, 226
  treatment, 227–229
Submucosal tumours, 98
  carcinoid tumour, 98
  duplication cysts, 99
  gastrointestinal stromal tumours, 99–100
  granular cell tumours, 98
  lipoma, 98
Suppurative gastritis (SG). See Phlegmonous gastritis (PG)
Surgical reanastamosis, 475
Swallowing
  dermatomyositis, 14
  dysphagia, 11–14
  lower esophageal sphincter and, 7–10
  physiology of
    esophagus, 4t–5t
    larynx, 4
    mouth/tongue, 3
    oropharynx, 3
    peristalsis, 5–6
    skeletal muscle, 6
    smooth muscle, 6–7

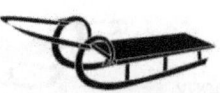

643

 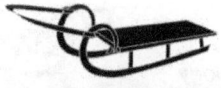

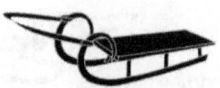

Mastering the Boards: Gastroenterology   A.B.R. Thomson

refractory, 198
risk factors, 197
treatment, 198–199, 199t

W
Whipple disease
  causes/associations, 286
  clinical, 286–287
  definition, 286
  diagnostic imaging, 287
  histopathology, 287–288
  immunopathogenesis, 286
  laboratory, 287
  treatment, 288
Whirl sign, 354

Z
ZD. See Zenker diverticulum
Zenker diverticulum (ZD)
  definition, 68
  diagnostic imaging, 69
  pathophysiology, 69
  treatment, 69
ZES. See Zollinger-Ellison syndrome
Zollinger-Ellison syndrome (ZES)
  clinical features of, 158
  diagnostic imaging, 159–160
  endoscopy for, 159
  gastrin test in, 160
  laboratory tests, 159
  multiple endocrine neoplasia type I (MEN-1) gastrinomas, 160–162
  presentations of, 178
  provocative tests, 159

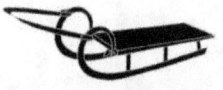

www.ingramcontent.com/pod-product-compliance
Lightning Source LLC
Chambersburg PA
CBHW080632180526
45168CB00008B/3145